DRUG EFFICACY, SAFETY, AND BIOLOGICS DISCOVERY

Wiley Series on Technologies for the Pharmaceutical Industry

Sean Ekins, Series Editor

Computational Toxicology: Risk Assessment for Pharmaceutical and Environmental Chemicals
Edited by Sean Ekins

Pharmaceutical Applications of Raman Spectroscopy
Edited by Slobodan Šašić

Pathway Analysis for Drug Discovery: Computational Infrastructure and Applications
Edited by Anton Yuryev

Drug Efficacy, Safety, and Biologics Discovery: Emerging Technologies and Tools
Edited by Sean Ekins and Jinghai J. Xu

DRUG EFFICACY, SAFETY, AND BIOLOGICS DISCOVERY

Emerging Technologies and Tools

SEAN EKINS
JINGHAI J. XU

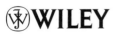**WILEY**

A JOHN WILEY & SONS, INC., PUBLICATION

Cover designs by Sean Ekins from images from Chapters 3 and 4.

Published by John Wiley & Sons, Inc., Hoboken, New Jersey
Published simultaneously in Canada

For general information on our other products and services or for technical support, please contact our Customer Care Department within the United States at (800) 762-2974, outside the United States at (317) 572-3993 or fax (317) 572-4002.

Wiley also publishes its books in a variety of electronic formats. Some content that appears in print may not be available in electronic formats. For more information about Wiley products, visit our web site at www.wiley.com.

Library of Congress Cataloging-in-Publication Data:
Drug efficacy, safety, and biologics discovery : emerging technologies and tools / [edited by] Sean Ekins, Jinghai J. Xu.
    p. ; cm.
  Includes bibliographical references and index.
  ISBN 978-0-470-22555-4 (cloth)
  1. Drug development–Technological innovations. 2. Pharmaceutical technology. 3. Biological products. I. Ekins, Sean. II. Xu, Jinghai J.
  [DNLM: 1. Drug Evaluation–trends. 2. Biological Products. 3. Drug Design. 4. Drug Toxicity. 5. Technology, Pharmaceutical–trends. QV 771 D7943 2009]
  RS192.D82 2009
  615'.19--dc22

                    2008036264

Printed in the United States of America

10 9 8 7 6 5 4 3 2 1

To Enya, Elisa, and Penelope

Biotechnology is likely to be the main driving force of change in human affairs for the next hundred years.

Freeman J. Dyson, *A Many Colored Glass*, University of Virginia Press, 2007

Hopes of realizing the optimistic forecasts about the benefits that molecular biology will bring to pharmacology are likely, I believe, to be circumscribed by the state of physiological knowledge, models, and concepts.

Sir James Black, Foreword in *The Logic of Life*, edited by C. A. R. Boyd and D. Noble, Oxford University Press, 1993

CONTENTS

PREFACE

Most drugs fail at the critical and expensive stage of clinical development due to inadequate prediction of efficacy and/or safety. Today new technologies that enable us to be more systematic and proficient at deciphering the complex interactions between biology and medicine are one of our best hopes in achieving a better therapeutic index. The goal of this book is to educate the readers in aspects of several key emerging technologies and how they have substantially impacted drug discovery, while stimulating thinking on how to better address safety and efficacy for drug research and development.

Systems biology, stem cells, RNAi, biomarker discovery and new models in vivo, are already influencing our predictions of drug efficacy. Automated data mining, computational (in silico) approaches, high-throughput screening and high-content screening, will continue to impact our predictions of drug safety. Finally, several key technological advances in nanotechnology, biologics, and complex drug discovery will be presented in the same forum to foster the cross-fertilization of ideas between the fields of small molecule and larger molecule discovery. Indeed the breakdown of disciplinary silos and systematic application of the four modalities (manipulate, measure, mine, and model) are the central theme of this book. It is envisioned that the cross-disciplinary collaborations that are implicit in integrating these technologies with drug discovery operations will fuel the engine for future innovations. This book cuts across multiple areas of drug discovery. These areas are each presented by pioneers in the field, and they should have a broad appeal to many biological scientists and interdisciplinary technologists interested in drug research.

The book is not intended to be a *how to* book but rather to enhance knowledge of concepts and provide perspectives on drug discovery applications of new technologies. Many of the chapters include case studies of how such technologies impact drug research and development. The reader should be able to take away from the book what the new technology is about, and how it enabled drug research and development that previous or conventional technology was not able to.

The book is divided into three sections:

Part I.   Drug Efficacy and Safety Discovery
Part II.   Biologics Technology
Part III.   Future Perspective

Among the topics addressed are:

- High throughput protein-based technologies and computational models for drug development, efficacy, and toxicity.
- Systems pharmacology, biomarkers, and biomolecular networks.
- Computational systems biology modeling of dosimetry and cellular response pathways.
- Nanotechnology to improve drug delivery.
- Modeling efficacy and safety of engineered biologics.

The book's authors from pharmaceutical and biotechnology companies and academe have aimed to present an accessible volume for scientists at every level pursing drug research and development. Each chapter has been edited to ensure consistency with explanatory figures and key references for readers who want to find out more about a topic. We hope that this book will prove to be a valuable reference resource on emerging technologies and tools and will enhance research productivity, which we show to be based on the modalities of manipulation, measuring, mining, and modeling.

ACKNOWLEDGMENTS

We sincerely thank Jonathan Rose and in particular Danielle Lacourciere, as well as and the team at Wiley for providing assistance and advice in developing this book. Our anonymous proposal reviewers are also kindly acknowledged for their helpful suggestions.

This book would not have been brought to fruition without the many authors of the chapters who agreed to contribute their time and effort in writing chapters. We thank them for allowing us to edit their work and making this such an enjoyable and rewarding endeavor.

J.J.X. would like to thank all his collaborators, teachers, and mentors in drug discovery and development. I am grateful to my parents and my family for encouraging me to follow my own path, and for being so supportive along the way.

S.E. would like to thank the editorial board and all the authors involved in creating this book series. I would like to acknowledge my family and Maggie for encouraging me to read, type, and pursue science topics of interest whenever I can.

Sean Ekins,
Jenkintown, Pennsylvania
May 2008

Jinghai J. Xu,
North Wales, Pennsylvania
May 2008

CONTRIBUTORS

Aram S. Adourian, BG Medicine, Inc., 610N Lincoln Street, Waltham, Massachusetts, USA. (aadourian@bg-medicine.com).

Noubar B. Afeyan, BG Medicine, Inc., 610N Lincoln Street, Waltham, Massachusetts, USA.

Leonidas G. Alexopoulos, Department of Systems Biology, Harvard Medical School, Boston, Massachusetts, USA and Department of Biological Engineering, Massachusetts Institute of Technology, Cambridge, Massachusetts, USA. Current address: Department of Mechanical Engineering, National Technical University of Athens, Heroon Polytechniou 9, 15780 Zografou, Athens, Greece. (leo@mail.ntua.gr)

Mansoor M. Amiji, Department of Pharmaceutical Sciences, School of Pharmacy, Northeastern University, 110 Mugar Life Sciences Building, Boston, Massachusetts, USA. (m.amiji@neu.edu)

Melvin E. Andersen, Division of Computational Biology, The Hamner Institutes for Health Sciences, Research Triangle Park, North Carolina, USA. (MAndersen@thehamner.org)

Raji Balasubramanian, BG Medicine, Inc., 610N Lincoln Street, Waltham, Massachusetts, USA.

Sudin Bhattacharya, Division of Computational Biology, The Hamner Institutes for Health Sciences, Research Triangle Park, North Carolina, USA.

Mayank D. Bhavsar, Department of Pharmaceutical Sciences, School of Pharmacy, Northeastern University, 110 Mugar Life Sciences Building, Boston, Massachusetts, USA.

Jeffrey R. Chabot, Pfizer, Research and Technology Center, 620 Memorial Drive, Cambridge, Massachusetts, USA. (Jeffrey.Chabot2@pfizer.com)

Julio C. Davila, Pfizer, Inc., PGRD, Drug Safety Research and Development, Saint Louis Laboratories, St. Louis, Missouri, USA. (Julio.c.davila@pfizer.com)

Sean Ekins, Collaborations in Chemistry, 601 Runnymede Avenue, Jenkintown, PA 19046. USA; ACT LLC, 1 Penn Plaza-36th Floor, New York, New York, USA; Department of Pharmaceutical Sciences, University of Maryland, 20 Penn Street, Baltimore, Maryland, USA; Department of Pharmacology, University of Medicine and Dentistry of New Jersey, Robert Wood Johnson Medical School, 675 Hoes Lane, Piscataway, New Jersey, USA. (ekinssean@yahoo.com)

Sandra J. Engle, Pfizer, Inc., PGRD, Genetically Modified Mice, Eastern Point Road, Groton, Connecticut, USA.

Christopher W. Espelin, Pfizer, Research and Technology Center, 620 Memorial Drive, Cambridge, Massachusetts, USA.

Bruce Gomes, Pfizer, Research and Technology Center, 620 Memorial Drive, Cambridge, Massachusetts, USA.

Albert Gough, Cellumen, Inc., 3180 William Pitt Way, Pittsburgh, Pennsylvania, USA.

Kenneth A. Giuliano, Cellumen, Inc., 3180 William Pitt Way, Pittsburgh, Pennsylvania, USA. (kgiuliano@cellumen.com)

Jan van der Greef, BG Medicine, Inc., 610N Lincoln Street, Waltham, Massachusetts, USA, and Analytical Sciences Department, TNO Quality of Life, PO Box 360, Zeist, The Netherlands.

Roman Herrara, Pfizer, Research and Technology Center, 620 Memorial Drive, Cambridge, Massachusetts, USA.

William Irwin, Cellumen, Inc., 3180 William Pitt Way, Pittsburgh, Pennsylvania, USA.

Shardool Jain, Department of Pharmaceutical Sciences, School of Pharmacy, Northeastern University, 110 Mugar Life Sciences Building, Boston, Massachusetts, USA.

Ezra G. Jennings, BG Medicine, Inc., 610N Lincoln Street, Waltham, Massachusetts, USA.

Kate Johnston, Cellumen, Inc., 3180 William Pitt Way, Pittsburgh, Pennsylvania, USA.

Douglas Lauffenburger, Massachusetts Institute of Technology, Department of Biology, 77 Massachusetts Avenue, Cambridge, Massachusetts, USA. (lauffen@mit.edu)

Shuo Lin, Laboratory of Chemical Genomics, Shenzhen Graduate School, Peking University, Shenzhen, China, and Department of Molecular, Cell, and Developmental Biology, University of California, Los Angeles, California, USA. (shuolin@ucla.edu)

Ning-Ai Liu, Cedars-Sinai Medical Center, Los Angeles, California, USA.

Stephen Martin, BG Medicine, Inc., 610N Lincoln Street, Waltham, Massachusetts, USA. (aadourian@bg-medicine.com)

Robert N. McBurney, BG Medicine, Inc., 610N Lincoln Street, Waltham, Massachusetts, USA.

Michael McGlashen, Pfizer, Research and Technology Center, 620 Memorial Drive, Cambridge, Massachusetts, USA. (Michael.McGlashen@pfizer.com)

Pieter Muntendam, BG Medicine, Inc., 610N Lincoln Street, Waltham, Massachusetts, USA.

Thomas N. Plasterer, BG Medicine, Inc., 610N Lincoln Street, Waltham, Massachusetts, USA.

Howard I. Pryor II, Harvard Medical School Center for Regeneration Medicine, Massachusetts General Hospital, Boston, Massachusetts, USA.

Julio Saez Rodriguez, Department of Systems Biology, Harvard Medical School, Boston, Massachusetts, USA and Department of Biological Engineering, Massachusetts Institute of Technology, Cambridge, Massachusetts, USA.

Ram Sasisekharan, Department of Biological Engineering, Massachusetts Institute of Technology, 77 Massachusetts Avenue 16-561, Cambridge, Massachusetts, USA. (rams@mit.edu).

Josef Scheiber, Lead Finding Platform, Novartis Institutes for BioMedical Research Inc., 250 Massachusetts Ave., Cambridge, Massachusetts, USA.

Donald B. Stedman, Pfizer, Inc., PGRD, Developmental and Reproductive Toxicology, Eastern Point Rd, Groton, Connecticut, USA.

Yu-Mei Tan, Division of Computational Biology, The Hamner Institutes for Health Sciences, Research Triangle Park, North Carolina, USA.

D. Lansing Taylor, Cellumen, Inc., 3180 William Pitt Way, Pittsburgh, Pennsylvania, USA. (ltaylor@cellumen.com).

Eric Tien, Pfizer, Research and Technology Center, 620 Memorial Drive, Cambridge, Massachusetts, USA. (Eric.Tien@pfizer.com)

Joseph P. Vacanti, Harvard Medical School Center for Regeneration Medicine, Co-Director, Harvard Stem cell Institute, Massachusetts General Hospital, Boston, Massachusetts, USA.

Lawrence Vernetti, Cellumen, Inc., 3180 William Pitt Way, Pittsburgh, Pennsylvania, USA.

Karthik Viswanathan, Department of Biological Engineering, Massachusetts Institute of Technology, 77 Massachusetts Avenue 16-561, Cambridge, Massachusetts, USA.

Shunguang Wang, BG Medicine, Inc., 610N Lincoln Street, Waltham, Massachusetts, USA.

Jinghai J. Xu, Pfizer, Research and Technology Center, 620 Memorial Drive, Cambridge, Massachusetts, USA. Current Address: Department of Automated Biotechnology, Merck and Co., 140 Wissahickon Avenue, North Wales, Pennsylvania, USA. (jimxu2@gmail.com)

Yi Yang, Novartis Pharmaceuticals Corp., 406-137, East Hanover, New Jersey, USA. (yi1.yang@novartis.com)

Li J. Yu, Drug Safety and Disposition, Millennium Pharmaceuticals, Inc., 45–5 Sidney Street., Cambridge, Massachusetts, USA. (li.yu@mpi.com)

Qiang Zhang, Division of Computational Biology, The Hamner Institutes for Health Sciences, Research Triangle Park, North Carolina, USA.

Hanbing Zhong, Laboratory of Chemical Genomics, Shenzhen Graduate School, Peking University, Shenzhen, China.

PART I

DRUG EFFICACY AND SAFETY TECHNOLOGY

1

FOCUS ON THE FUNDAMENTALS: TOWARD BETTER THERAPEUTIC INDEX PREDICTION

Jinghai J. Xu and Li J. Yu

Contents

1.1 INTRODUCTION

"What is there that is not poison? Everything can be poison. What differentiates a poison from a medicine is its dose" [1]. This is the famous revelation of Paracelsus (1493–1541), the father of modern medicine. Modern

Drug Efficacy, Safety, and Biologics Discovery: Emerging Technologies and Tools,
Edited by Sean Ekins and Jinghai J. Xu
Copyright © 2009 by John Wiley & Sons, Inc.

pharmaceutical scientists have refined the concept of dose with concentration, and added a time variable [2]. Successful drug therapy relies on not drug potency per se but on a wide enough safety margin between toxicity and efficacy, the so-called sufficient therapeutic index (TI) [3]. This safety margin is exemplified by the lipid-lowering drug class hydroxymethylglutaryl-CoA (HMG-CoA) reductase inhibitors known as statins. Cerivastatin is a potent statin with therapeutic exposure levels that are an order of magnitude lower than other statins. However, it was withdrawn from the market after widespread prescription because of a significantly higher incidence and severity of muscle toxicity [4]. The challenge facing all of us in the pharmaceutical research and development field is how to establish robust screening paradigms and predictive strategies to (1) proactively identify drugs with narrow therapeutic indexes, before they are administered to humans, and (2) select drug candidates with sufficient safety margins that can withstand the test of time and widespread use.

Traditionally drug safety evaluation is conducted in the later stages of development when the entire development program is focusing on a single new chemical entity (NCE). In this mode of compound testing, the safety evaluation of the NCE is composed of preclinical animal toxicology, pathology, and safety pharmacology studies followed by phased human clinical tests (i.e., phases I, II, III, and postmarketing surveillance). In the event that severe toxicity occurs without a sufficient TI, it can lead to abandonment of such development programs or severe restrictions on the utility of such an NCE (Figure 1.1). It is now widely recognized that drug toxicity is the leading cause of drug candidate attrition in development [5], as well as drug withdrawals

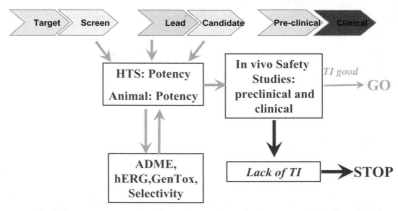

Traditional Discovery and Development

Q: Why not screen against the end goal: therapeutic index (TI)?

Figure 1.1 Role of therapeutic index (TI) screening in drug discovery and development.

from the market after they were initially approved by the drug regulatory agencies [6]. Approximately one-third of drug attrition is due to preclinical drug toxicity or clinical safety [7]. These statistics, however, may underestimate the contribution of toxicity to overall drug attrition. "Lack of efficacy" has been the other leading cause of drug attrition. However, among the drug candidates that have exhibited poor efficacy, there is evidence that for a significant number of these candidates, the clinical dosing regimen was limited or restricted by dose-limiting toxicity. In other words, the proof of clinical efficacy could not be fully achieved if an NCE did not have a sufficient TI (e.g., [8]). Hence an additional fraction of the "lack of efficacy" group also contained an underlying drug safety cause. If one would introduce a category called "lack of sufficient therapeutic index," this category would certainly occupy the largest cohort of drug attrition [9].

If lack of sufficient TI is the major hurdle of pharmaceutical research and development (R&D), the obvious question is, why not focus on this key parameter by applying emerging technologies to screen for improved TI in key transitioning steps during prolonged R&D programs? If this screening strategy is applied early enough in the drug discovery stage (e.g., right after cell-based efficacy screens), the data could help the drug discovery teams proactively identify and select drug candidates with an increasing probability of improved TI in vivo. The remainder of this chapter will discuss emerging technologies that could make this happen, and provide the authors' perspectives on challenges in the field.

1.2 GENERAL APPROACHES IN PREDICTING THE THERAPEUTIC INDEX

Predicting a therapeutic index is intrinsically a systems pharmacology and systems toxicology challenge. This exercise no longer deals with a single enzyme or receptor, but with a multiple-component system that includes competing endogenous ligands, co-factors, off-targets, multiple cell types, organs, and tissues. Many scientists view systems biology as an "integrated" *omics*. While there is a need to integrate all the *omic* data to generate a "pathways view" of biology, this per se does not allow quantitative prediction of a therapeutic index. To translate biological knowledge into an effective therapy, one needs to quantitatively predict the fundamental attributes of drugs, for example, the intrinsic TI of a drug and different ways to optimize TI in vivo. This necessitates an accurate prediction of both efficacious and toxic concentrations (Figure 1.2). Hence the in vitro–in vivo correlations for cellular models, biomarkers, and concentrations need to be established for both drug efficacy and drug toxicity. Furthermore drug disposition and pharmacokinetic (PK) properties need to be taken into consideration for the final calculation of therapeutic index. In this sense, systems pharmacology and systems toxicology build on basic biological knowledge derived from systems biology, but

Therapeutic Index Screening

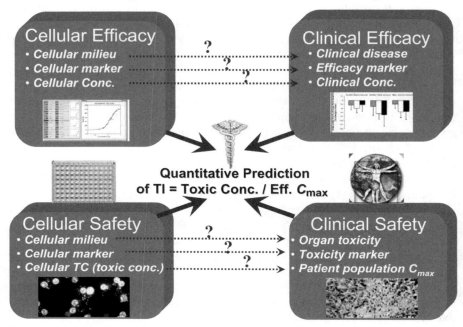

Figure 1.2 Therapeutic index (TI) screening requires the quantitative prediction of clinical efficacy and safety by a combination of cellular models, biomarkers, and in vivo relevant concentrations.

additionally integrate that with in vitro–in vivo correlation, PK measurements, pharmacodynamic prediction, and knowledge about mechanisms of chemical toxicity and its reversibility.

1.3 PREDICTING EFFICACIOUS EXPOSURE

A major challenge in predicting drug efficacious exposure is the apparent "loss of efficacy" through the translation of model systems. Such "loss of efficacy" may happen when transitioning from the isolated enzyme or receptor screens to whole cell assays, from whole cell assays to animal models, from animal models to human proof-of-concept (POC) studies, from human POC studies to large-scale and/or longer term human patient trials. Since such "loss of efficacy" leads to negative results, and negative results are typically considered less interesting to publish, our systematic understanding of the mechanisms behind such a "loss of efficacy" are relatively poor. This is unfortunate since more productive strategies of drug R&D cannot be devised unless we understand such mechanisms. After all, the number of negative results by far exceeds the successful NCE launches in the R&D endeavor [7].

While there are few systematic studies on the mechanisms of such apparent "loss of efficacy," anecdotally several reasons have been postulated: (1) preclinical efficacy models do not correlate with clinical diseases, (2) preclinical efficacy biomarkers do not correlate with disease regression, and (3) in vitro effective concentrations do not correlate with in vivo concentrations. Fundamentally too much emphasis on the isolated disease target and the reductionist approach of drug discovery has driven us away from a more holistic understanding of disease pathophysiology in an "open system" in vivo. Translational medicine, which focuses on the quantitative correlation between in vitro and in vivo, between animals and humans, aims to bridge this gap. In this section we will use case studies to highlight certain key principles of such translation and present emerging technological approaches that could address this challenge.

1.3.1 Clinically Relevant Endpoint

An example of a "loss of efficacy" during preclinical to clinical transition is the case of acyl-CoA cholesterol acyltransferase (ACAT) inhibitors. ACAT converts free cholesterol to cholesterol esters; hence it catalyses the reverse reaction of cholesteryl ester hydrolase (CEH). The original hypothesis was that if ACAT in peripheral cells such as foamy microphages was inhibited, more cholesterol would stay in the form of free cholesterol instead of cholesterol esters. Since it was thought that only free cholesterol could leave the foamy microphages, it was hypothesized that inhibition of ACAT could drive the efflux of cholesterol from these cells, and ultimately up-regulate the rate of reverse cholesterol transport (RCT) back to liver for subsequent clearance (Figure 1.3). In cellular efficacy models it was found that ACAT inhibitor

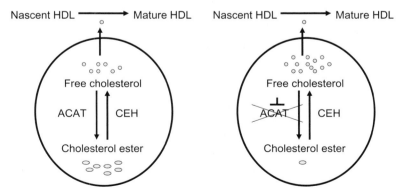

Figure 1.3 Role of acyl-CoA cholesterol acyltransferase (ACAT) and ACAT inhibitors in reverse cholesterol transport from peripheral cells.

significantly inhibited cholesterol esterification in rat aortic smooth muscle cells and macrophages. It reduced cholesterol ester by 97% and increased the cellular free cholesterol by approximately twofold [10]. In the cholesterol-fed rabbit model, the ACAT inhibitor was shown to prevent the formation of atherosclerosis and even accelerate its regression [11]. In fact several ACAT inhibitors that were tested in this animal model have showed some degree of anti-atheroscerotic effects [11–21].

To date two ACAT inhibitors, avasimibe and pactimibe, have been tested in large-scale human clinical trials. However, both trials showed lack of efficacy or even exacerbated the atheroma outcome compared to the current standard of care (i.e., statin therapy). In the Avasimibe and Progression of Lesions on Ultrasound (A-PLUS) trial, over 600 patients with coronary atherosclerosis were randomized to receive a statin or statin plus avasimibe for a period of two years [22]. The primary outcome was plaque burden, as measured by intravascular ultrasonography (IVUS) in all patients. At the end of the trial, the percent atheroma volume increased or worsened by 0.4% to 1% compared with placebo (statin alone) in a dose-dependant manner in the dose-escalating avasimibe plus statin groups [22]. In the ACAT Intravascular Atherosclerosis Treatment Evaluation (ACTIVATE) trial, over 400 patients with coronary atherosclerosis were randomized to receive statin or statin plus pactimibe, another ACAT inhibitor, for 18 months [23]. The primary outcome was also plaque burden, as measured by IVUS. In this study the atheroma volume in the most diseased 10-mm segment regressed by $3.2\,mm^3$ in the placebo (i.e., statin) group, as compared with a decrease of only $1.3\,mm^3$ in the pactimibe group ($P = 0.01$) [23].

The fact that both trials with two different ACAT inhibitors showed less than the expected atheroma outcomes compared to statin alone, showed a lack of correlation between the clinically relevant endpoint, in this case IVUS imaging, and previously measured endpoints in vitro (e.g., inhibition of ACAT per se). It is possible that direct measurements of the rate of cholesterol efflux from cholesterol-filled human macrophages could be a much more clinically relevant endpoint to measure in vitro. Indeed pre-incubation of THP-1 macrophages with atorvastatin, a widely-prescribed statin, dose dependently stimulated cholesterol efflux to apolipoprotein AI (apoAI) and high density lipoprotein (HDL) [24]. This was confirmed by ex vivo cellular cholesterol efflux studies in patients treated with atorvastatin [25]. In the future such cholesterol efflux studies (both in vitro *and* ex vivo) should be conducted to compare the effects of the statin alone with the statin plus an ACAT inhibitor. Since statin treatment already inhibits cholesteryl ester accumulation in macrophages challenged with atherogenic hypertriglyceridemic very low density lipoproteins (VLDL) [24], it is possible that any further reduction of cholesteryl ester content by avasimibe or pactimibe did not result in any additional increase in the rate of reverse cholesterol transfer (i.e., ACAT no longer being the rate-limiting step of reverse cholesterol transfer).

An analogous situation exists in the debate about which is more important in vivo, high-density lipoprotein (HDL) concentration or HDL function? Since current clinically accepted measurements are IVUS imaging of plaque burden in phase 2 or 3 trials, the HDL function on reverse cholesterol transfer is likely to be a more important translational biomarker. Indeed the ApoA-1 (Milano) carriers originally identified in northern Italy have very low HDL levels [26]. But they also have exceptional longevity with apparent protection from atherosclerosis [26,27]. The putative "HDL functions" can be measured both in vitro and ex vivo by (1) the ability to induce cholesterol efflux in aortic smooth muscle cells and macrophages, (2) the apoA-1 level, (3) paraoxonase 1 (PON1) activity, (4) reactive oxygen species (ROS) content, and (5) the ability to prevent low-density lipoprotein (LDL) oxidation. Since many clinically effective anti-atherosclerosis medicines have been shown to improve one or more of these "HDL functions," it is anticipated that a composite index of "HDL function" is a better biomarker for atherosclerosis risk than HDL levels [28–30]. It is of interest to note that physiologically relevant assays to measure all of these five HDL functions are available [30]. Therefore future HDL-targeted therapies should include these functional assays as part of their screening paradigm.

1.3.2   Simulated In Vivo Milieu

An apparent "loss of efficacy" can occasionally be obscured by a lack of in vitro–in vivo concentration correlation. In the current drug discovery paradigm, initial lead compounds are often identified from in vitro high-throughput screens (HTS), for example, an inhibition assay against a target enzyme or receptor. It is often hoped that the in vitro potency (e.g., IC_{50}) measured can be used to predict the in vivo pharmacological activity (e.g., EC_{50}). When such a correlation does not exist, there is added uncertainty as to the validity of the pharmacological target and/or the in vitro screening strategy. Also the HTS cannot be relied upon to drive the structure activity relationship (SAR), and quantitative predictions of TI become impossible to derive. Hence establishment of a correlation between in vitro potency and in vivo activity is crucial in selecting drug candidates with an optimal therapeutic window.

Theoretically the average free efficacious concentration at the steady state in vivo should be correlated with the free efficacious concentration determined from an in vitro assay as described by Recant and Riggs [31]. The Recant equation constitutes a fundamental free ligand hypothesis and has been supported by many researchers [32–35]. In practice, however, this relationship is often obscured or confounded due to a variety of factors. For example, nonphysiological conditions and nonspecific binding within in vitro systems may yield an inaccurate estimate of true intrinsic potency. In addition complex PK–PD relationships arising from indirect effects or target site disequilibrium may result in inappropriate determination of potency in vivo.

This was the case for the initial lack of correlation between in vitro potency and in vivo activity for human liver glycogen phosphorylase a (GPa) inhibitors [36]. Inhibition of liver GPa blocks the glycogenolysis pathway and therefore leads to reduction of hepatic glucose production [37,38], an effect that may be beneficial for treating type 2 diabetes mellitus. Initially, among 13 GPa reversible inhibitors (GPIs), no obvious correlation was observed between in vitro GPa enzyme IC_{50}s and any in vivo measurements such as the minimum efficacious dose (MED), or plasma or liver total and free drug concentrations at MED. It was hypothesized that the IC_{50} values obtained from HTS was probably determined under nonphysiological conditions because of the absence of adequate amounts of important cofactors or modulators present in vivo, such as AMP, ATP, and other unknown factors. Indeed there is evidence that some of these cofactors affect the binding affinity of a GPI to a GPa in vivo [39–41].

Theoretically the in vivo activity should be driven by the amount of enzyme bound to the administered inhibitor, which in turn is determined by the intrinsic dissociation constant (K_d) and the free enzyme concentration at the target site. However, accurate measurement of K_d for a target enzyme under physiological conditions can be complicated and time-consuming [35,42]. A robust method was developed to determine the intrinsic K_d of inhibitors for a purified human enzyme in the presence of organ homogenate using a previously validated 96-well equilibrium dialysis apparatus [43,44]. These conditions were supposed to mimic those in vivo better than the conventional assay [38] because most, if not all, cofactors are present in the organ homogenate (in this case, liver). The method utilizes three 96-well equilibrium dialysis apparatus in the following configurations (Figure 1.4): (1) liver homogenate against the target enzyme (in this case, GPa), (2) liver homogenate against the buffer, and (3) the target enzyme against the buffer. In the parallel dialysis setups 1 and 2, small cofactors that exist in the liver homogenate can pass the dialysis membrane and reach the enzyme chamber or buffer chamber, respectively. To facilitate rapid equilibrium, the inhibitor was added to both chambers at concentration of 250 ng/mL (~0.5 μM). At the end of dialysis (7 h), total concentrations of inhibitor at both sides of the chambers were determined by LC/MS/MS measurements [36].

By this highly parallel equilibrium dialysis technology, a significantly improved in vitro–in vivo correlation was found between the free K_d determined in the presence of liver homogenate and the free inhibitor liver concentration at the MED [36]. In addition, by this method, the concentration ratio of an inhibitor bound to the target enzyme over the total inhibitor concentration in the liver ($[I]_{b\text{-GPa}}/[I]_{t\text{-liver}}$) was estimated. This ratio has several important implications: (1) it can predict the total liver exposure in vivo at the MED, (2) it is useful in estimating the amount of target enzyme bound to an inhibitor at the MED, (3) the higher this ratio is, the more "selective" an inhibitor is for the target enzyme as opposed to the other "off-target" components in liver, and (4) this ratio represents the target efficiency of local drug

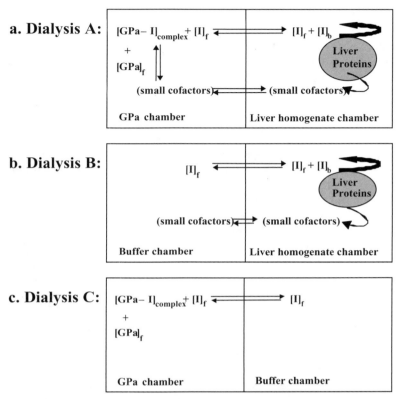

Figure 1.4 Setup of three parallel 96-well equilibrium dialysis assay configurations for the quantitative prediction of in vivo efficacy of inhibiting glycogen phosphorylase a (GPa): (*a*) liver homogenate versus the target enzyme (here, GPa), (*b*) liver homogenate versus buffer, (*c*) the target enzyme versus buffer.

disposition in this particular organ. One may extend this methodology to include a second organ, in order to estimate the relative drug disposition between two different organs. Such local drug disposition studies may have important implications in predicting TI. After all, it is the local drug concentration and ultimately local enzyme/receptor occupancy that drives drug efficacy.

This example highlights the importance of evaluating in vitro drug potency in the relevant in vivo milieu. This can be done using the appropriate endogenous ligands and co-factors at in vivo relevant concentrations. When such information is not known, whole organ lysates may be used instead. In general, a better understanding of local drug disposition studies within the target organ is an important consideration for drugs that target intracellular enzymes.

1.3.3 Kinetics Rule

The previous example relies on the thermodynamic dissociation constant, K_d (or K_i), as the primary measure of drug–target potency. However, there is also an underlying need to study kinetic properties of drug candidates using in vitro approaches, and the resulting data to make efficacy predictions [45–47]. In particular, since every drug will eventually be cleared from the body, the dissociation kinetics of a drug candidate from its target enzyme needs to be evaluated and placed into the context of its pharmacokinetic and disposition properties. Until now, few researchers have made the effort to systematically study compound SAR on the basis of on-rate and off-rate determinations, and fewer still have translated this information into in vivo effects [48].

One exception is an in vitro–in vivo correlation study on three neurokinin 1 receptor (NK-1R) antagonists [49]. In preclinical animal models the NK-1R was shown to be involved in emesis, asthma, psychiatric disorders, gastrointestinal disorders, pain, migraine, inflammation, and urinary bladder disorders (reviewed by [50]). However, to date only aprepitant has reached the market for treatment of chemotherapy-induced emesis, despite prolonged and extensive efforts by many pharmaceutical companies [51]. In a proof of concept study three different NK-1R antagonists were compared with respect to their functional dissociation kinetics to NK-1R. The study was performed in U373MG human astrocytoma cells endogenously expressing the human NK-1R. Substance P-induced mobilization of intracellular calcium (Ca^{2+}) was measured by the fluorescent calcium-sensitive dye Fluo-4, which provided the kinetic readouts of the functional interaction to NK-1R. Cells were pre-loaded with $4\,\mu M$ Fluo-4 together with $10\,nM$ of each antagonist or buffer. After 30 minutes of incubation, the cells were washed three times in assay buffer, and the "functional dissociation kinetics" of each antagonist from the NK-1R was determined by the residual Fluo-4 dye fluorescence upon substance P stimulation at various time points post–drug removal [49]. The inhibitory effect of CP-99994 was abolished within 30 minutes, whereas for ZD6021, 50% inhibition still persisted after 60 minutes. In contrast, aprepitant produced maximal inhibition lasting more than an hour. The "functional dissociation kinetics" measurement correlated very well with the duration of efficacy in the preclinical in vivo animal models of NK-1R antagonism. Slow functional reversibility of aprepitant was associated with long-lasting efficacy in vivo, whereas the efficacy of compounds with rapid reversibility closely mimicked their pharmacokinetic profiles in vivo [49].

The three examples highlighted here serve to remind us that drugs in vivo interact with complex systems including endogenous ligands and co-factors, other "off-targets," and other binding parties. A successful prediction of in vivo efficacious concentration requires a renewed thinking of in vivo-relevant endpoints, cell milieu, concentrations, dissociation kinetics, pharmacokinetic and disposition properties. Key considerations to correlate in vitro potency to in vivo activity include (1) the in vitro endpoint measured is not limited to the known activity of the target enzyme or receptor but resembles relevant in vivo clinical endpoints, (2) the in vitro milieu utilized closely resembles the in vivo milieu, (3) the in vitro dissociation kinetics is studied and integrated with the in vivo pharmacokinetic measurements and simulations. The approaches presented here can be applied to many drugs in pharmacology studies where there is a need to use preclinical efficacious concentrations (C_{eff}) to predict in vivo C_{eff}, and duration of effects.

Finally, it is important to reiterate that the drug efficacy consideration alone is not sufficient for a reliable TI prediction. For example, if a drug-induced side effect is directly linked to hyperantagonism of a target enzyme (as is the case for cerivastatin), a slow dissociation rate and long residence time can potentially exacerbate such a side effect (especially upon repeated drug dosing). While it is likely that poor efficacy could stem from rapid drug dissociation from its efficacy target, toxicity could result from slow drug dissociation from its "toxicity target." This can explain why drug-induced organ toxicity typically takes repeated dosing and manifests over longer period of time, as intracellular drug concentrations can reach a toxic level. Therefore it is important to assess whether toxicity is likely to occur at supratherapeutic levels during drug candidate selection.

1.4 PREDICTING SIDE EFFECTS/TOXICITY EXPOSURE

We now turn to the prediction of drug exposure levels where toxicity is likely to be experienced in vivo, as therapeutic index is defined as the ratio between toxic and efficacious concentrations. Major dose-limiting toxicities encountered by pharmaceutical products include cardiac toxicity [52], hepatotoxicity [53,54], muscle toxicity [55], hematotoxicity [56], genetic toxicity [57], and teratogenecity [58]. While many studies have been published on a particular drug and its associated organ toxicity, what is still needed at the drug discovery stage is a robust quantitative model that can predict across multiple drugs the exposure of a toxic drug level compared to a nontoxic drug level. Due to space limitations not all organ toxicities will be covered in detail in this chapter. The examples provided in this chapter will instead aim to highlight the key strategies and challenges in predicting toxicity exposure.

1.4.1 Cardiac Toxicity

Human life heavily depends on a functional human heart. Hence it is critical to predict and evaluate the safety margin for cardiac side effects for all drugs. In particular, the potential proarrhythmic risk of new drug candidates is a major subject of concern and needs to be carefully addressed before treatment of human volunteers or patients takes place [59]. The prolongation of the time interval between Q and T waves in an electrocardiogram (i.e., QT prolongation), is now a well-recognized biomarker for a life-threatening form of arrhythmia, called torsade de pointes (or twisting of points in an electrocardiogram) [60]. The molecular mechanisms of drug-induced QT prolongation have been well characterized. Many drugs that prolong the QT interval also block the hERG (human ether-a-go-go-related gene) potassium channel (I_{Kr} channel) (reviewed by [61,62]). Drug regulators now routinely require ligand binding studies for the I_{Kr} channel, and thorough QT assessment in preclinical species and in clinical trials [63]. Indeed the I_{Kr} channel binding assay and QT prolongation evaluations are probably the best characterized drug safety tests developed in the past decade. The collaborative work among scientists from several pharmaceutical companies suggested a provisional safety margin of 30 times the drug's efficacious exposure for in vitro hERG I_{Kr} channel binding assays [64]. However, significant gaps and challenges still exist. They include (1) estimation of efficacious exposure (related to the "loss of efficacy" when transitioning from one drug efficacy model to the next) and (2) whole systems' understanding of the interactions among multiple ion channels of the heart.

In one example, a compound that was inactive at hERG channels produced no significant QT changes in preclinical dog studies or in phase I trials with healthy human volunteers. However, prolongation of QT occurred in osteoarthritis and diabetic neuropathy patients in phase II trials, as a result of a significantly higher systemic exposure in these patients, compared with healthy volunteers [65]. This case study illustrated the importance of verifying exposure values and hence safety margins as new clinical pharmacokinetic data are available.

Small molecules can interact with not just one ion channel, but multiple ion channels of the heart. Such interactions can either "cancel" or exacerbate its proarrhythmic risk. More thorough studies should be performed to systematically characterize the interactions of such small drug molecules with several well-known cardiac ion channels. The systems biology modeling efforts to integrate the sustained $I_{(Na+)}$ and L-type $I_{(Ca2+)}$, in addition to I_{Kr} inhibition values hold promise to provide more holistic predictions of cardiac tissue's arrhythmic outcome in the future [66,67].

1.4.2 Hepatotoxicity

Since the liver is a highly perfused and the "first-pass" organ for any orally administered xenobiotic, it is a frequent site of toxicity of pharmaceuticals in humans [53,68]. Indeed drug-induced liver injury (DILI) is the number one reason why drugs were not approved in the first place, and why some of them were withdrawn from the market after approval [9]. The physiological location and drug-clearance function of the liver dictate that for an orally administered drug, the drug exposure or drug load that the liver "sees" is higher than what is being measured systemically at peripheral blood [69]. Hence we hypothesized that for DILI, a higher safety margin than QT prolongation may be needed.

To test this hypothesis, we assembled a list of more than 300 drugs and chemicals with a classification scheme based on clinical data for hepatotoxicity. Our DILI positive drugs include those (1) withdrawn from the market mainly due to hepatotoxicity (e.g., troglitazone [70]), (2) not marketed in the United States due to hepatotoxicity (e.g., nimesulide [71]), (3) receiving black box warnings from the FDA due to hepatotoxicity (e.g., dantrolene [72]), (4) marketed with hepatotoxicity warnings in their labels (e.g., zileuton [73]), (5) others (mostly old drugs) that have well-known associations with liver injury and have a significant number (>10) of independent clinical reports of hepatotoxicity (e.g., diclofenac [74]). Drugs that do not meet any of the positive criteria above are classified as DILI negatives. Since every drug can exhibit some toxicity at high enough exposure (i.e., the notion of "dose makes a poison" by Paracelsus), we searched therapeutic exposure levels through a variety of databases (Physicians' Desk Reference, PubMed, Pharmapendium™, Prous™) and collated the therapeutically active average plasma maximum concentration (C_{max}) values upon single-dose administration at commonly recommended median therapeutic doses.

To evaluate these drugs for their potential to induce hepatocyte damage, we utilized primary human hepatocytes cultured in a sandwiched configuration and multi-parameter image-based technology. Human hepatocytes cultured in the sandwiched configuration express liver-specific metabolizing enzymes [75–77], uptake and efflux transporters [78–80], and predict drug clearance via the hepatobiliary route [81]. Cryopreserved human hepatocytes were obtained commercially from CellzDirect (http://www.cellzdirect.com/). The cells were plated on collagen-coated 96-well plates (BD Biosciences) in hepatocyte plating medium (Dulbecco's Minimal Essential Medium with 5% fetal bovine serum; all media obtained from CellzDirect). Upon cell attachment, the medium was changed to hepatocyte culturing medium (Williams E medium). On the second day, the hepatocytes were sandwiched by applying an overlay of Matrigel™ (BD Biosciences). On the third day, the cells underwent a medium change with hepatocyte culturing medium. On the fourth day, the cells were treated overnight with the compound of interest or vehicle (0.1% DMSO). All compounds were initially solubilized in DMSO and diluted in culturing medium containing 5% fetal bovine serum to a final DMSO concentration of 0.1%. After 24 hours of incubation (37°C, 5% CO_2, 100% humidity) media were removed and the cells were stained by fluorescent probes in the same culturing medium lacking serum. The fluorescent probes were tetramethyl rhodamine methyl ester for mitochondrial membrane potential (TMRM; 0.02 μM, 1 h), 1,5-bis[[2-(dimethylamino)ethyl]amino]-4,8-dihydroxyanthracene-9,10-dione for nuclei and lipids DNA (DRAQ5; 45 μM, 30 min), 5-(and-6)-chloromethyl-2′7′-dichlorodihydrofluorescein diacetate acetyl ester for reactive oxygen species (CM-H_2DCFDA; 10 μM, 30 min), and finally monochlorobimane for glutathione (mBCl; 80 μM, 5 min). Automated live-cell multispectral image acquisition was performed on a Kinetic Scan Reader (Cellomics (http://www.cellomics.com/) using a 20× objective and an XF93 filter. The fluorescent images were captured according to the excitation and emission wavelengths of each probe. To capture enough cells (>500) for analysis, six image fields starting from the center of each well were collected. Image analysis was performed using ImagePro Plus (Media Cybernetics, Bethesda, MD).

It was found that the 100-fold C_{max} scaling factor represented a reasonable threshold to differentiate safe from toxic drugs, for an orally dosed drug and with regard to hepatotoxicity (Table 1.1). The first 11 drugs in Table 1.1 were known to cause idiosyncratic hepatotoxicity in humans. These drugs induced changes in the human hepatocyte imaging assays in concordance with many of their known mechanisms of hepatotoxicity. Perhexiline was reported to induce nonalcoholic steatohepatitis (NASH) in humans [82]. The mechanism of perhexiline-induced NASH involves mitochondrial injury, which causes steatosis due to impaired beta-oxidation of fatty acids, and leads to the generation of reactive oxygen species and ATP depletion [82,83]. In our imaging assay, perhexiline increased ROS and lipid intensity, and decreased mitochondrial membrane potential, GSH content, and GSH area. Troglitazone, a diabetic drug that was withdrawn from the market due to idiosyncratic liver injury, was known to cause mitochondrial damage in the literature [84,85], and completely depleted mitochondrial membrane potential in our assay (Table 1.1). In addition troglitazone also increased lipid intensity, and decreased GSH content in the hepatocytes. Nefazodone, an antidepressant that was withdrawn from the market due to hepatotoxicity [86], exhibited substantially higher frequency and severity of hepatic injury compared to other prescribed antidepressants. The hepatocyte imaging assay points to mitochondrial damage as a potential target underlying its side effects. Tetracycline, an antibiotic that was frequently associated with liver injury, was reported to induce oxidative stress both in vitro and in vivo [87–89]. As expected, the ROS signal was substantially increased in our assay. Tetracycline is also known to cause steatosis and affect mitochondria both in vitro and in vivo [90,91], and this was confirmed in the imaging assay by measurements of lipid and mitochondrial membrane potential. Nimesulide is a nonsteroidal antiinflammatory drug (NSAID) associated with a higher risk of hepatotoxicity compared to other NSAIDs [92]. Even though in vitro studies have suggested mitochondria as a potential target of toxicity, this has not been substantiated by in vivo studies [93]. Indeed, in human hepatocytes, nimesulide increased ROS and lipid intensity without affecting mitochondrial health. Likewise, sulindac and diclofenac, the other two NSAIDs with a higher risk of hepatotoxicity in the NSAID class of drugs [92], also increased ROS in our model, suggesting oxidative stress as a common mechanism of NSAID-induced liver injury (Table 1.1). Our assay technology also identified mechanisms of toxicity for those drugs that caused severe clinical DILI, but with unknown mechanisms thus far. Zileuton, a 5-lipoxygenase inhibitor approved for the treatment of asthma in adults and children, is known to cause idiosyncratic hepatocellular damage [73]. The imaging assay results suggested an increased level of oxidative stress and intracellular lipids

TABLE 1.1 High Content Image Analysis Output from the Human Hepatocyte Imaging Assay Technology (HIAT)

Drug	DILI Label	Nuclei Count (<0.4 = Positive)	Nuclei Area (<0.4 = Positive)	ROS Intensity (>2.5 = Positive)	TMRM Intensity (<0.4 = Positive)	Lipid Intensity (>2 = Positive)	GSH Content (<0.4 = Positive)	GSH Area (<0.4 = Positive)	Test Score (Logical OR of All Results)
Perhexiline	**P**	0.96	1.07	**24.0**	**0.04**	**2.48**	**0.01**	**0.02**	**P**
Troglitazone	**P**	0.71	0.85	0.00	**0.01**	**2.90**	**0.01**	**0.02**	**P**
Nefazodone	**P**	0.45	0.52	0.00	**0.04**	1.81	**0.01**	**0.03**	**P**
Tetracycline	**P**	1.04	1.06	**430**	**0.10**	**2.90**	1.13	0.82	**P**
Nimesulide	**P**	0.96	0.92	**27.3**	1.43	**2.86**	0.88	0.98	**P**
Sulindac	**P**	1.14	1.08	**14.2**	0.69	0.79	0.63	0.81	**P**
Zileuton	**P**	1.08	1.01	**4.83**	1.32	**3.46**	0.92	0.67	**P**
Labetalol	**P**	0.89	0.81	**4.88**	0.70	**5.10**	1.41	0.97	**P**
Diclofenac	**P**	0.61	0.70	**35.3**	0.98	1.86	1.91	1.22	**P**
Chlorzoxazone	**P**	0.48	0.74	**8.39**	0.78	1.70	1.01	1.65	**P**
Dantrolene	**P**	0.72	0.78	**8.54**	1.23	1.58	1.57	1.17	**P**
Amitriptyline	N	0.96	1.00	0.30	1.26	1.36	1.06	0.97	N
Pioglitazone	N	1.13	1.11	0.88	1.69	1.38	0.57	0.87	N
Rosiglitazone	N	0.66	0.79	0.44	1.04	1.66	1.52	1.38	N
Primidone	N	0.96	0.91	0.62	0.90	1.19	0.75	0.95	N
Aspirin	N	1.04	1.00	0.58	1.25	0.87	0.62	0.94	N
Penicillin	N	0.91	0.98	0.29	1.31	1.32	0.67	1.07	N
Melatonin	N	0.97	0.96	0.68	0.95	0.93	0.91	1.00	N
Nadolol	N	0.95	0.99	0.44	2.07	0.92	0.91	1.04	N
Ketotifen	N	1.02	1.01	0.60	1.00	0.88	0.90	0.94	N
Paromomycin	N	1.00	1.02	1.02	1.66	0.93	1.23	0.99	N
Sumatriptan	N	1.13	1.10	0.26	1.18	0.86	0.76	0.87	N
Famotidine	N	1.20	1.15	0.47	1.15	0.89	0.96	0.84	N
Fluoxetine	N	1.05	1.07	1.46	0.79	0.84	0.59	0.91	N

Note: In the "DILI Label" column, P = DILI positive, or hepatotoxic in humans; N = DILI negative, or nonhepatotoxic in humans according to the drug classification scheme described in the main text (see page 15). In the HIAT results columns, the test "positives" were produced by the following thresholds: reduction in nuclei count, nuclei area, TMRM intensity, GSH content, and GSH area to 40% or less of the sample treated by the vehicle control; as well as by ROS intensity that was 250% or above, or lipid intensity that was 200% or above the vehicle-treated control. The last "Test Score" column is a logical OR of the previous seven experimental results (i.e., a positive in any measurement would classify that drug as positive). Both DILI Label positives and Test Score positives were shown in bold. All these drugs were tested at 100-fold of the therapeutically active average single-dose plasma maximum concentrations (C_{max}) for 24 hours in sandwich-cultured primary human hepatocytes.

as potential mechanisms. Labetalol, an antihypertensive agent known to cause hepatotoxicity in some patients [94], increased oxidative stress and intracellular lipids in our human hepatocyte assay. Increased oxidative stress was also observed for chlorzoxazone and dantrolene, two muscle relaxants known to be associated with idiosyncratic but serious hepatotoxicity in the clinic [95]. In comparison, the bottom 13 drugs in Table 1.1 did not induce the same frequency of hepatotoxicity as the first 11 drugs, and they did not induce any significant changes in the human hepatocyte imaging assays. Among these 13 drugs were antidiabetic drugs pioglitazone and rosiglitazone, antidepressants amitriptyline and fluoxetine, NSAIDs aspirin and ketotifen, and antibiotics penicillin and paromomycin. These drugs have relatively safer clinical profiles with regard to hepatotoxcity compared to others within their respective therapeutic classes, as discussed earlier. The overall concordance of the human hepatocyte imaging assay technology (HIAT), when applied to over 300 drugs and chemicals, is about 75% with regard to clinical hepatotoxicity, with very few false-positives. The fact this relatively simple and high-throughput hepatocyte imaging assay can uncover so many common hepatotoxicity mechanisms previously reported in the literature made this technology especially attractive as a preclinical in vitro assay system to select drug candidates with improved TI for clinical hepatotoxicity.

1.4.3 Muscle Toxicity

Because of its high dependence on intracellular energy levels, muscle can be another major site of toxicity for pharmaceuticals [55]. As referenced in the beginning of this chapter, cerivastatin is a structurally distinct HMG-CoA reductase inhibitor. It effectively decreases LDL cholesterol at 1% to 3% of the doses and about 10% of the C_{max} levels of previously available statins [96]. In preclinical safety evaluation in rats, mice, minipigs, dogs, and monkeys, cerivastatin exhibited a similar toxicologic profile to other statins and is well tolerated [97]. However, in postmarket adverse event reports (AERs) submitted to the US Food and Drug Administration (FDA), cerivastatin showed a higher propensity to cause muscle toxicity, especially when co-administered with fibric acid derivatives to lower both cholesterol and triglyceride levels [98]. This led to the market withdrawal of cerivastatin [99]. Reporting rates for all statins, except for cerivastatin, were similar and much lower than 1 per 100,000 prescriptions. The cerivastatin reporting rate was much higher at 4.24/100,000 prescriptions [98]. Could such a subtle, but important, difference be predicted by a therapeutic index screening approach, at least retrospectively?

The comparative cytotoxicity effects of a panel of statins on human skeleton muscle cells (HSkMCs) were studied in vitro [100]. These HSkMCs were derived from normal human fetal skeleton muscle, and were positive for sarcomeric myosin and were fused into multinucleated myotubes (Cell

Applications, Inc.). HSkMCs were cultured in 24-well culture plates and grown to semiconfluence. They were induced to differentiate by changing the growth medium to differentiation medium (Cell Applications, Inc.). Three days later, various concentrations of drugs were added and the cultures were incubated for 24 hours. Under the light microscope, cerivastatin induced significant cell damage in cultured HSkMCs at 0.1 to 1 μM [100], while other statins induced similar damage only at 10 μM or higher. The cell damage induced by cerivastatin was abolished by the addition of mevalonolactone, suggesting the mechanism of toxicity may be linked to excessive antagonism of the HMG-CoA reductase activity in the HSkMCs. It was known that after a single oral 0.8 mg dose of cerivastatin, the C_{max} of total cerivastatin is about 8 μg/L, or 0.016 μM [101]. Thus, based on this limited HSkMC culture studies, a provisional safety margin of 30 times the efficacious C_{max} is needed to minimize the risk of muscle toxicity by cerivastatin and possibly other statin drugs. In several comparative studies among several statins, a consistent trend is that cerivastatin is the one with an exceptionally low TI in those in vitro test systems [100,102–104].

1.4.4 Is Dose Escalation a Common Theme in Estimating Toxic Exposure?

As noted above, a provisional safety margin of 30- to 100-fold has been proposed for cardiac toxicity and hepatic toxicity respectively, and possibly 30-fold for myopathy. The requirement for an elevated exposure in the in vitro setting to identify deleterious organ effects of drugs may be due to a combination of (1) liver exposure to an orally dosed drug can be higher than its systemic exposure; (2) population PK variability due to age, genetics (including drug metabolism and transporters), and drug–drug interactions could further exacerbate local drug exposure and toxicity; (3) idiosyncratic organ history (including disease and previous drug exposures); (4) onset of toxicity in vivo is typically much longer than in vitro, thus requiring dose escalation in most short-term in vitro systems. Hence it is likely that dose escalation may be a common theme in estimating toxic exposure in the drug discovery stage. In the future, when all the variables in PK and pharmacodynamics can be accounted for and simulated a priori, a more precise estimation of TI may be possible.

Another theme is that the predictive safety margin of each in vitro system needs to be "calibrated" retrospectively using both toxic drugs and "clean" drugs in approaches similar to the examples given above. This is a prerequisite of building enough confidence that such predictions can be applied to new chemical entities for the same therapeutic target or targets. In the drug discovery stage, a TI prediction strategy needs to be practical to be applied broadly. Specifically at this stage, the volume of compounds that are generated and need to be evaluated typically exceeds several dozens to hundreds or thousands, the actual amount of compounds that are available for testing often less than 100 mg, the time window for decision making is often limited to a few days to weeks. In these scenarios human and animal cellular systems cultured in well-characterized ways to recapitulate the relevant in vivo responses, coupled with high-throughput and high-content screening technologies, have the best potential for an efficient prediction of TI in the drug discovery stage.

1.5   FUTURE PERSPECTIVES

As illustrated in this chapter, the choices of cellular models, biomarkers being investigated, and the concentration–effect responses being measured have a profound effect on the therapeutic index prediction. Future efforts to improve TI prediction should therefore focus on these directions: (1) cellular models that better mimic the in vivo situation, (2) more accurate concentration measurement, and (3) systems based pharmacokinetic and pharmacodynamic prediction.

Although cellular models have been used in pharmacology and toxicology research for decades, it is only recently that the *omics* technology has been applied to the characterization of cell culture models [77,105,106] and the cell engineering field [107,108]. Primary cells cultured under defined conditions to better mimic the disease situation will be increasingly used as the result of better isolation, culturing, and characterization techniques. In particular, primary cells that maintain tissue-specific metabolic functions will be in increasing demand (primary neurons, beating cardiomyocytes, drug-metabolizing and polarized hepatocytes and nephrons, etc.). Stem cell technology promises to deliver unlimited sources of differentiated primary cells without the need to wait for donor availability [109,110]. Tissue engineering is an emerging field that can provide us with more physiological cell–cell interactions, endogenous functions, and well-defined fluid dynamics [111–113]. Taken together, these technologies promise to decrease the gaps between the in vitro and in vivo world.

However, technology alone cannot bring us closer to improved TI prediction without the sound principle of pharmacology and appropriate design of toxicological studies. Bioanalytical quantification of the actual "total" and "free" in vitro drug concentration in both whole cell efficacy and toxicity tests, and better PK prediction to project both efficacy and toxicity concentrations in vivo are still needed for any TI prediction. Recently human PK predictions based on in vitro systems have become more realistic [114,115]. This had led to the hope that in silico predictions of PK are not too far in the future [116–118]. Regarding pharmacodynamic predictions, mathematical simulations based on our understanding of human pathophysiology will become an integral part of any future drug R&D strategy [119–121]. With these technological advances, the science of projecting in vivo therapeutic index based on integrated in silico, in vitro, and in vivo approaches will flourish.

REFERENCES

1. Deichmann WB, Henschler D, Holmsted B, Keil G. What is there that is not poison? A study of the *Third defense* by Paracelsus. *Arch Toxicol* 1986;58:207–13.

2. Rozman KK. Quantitative definition of toxicity: a mathematical description of life and death with dose and time as variables. *Med Hypotheses* 1998;51:175–8.

3. Fitzgerald JB, Schoeberl B, Nielsen UB, Sorger PK. Systems biology and combination therapy in the quest for clinical efficacy. *Nat Chem Biol* 2006;2:458–66.

4. Cziraky MJ, Willey VJ, McKenney JM, Kamat SA, Fisher MD, Guyton JR, et al. Statin safety: an assessment using an administrative claims database. *Am J Cardiol* 2006;97:61C–8C.

5. Kramer JA, Sagartz JE, Morris DL. The application of discovery toxicology and pathology towards the design of safer pharmaceutical lead candidates. *Nat Rev Drug Discov* 2007;6:636–49.

6. Giacomini KM, Roden KR, Eichelbaum DM, Hayden MR, Nakamura Y. When good drugs go bad. *Nature* 2007;446:975–7.

7. Kola I, Landis J. Can the pharmaceutical industry reduce attrition rates? *Nat Rev Drug Discov* 2004;3:711–6.

8. Nissen SE, Tardif JC, Nicholls SJ, Revkin JH, Shear CL, Duggan WT, et al. Effect of torcetrapib on the progression of coronary atherosclerosis. *N Engl J Med* 2007;356:1304–16.

9. Schuster D, Laggner C, Langer T. Why drugs fail—a study on side effects in new chemical entities. *Curr Pharm Des* 2005;11:3545–59.

10. Nicholson AC, Pomerantz KB, Fujimori T, Hajjar DP. Inhibition of cholesterol esterification in macrophages and vascular smooth muscle foam cells: evaluation of E5324, an acyl-CoA cholesterol acyltransferase inhibitor. *Lipids* 1995;30:771–4.

11. Aragane K, Kojima K, Fujinami K, Kamei J, Kusunoki J. Effect of F-1394, an acyl-CoA:cholesterol acyltransferase inhibitor, on atherosclerosis induced by high cholesterol diet in rabbits. *Atherosclerosis* 2001;158:139–45.

12. Aragane K, Fujinami K, Kojima K, Kusunoki J. ACAT inhibitor F-1394 prevents intimal hyperplasia induced by balloon injury in rabbits. *J Lipid Res* 2001;42:480–8.

13. Asami Y, Yamagishi I, Murakami S, Araki H, Tsuchida K, Higuchi S. HL-004, the ACAT inhibitor, prevents the progression of atherosclerosis in cholesterol-fed rabbits. *Life Sci* 1998;62:1055–63.

14. Azuma Y, Date K, Ohno K, Matsushiro S, Nobuhara Y, Yamada T. NTE-122, an acyl-coa:cholesterol acyltransferase inhibitor, prevents the progression of atherogenesis in cholesterol-fed rabbits. *Jpn J Pharmacol* 2001;86:120–3.

15. Azuma Y, Kawasaki T, Ikemoto K, Obata K, Ohno K, Sajiki N, et al. Cholesterol-lowering effects of NTE-122, a novel acyl-CoA:cholesterol acyltransferase (ACAT) inhibitor, on cholesterol diet-fed rats and rabbits. *Jpn J Pharmacol* 1998;78:355–64.

16. Ioriya K, Noguchi T, Muraoka M, Fujita K, Shimizu H, Ohashi N. Effect of SMP-500, a novel acyl-coA:cholesterol acyltransferase inhibitor, on the cholesterol

esterification and its hypocholesterolemic properties. *Pharmacology* 2002;65: 18–25.

17. Ishii I, Yokoyama N, Yanagimachi M, Ashikawa N, Hata M, Murakami S, et al. Stimulation of cholesterol release from rabbit foam cells by the action of a new inhibitor for acyl CoA:cholesterol acyltransferase (ACAT), HL-004. *J Pharmacol Exp Ther* 1998;287:115–21.

18. Junquero D, Oms P, Carilla-Durand E, Autin J, Tarayre J, Degryse A, et al. Pharmacological profile of F 12511, (S)-2′,3′, 5′-trimethyl-4′-hydroxy-alpha-dodecylthioacetanilide a powerful and systemic acylcoenzyme A: cholesterol acyltransferase inhibitor. *Biochem Pharmacol* 2001;61:97–108.

19. Matsui Y, Horiuchi K, Yamamoto K, Kanai K. Pharmacological properties of R-755, a novel acyl-CoA:cholesterol acyltransferase inhibitor, in cholesterol-fed rats, hamsters and rabbits. *Jpn J Pharmacol* 2001;85:423–33.

20. Nakamura S, Kamiya S, Shirahase H, Kanda M, Yoshimi A, Tarumi T, et al. Hypolipidemic and antioxidant activity of the novel acyl-CoA:cholesterol acyltransferase (ACAT) inhibitor KY-455 in rabbits and hamsters. *Arzneimittelforschung* 2004;54:102–8.

21. Yamaguchi J, Hachiuma K, Kimura Y, Ogawa N, Higuchi S. Highly sensitive determination of TS-962 (HL-004), a novel acyl-CoA:cholesterol acyltransferase inhibitor, in rat and rabbit plasma by liquid chromatography and atmospheric pressure chemical ionization-tandem mass spectrometry combined with a column-switching technique. *J Chromatogr B Biomed Sci Appl* 2001;750:99–108.

22. Tardif JC, Gregoire J, L'Allier PL, Anderson TJ, Bertrand O, Reeves F, et al. Effects of the acyl coenzyme A:cholesterol acyltransferase inhibitor avasimibe on human atherosclerotic lesions. *Circulation* 2004;110:3372–7.

23. Nissen SE, Tuzcu EM, Brewer HB, Sipahi I, Nicholls SJ, Ganz P, et al. Effect of ACAT inhibition on the progression of coronary atherosclerosis. *N Engl J Med* 2006;354:1253–63.

24. Argmann CA, Edwards JY, Sawyez CG, O'Neil CH, Hegele RA, Pickering JG, et al. Regulation of macrophage cholesterol efflux through hydroxymethylglutaryl-CoA reductase inhibition: a role for RhoA in ABCA1-mediated cholesterol efflux. *J Biol Chem* 2005;280:22212–21.

25. Guerin M, Egger P, Soudant C, Le Goff W, van Tol A, Dupuis R, et al. Dose-dependent action of atorvastatin in type IIB hyperlipidemia: preferential and progressive reduction of atherogenic apoB-containing lipoprotein subclasses (VLDL-2, IDL, small dense LDL) and stimulation of cellular cholesterol efflux. *Atherosclerosis* 2002;163:287–96.

26. Gomaraschi M, Baldassarre D, Amato M, Eligini S, Conca P, Sirtori CR, et al. Normal vascular function despite low levels of high-density lipoprotein cholesterol in carriers of the apolipoprotein A-I(Milano) mutant. *Circulation* 2007;116: 2165–72.

27. Kaul S, Shah PK. ApoA-I Milano/phospholipid complexes emerging pharmacological strategies and medications for the prevention of atherosclerotic plaque progression. *Curr Drug Targets Cardiovasc Haematol Disord* 2005;5:471–9.

28. Navab M, Anantharamaiah GM, Reddy ST, Van Lenten BJ, Ansell BJ, Fogelman AM. Mechanisms of disease: proatherogenic HDL—an evolving field. *Nat Clin Pract Endocrinol Metab* 2006;2:504–11.

29. Navab M, Ananthramaiah GM, Reddy ST, Van Lenten BJ, Ansell BJ, Hama S, et al. The double jeopardy of HDL. *Ann Med* 2005;37:173–8.

30. Narasimha A, Watanabe J, Lin JA, Hama S, Langenbach R, Navab M, et al. A novel anti-atherogenic role for COX-2—potential mechanism for the cardio-vascular side effects of COX-2 inhibitors. *Prostaglandins Other Lipid Mediat* 2007;84:24–33.

31. Recant L, Riggs DS. Thyroid function in nephrosis. *J Clin Invest* 1952;31:789–97.

32. Wagner JG. Simple model to explain effects of plasma protein binding and tissue binding on calculated volumes of distribution, apparent elimination rate constants and clearances. *Eur J Clin Pharmacol* 1976;10:425–32.

33. Wagner JG, Northam JI, Alway CD, Carpenter OS. Blood levels of drug at the equilibrium state after multiple dosing. *Nature* 1965;207:1301–2.

34. DeGuchi Y, Terasaki T, Yamada H, Tsuji A. An application of microdialysis to drug tissue distribution study: in vivo evidence for free-ligand hypothesis and tissue binding of beta-lactam antibiotics in interstitial fluids. *J Pharm Dyn* 1992;15:79–89.

35. Wright JD, Boudinot FD, Ujhelyi MR. Measurement and analysis of unbound drug concentrations. *Clin Pharmacokinet* 1996;30:445–62.

36. Yu LJ, Chen Y, Treadway JL, McPherson RK, McCoid SC, Gibbs EM, et al. Establishment of correlation between in vitro enzyme binding potency and in vivo pharmacological activity: application to liver glycogen phosphorylase a inhibitors. *J Pharmacol Exp Ther* 2006;317:1230–7.

37. Treadway JL, Mendys P, Hoover DJ. Glycogen phosphorylase inhibitors for treatment of type 2 diabetes mellitus. *Expert Opin Invest Drugs* 2001;10:439–54.

38. Martin WH, Hoover DJ, Armento SJ, Stock IA, McPherson RK, Danley DE, et al. Discovery of a human liver glycogen phosphorylase inhibitor that lowers blood glucose in vivo. *Proc Natl Acad Sci USA* 1998;95:1776–81.

39. Monanu MO, Madsen NB. Distinction between substrate- and enzyme-directed effects of modifiers of rabbit liver phosphorylase a phosphatases. *Biochem Cell Biol* 1987;65:293–301.

40. Ercan-Fang N, Gannon MC, Rath VL, Treadway JL, Taylor MR, Nuttall FQ. Integrated effects of multiple modulators on human liver glycogen phosphorylase a. *Am J Physiol Endocrinol Metab* 2002;283:E29–37.

41. Ercan-Fang NG, Taylor MR, Gannon MC, Treadway JL, Rath VL, Nuttall FQ. Regulation of human liver glycogen phosphorylase a by multiple modulators in the presence of an indole-site inhibitor. American Diabetes Association 62nd Annual Meeting and Scientific Sessions 2002:1412-P. Diabetes 51 Suppl 2.

42. Romer J, Bickel MH. A method to estimate binding constants at variable protein concentrations. *J Pharm Pharmacol* 1979;31:7–11.

43. Banker MJ, Clark TH, Williams JA. Development and validation of a 96-well equilibrium dialysis apparatus for measuring plasma protein binding. *J Pharm Sci* 2003;92:967–74.

44. Cory Kalvass J, Maurer TS. Influence of nonspecific brain and plasma binding on CNS exposure: implications for rational drug discovery. *Biopharm Drug Dispos* 2002;23:327–38.

45. Shuman CF, Vrang L, Danielson UH. Improved structure-activity relationship analysis of HIV-1 protease inhibitors using interaction kinetic data. *J Med Chem* 2004;47:5953–61.

46. Vestergaard HT, Cannillo C, Frolund B, Kristiansen U. Differences in kinetics of structurally related competitive GABA(A) receptor antagonists. *Neuropharmacology* 2007;52:873–82.

47. Markgren PO, Schaal W, Hamalainen M, Karlen A, Hallberg A, Samuelsson B, et al. Relationships between structure and interaction kinetics for HIV-1 protease inhibitors. *J Med Chem* 2002;45:5430–9.

48. Copeland RA, Pompliano DL, Meek TD. Drug-target residence time and its implications for lead optimization. *Nat Rev Drug Discov* 2006;5:730–9.

49. Lindstrom E, von Mentzer B, Pahlman I, Ahlstedt I, Uvebrant A, Kristensson E, et al. Neurokinin 1 receptor antagonists: correlation between in vitro receptor interaction and in vivo efficacy. *J Pharmacol Exp Ther* 2007;322:1286–93.

50. Quartara L, Altamura M. Tachykinin receptors antagonists: from research to clinic. *Curr Drug Targets* 2006;7:975–92.

51. Alvaro G, Di Fabio R. Neurokinin 1 receptor antagonists—current prospects. *Curr Opin Drug Discov Devel* 2007;10:613–21.

52. Sereno M, Brunello A, Chiappori A, Barriuso J, Casado E, Belda C, et al. Cardiac toxicity: old and new issues in anti-cancer drugs. *Clin Transl Oncol* 2008;10: 35–46.

53. Kaplowitz N. Idiosyncratic drug hepatotoxicity. *Nat Rev Drug Discov* 2005; 4:489–99.

54. Navarro VJ, Senior JR. Drug-related hepatotoxicity. *N Engl J Med* 2006;354: 731–9.

55. Owczarek J, Jasinska M, Orszulak-Michalak D. Drug-induced myopathies: an overview of the possible mechanisms. *Pharmacol Rep* 2005;57:23–34.

56. Pessina A, Malerba I, Gribaldo L. Hematotoxicity testing by cell clonogenic assay in drug development and preclinical trials. *Curr Pharm Des* 2005;11:1055–65.

57. Kasper P, Uno Y, Mauthe R, Asano N, Douglas G, Matthews E, et al. Follow-up testing of rodent carcinogens not positive in the standard genotoxicity testing battery: IWGT workgroup report. *Mutat Res* 2007;627:106–16.

58. Reamon-Buettner SM, Borlak J. A new paradigm in toxicology and teratology: altering gene activity in the absence of DNA sequence variation. *Reprod Toxicol* 2007;24:20–30.

59. Hanton G. Preclinical cardiac safety assessment of drugs. *Drugs RD* 2007;8: 213–28.

60. Steinbrecher UP, Fitchett DH. Torsade de pointes: a cause of syncope with atrioventricular block. *Arch Intern Med* 1980;140:1223–6.

61. Brown AM. HERG block, QT liability and sudden cardiac death. *Novartis Found Symp* 2005;266:118–31; discussion 31–5, 55–8.

62. Stansfeld PJ, Sutcliffe MJ, Mitcheson JS. Molecular mechanisms for drug interactions with hERG that cause long QT syndrome. *Expert Opin Drug Metab Toxicol* 2006;2:81–94.

63. Shah RR. Drugs, QTc interval prolongation and final ICH E14 guideline: an important milestone with challenges ahead. *Drug Saf* 2005;28:1009–28.

64. Redfern WS, Carlsson L, Davis AS, Lynch WG, MacKenzie I, Palethorpe S, et al. Relationships between preclinical cardiac electrophysiology, clinical QT interval prolongation and torsade de pointes for a broad range of drugs: evidence for a provisional safety margin in drug development. *Cardiovasc Res* 2003;58:32–45.

65. Hanton G, Tilbury L. Cardiac safety strategies. 25–26 October 2005, the Radisson SAS Hotel, Nice, France. *Expert Opin Drug Saf* 2006;5:329–33.

66. Bottino D, Penland RC, stamps A, Traebert M, Dumotier B, Georgiva A, et al. Preclinical cardiac safety assessment of pharmaceutical compounds using an integrated systems-based computer model of the heart. *Prog Biophys Mol Biol* 2006;90:414–43.

67. Crumb WJ, Jr, Ekins S, Sarazan RD, Wikel JH, Wrighton SA, Carlson C, et al. Effects of antipsychotic drugs on I(to), I (Na), I (sus), I (K1), and hERG: QT prolongation, structure activity relationship, and network analysis. *Pharm Res* 2006;23:1133–43.

68. Lee WM. Drug-induced hepatotoxicity. *N Engl J Med* 2003;349:474–85.

69. Ito K, Chiba K, Horikawa M, Ishigami M, Mizuno N, Aoki J, et al. Which concentration of the inhibitor should be used to predict in vivo drug interactions from in vitro data? *AAPS Pharm Sci* 2002;4:E25.

70. Parker JC. Troglitazone: the discovery and development of a novel therapy for the treatment of type 2 diabetes mellitus. *Adv Drug Deliv Rev* 2002;54:1173–97.

71. Macia MA, Carvajal A, del Pozo JG, Vera E, del Pino A. Hepatotoxicity associated with nimesulide: data from the Spanish Pharmacovigilance System. *Clin Pharmacol Ther* 2002;72:596–7.

72. Durham JA, Gandolfi AJ, Bentley JB. Hepatotoxicological evaluation of dantrolene sodium. *Drug Chem Toxicol* 1984;7:23–40.

73. Watkins PB, Dube LM, Walton-Bowen K, Cameron CM, Kasten LE. Clinical pattern of zileuton-associated liver injury: results of a 12-month study in patients with chronic asthma. *Drug Saf* 2007;30:805–15.

74. Boelsterli UA. Diclofenac-induced liver injury: a paradigm of idiosyncratic drug toxicity. *Toxicol Appl Pharmacol* 2003;192:307–22.

75. Wilkening S, Stahl F, Bader A. Comparison of primary human hepatocytes and hepatoma cell line Hepg2 with regard to their biotransformation properties. *Drug Metab Dispos* 2003;31:1035–42.

76. Hamilton GA, Jolley SL, Gilbert D, Coon DJ, Barros S, LeCluyse EL. Regulation of cell morphology and cytochrome P450 expression in human hepatocytes by extracellular matrix and cell–cell interactions. *Cell Tissue Res* 2001;306:85–99.

77. Olsavsky KM, Page JL, Johnson MC, Zarbl H, Strom SC, Omiecinski CJ. Gene expression profiling and differentiation assessment in primary human hepatocyte cultures, established hepatoma cell lines, and human liver tissues. *Toxicol Appl Pharmacol* 2007;222:42–56.

78. Bi YA, Kazolias D, Duignan DB. Use of cryopreserved human hepatocytes in sandwich culture to measure hepatobiliary transport. *Drug Metab Dispos* 2006;34:1658–65.

79. Marion TL, Leslie EM, Brouwer KL. Use of sandwich-cultured hepatocytes to evaluate impaired bile acid transport as a mechanism of drug-induced hepatotoxicity. *Mol Pharm* 2007;4:911–8.

80. Hoffmaster KA, Turncliff RZ, LeCluyse EL, Kim RB, Meier PJ, Brouwer KL. P-glycoprotein expression, localization, and function in sandwich-cultured primary rat and human hepatocytes: relevance to the hepatobiliary disposition of a model opioid peptide. *Pharm Res* 2004;21:1294–302.

81. Ghibellini G, Vasist LS, Leslie EM, Heizer WD, Kowalsky RJ, Calvo BF, et al. In vitro–in vivo correlation of hepatobiliary drug clearance in humans. *Clin Pharmacol Ther* 2007;81:406–13.

82. Farrell GC. Drugs and steatohepatitis. *Semin Liver Dis* 2002;22:185–94.

83. Fromenty B, Pessayre D. Inhibition of mitochondrial beta-oxidation as a mechanism of hepatotoxicity. *Pharmacol Ther* 1995;67:101–54.

84. Masubuchi Y, Kano S, Horie T. Mitochondrial permeability transition as a potential determinant of hepatotoxicity of antidiabetic thiazolidinediones. *Toxicology* 2006;222:233–9.

85. Ong MM, Latchoumycandane C, Boelsterli UA. Troglitazone-induced hepatic necrosis in an animal model of silent genetic mitochondrial abnormalities. *Toxicol Sci* 2007;97:205–13.

86. Choi S. Nefazodone (Serzone) withdrawn because of hepatotoxicity. *CMAJ* 2003;169:1187.

87. Kikkawa R, Fujikawa M, Yamamoto T, Hamada Y, Yamada H, Horii I. In vivo hepatotoxicity study of rats in comparison with in vitro hepatotoxicity screening system. *J Toxicol Sci* 2006;31:23–34.

88. Yamamoto T, Kikkawa R, Yamada H, Horii I. Identification of oxidative stress-related proteins for predictive screening of hepatotoxicity using a proteomic approach. *J Toxicol Sci* 2005;30:213–27.

89. Yamamoto T, Kikkawa R, Yamada H, Horii I. Investigation of proteomic biomarkers in in vivo hepatotoxicity study of rat liver: toxicity differentiation in hepatotoxicants. *J Toxicol Sci* 2006;31:49–60.

90. Amacher DE, Martin BA. Tetracycline-induced steatosis in primary canine hepatocyte cultures. *Fundam Appl Toxicol* 1997;40:256–63.

91. Letteron P, Sutton A, Mansouri A, Fromenty B, Pessayre D. Inhibition of microsomal triglyceride transfer protein: another mechanism for drug-induced steatosis in mice. *Hepatology* 2003;38:133–40.

92. Aithal GP, Day CP. Nonsteroidal anti-inflammatory drug-induced hepatotoxicity. *Clin Liver Dis* 2007;11:563–75, vi–vii.

93. Moreno AJ, Oliveira PJ, Nova CD, Alvaro AR, Moreira RA, Santos SM, et al. Unaltered hepatic oxidative phosphorylation and mitochondrial permeability transition in wistar rats treated with nimesulide: relevance for nimesulide toxicity characterization. *J Biochem Mol Toxicol* 2007;21:53–61.

94. Stumpf JL. Fatal hepatotoxicity induced by hydralazine or labetalol. *Pharmacotherapy* 1991;11:415–8.

95. Chou R, Peterson K, Helfand M. Comparative efficacy and safety of skeletal muscle relaxants for spasticity and musculoskeletal conditions: a systematic review. *J Pain Symptom Manage* 2004;28:140–75.

96. Davignon J, Hanefeld M, Nakaya N, Hunninghake DB, Insull W, Jr, Ose L. Clinical efficacy and safety of cerivastatin: summary of pivotal phase IIb/III studies. *Am J Cardiol* 1998;82:32J–9J.

97. von Keutz E, Schluter G. Preclinical safety evaluation of cerivastatin, a novel HMG-CoA reductase inhibitor. *Am J Cardiol* 1998;82:11J–7J.

98. Chang JT, Staffa JA, Parks M, Green L. Rhabdomyolysis with HMG-CoA reductase inhibitors and gemfibrozil combination therapy. *Pharmacoepidemiol Drug Saf* 2004;13:417–26.

99. Holoshitz N, Alsheikh-Ali AA, Karas RH. Relative safety of gemfibrozil and fenofibrate in the absence of concomitant cerivastatin use. *Am J Cardiol* 2008;101:95–7.

100. Yamazaki H, Suzuki M, Aoki T, Morikawa S, Maejima T, Sato F, et al. Influence of 3-hydroxy-3-methylglutaryl coenzyme A reductase inhibitors on ubiquinone levels in rat skeletal muscle and heart: relationship to cytotoxicity and inhibitory activity for cholesterol synthesis in human skeletal muscle cells. *J Atheroscler Thromb* 2006;13:295–307.

101. Mazzu AL, Lasseter KC, Shamblen EC, Agarwal V, Lettieri J, Sundaresen P. Itraconazole alters the pharmacokinetics of atorvastatin to a greater extent than either cerivastatin or pravastatin. *Clin Pharmacol Ther* 2000;68:391–400.

102. Corpataux JM, Naik J, Porter KE, London NJ. The effect of six different statins on the proliferation, migration, and invasion of human smooth muscle cells. *J Surg Res* 2005;129:52–6.

103. Kaufmann P, Torok M, Zahno A, Waldhauser KM, Brecht K, Krahenbuhl S. Toxicity of statins on rat skeletal muscle mitochondria. *Cell Mol Life Sci* 2006;63: 2415–25.

104. Kobayashi M, Otsuka Y, Itagaki S, Hirano T, Iseki K. Inhibitory effects of statins on human monocarboxylate transporter 4. *Int J Pharm* 2006;317:19–25.

105. Jayaraman A, Yarmush ML, Roth CM. Evaluation of an in vitro model of hepatic inflammatory response by gene expression profiling. *Tissue Eng* 2005;11: 50–63.

106. Baudin B, Bruneel A, Bosselut N, Vaubourdolle M. A protocol for isolation and culture of human umbilical vein endothelial cells. *Nat Protoc* 2007;2:481–5.

107. Khoo SH, Al-Rubeai M. Metabolomics as a complementary tool in cell culture. *Biotechnol Appl Biochem* 2007;47:71–84.

108. Tyo KE, Alper HS, Stephanopoulos GN. Expanding the metabolic engineering toolbox: more options to engineer cells. *Trends Biotechnol* 2007;25:132–7.

109. McNeish JD. Stem cells as screening tools in drug discovery. *Curr Opin Pharmacol* 2007;7:515–20.

110. Gimble JM, Katz AJ, Bunnell BA. Adipose-derived stem cells for regenerative medicine. *Circ Res* 2007;100:1249–60.

111. Griffith LG, Swartz MA. Capturing complex 3D tissue physiology in vitro. *Nat Rev Mol Cell Biol* 2006;7:211–24.

112. Baudoin R, Corlu A, Griscom L, Legallais C, Leclerc E. Trends in the development of microfluidic cell biochips for in vitro hepatotoxicity. *Toxicol In vitro* 2007;21:535–44.

113. Khetani SR, Bhatia SN. Microscale culture of human liver cells for drug development. *Nat Biotechnol* 2008;26:120–6.

114. Cheng L, Tongtong L, Xiaoming C, Uss AS, Cheng KC. Development of in vitro pharmacokinetic screens using caco-2, human hepatocyte, and caco-2/human

hepatocyte hybrid systems for the prediction of oral bioavailability in humans. *J Biomol Screen* 2007;12:1084–91.

115. Hewitt NJ, Lecluyse EL, Ferguson SS. Induction of hepatic cytochrome P450 enzymes: methods, mechanisms, recommendations, and in vitro–in vivo correlations. *Xenobiotica* 2007;37:1196–224.

116. Dearden JC. In silico prediction of ADMET properties: how far have we come? *Expert Opin Drug Metab Toxicol* 2007;3:635–9.

117. Hunt CA, Ropella GE, Yan L, Hung DY, Roberts MS. Physiologically based synthetic models of hepatic disposition. *J Pharmacokinet Pharmacodyn* 2006; 33:737–72.

118. Zhang X, Shedden K, Rosania GR. A cell-based molecular transport simulator for pharmacokinetic prediction and cheminformatic exploration. *Mol Pharm* 2006;3:704–16.

119. Mager DE. Quantitative structure-pharmacokinetic/pharmacodynamic relationships. *Adv Drug Deliv Rev* 2006;58:1326–56.

120. Cavero I. Using pharmacokinetic/pharmacodynamic modelling in safety pharmacology to better define safety margins: a regional workshop of the Safety Pharmacology Society. *Expert Opin Drug Saf* 2007;6:465–71.

121. Dingemanse J, Appel-Dingemanse S. Integrated pharmacokinetics and pharmacodynamics in drug development. *Clin Pharmacokinet* 2007;46:713–37.

ACKNOWLEDGMENT

The authors extend profound gratitude to their past collaborators at Pfizer Global R&D, especially Margaret Dunn, Arthur Smith, Jeffrey Chabot, Peter Henstock, David de Graaf, Yue Chen, and Judith Treadway.

2

HIGH-THROUGHPUT PROTEIN-BASED TECHNOLOGIES AND COMPUTATIONAL MODELS FOR DRUG DEVELOPMENT, EFFICACY, AND TOXICITY

LEONIDAS G. ALEXOPOULOS, JULIO SAEZ-RODRIGUEZ, AND CHRISTOPHER W. ESPELIN

Contents

Drug Efficacy, Safety, and Biologics Discovery: Emerging Technologies and Tools,
Edited by Sean Ekins and Jinghai J. Xu
Copyright © 2009 by John Wiley & Sons, Inc.

2.1 INTRODUCTION

Major advances in high-throughput assay capability coupled with increasingly sophisticated computational methods for systematic data analysis have provided scientists with tools to better understand the complexity of biological systems. This potent combination of novel experimental and analytical approaches should in turn lead to more effective therapeutic design. Most high-throughput approaches can generally be categorized based on their readouts: genomic, transcriptomic, metabolomic or proteomic. However, despite the differences in the endpoints measured by each of these assays (DNA, mRNA, metabolites or proteins), the biological information they capture is often overlapping and complementary. Accordingly, the increasingly interdependent nature of science has also given rise to disciplines such as bioinformatics, systems biology and computational biology, which are charged with incorporating and interpreting the vast amounts of experimental data and generating hypotheses of biological significance. Scientists will therefore be increasingly required to understand the advantages and limitations of DNA, mRNA, metabolomic and proteomic capabilities and use them accordingly depending on the knowledge they wish to obtain. Especially critical for the pharmaceutical industry is the coupling of experimental approaches with computational algorithms. This integration has the potential to significantly impact discovery, reduce research and development costs, minimize drug failure by predicting efficacy and toxicity, and ultimately determine a company's competitiveness in the global market.

The primary objective of a therapeutic strategy is to selectively alter a targeted protein(s) or pathway(s) within diseased cells in order to ameliorate an undesired phenotype (unrestrained cell proliferation, inflammatory cytokine release, etc.). Ideally other pathways within the diseased cells, as well as all cellular functions in healthy cells, would remain unaffected by the therapeutic approach. Thus target selection is a multifaceted problem with several levels of complexity: (1) cellular pathway(s) or extracellular targets need to be selected; (2) associated biomarkers need to be identified that distinguish healthy and disease phenotypes and ideally are capable of reflecting pharmacological efficacy and safety; (3) the risk–benefit of different therapeutic approaches should be considered: small molecule inhibitors, biologics, siRNA-derived therapeutics (transcriptional targets), etc.; and (4) a selection criteria needs to be identified for screening compounds against a desired target. Addressing these initial issues, however, is just the beginning of the drug discovery process. Drug metabolism might render the pharmacologic approach ineffective, genetic and epigenetic person-to-person variability might cause *idiosyncratic toxicity* (i.e., a term that signifies the unknown cause of adverse drug effects), and the overlapping cellular pathway architecture might result in even very selective on-target compounds having unwanted effects on the same or different cells [1,2].

In this complicated world of drug discovery and development, high-throughput technologies (genomics, transcriptomics, metabolomics and proteomics) have become invaluable tools for tackling the complexity of the biological systems and optimizing therapeutic strategies. In the following section we explore different technologies and their niches in the area of drug development, efficacy, and toxicity.

2.1.1 Genomics Technologies

Several diseases are strongly correlated with specific genomic mutations (e.g. Huntington's disease, sickle cell anemia). As a general concept, cancer progression can be facilitated by gain-of-function mutations in oncogenes or loss-of-function mutations in tumor-supressor genes [3]. However, in many instances dozens of genomic aberrations are associated with the development of a single cancer type [4]. Specifically, in hepatocellular carcinoma (the most common type of liver cancer) genomic aberrations have been found in several proteins including TP53, TGFb, Ras, and Rb, EGFR, ERbB2, and members of the Wnt-signaling pathway [5–9]. Thus understanding the genomic basis for development of a disease can significantly impact the focus of pharmaceutical therapies. It is now evident that genomics has moved therapeutic strategies away from being phenotype specific (i.e., chemotherapy for highly proliferative cells), and focused them on pathway-specific targets (anti-EGFR or anti-VEGF treatments, etc.).

Specific examples of the role that interindividual genetic variability plays in drug efficacy have also been demonstrated in recent years. The epidermal growth factor receptor (EGFR) tyrosine kinase inhibitor Gefitinib represents just such a case. Gefitinib originally exhibited significant clinical response in only 10% of patients with non–small-cell lung cancer, a modest response rate [10]. However, when primary tumors from a group of patients were screened for EGFR gene mutations, eight of nine gefitinib-responsive patients had somatic mutations in the EGFR gene, representing a sub-population for which the drug was extremely effective [11]. This example of genomic information coupled with drug mechanism underscores the importance of understanding underlying genetic anomalies in order to better predict whether a therapy will be effective. Individual genetic variability of more general biological mechanisms involved in drug metabolism, distribution, and clearance can also influence drug efficacy. For example, polymorphisms in the P450 drug-metabolizing enzyme can generate significantly different profiles in drug metabolism [12,13].

Genomics approaches provide valuable information that can help us better understand and predict an individual's response to a drug therapy regarding:

- identification of critical genomic aberrations that strongly correlate with a specific disease and, in turn, implicate associated molecular pathways that may be appropriate for therapeutic intervention (i.e., targeted pathway(s) identification);

- identification of genetic variations among the population that indicate the likely success rate of a therapeutic intervention (i.e., treatment identification); and
- identification of genetic variations in the biological machinery required for drug metabolism, distribution, and clearance (impact on efficacy and toxicity).

The main approaches utilized for genomic discovery are *whole genome sequencing* (i.e., Sanger sequencing, 454 life sciences), which entail sequencing the entire genome without bias toward particular gene sequences, and *genotype analysis*, which is focused on specific genes or genomic locations. Moreover genotype analysis may succeed in evaluating the entire raw sequence of particular genes or, alternatively, lead to the identification of single nucleotide polymorphisms (SNPs) located at discrete genomic locations on a population level. New high-density DNA microarrays and bead-coupled universal Tag arrays have enabled SNP analysis to move toward a whole-genome approach [14]. For further details regarding the application of genomic technologies to drug development, we direct the reader to several reviews [4,15–18].

2.1.2 Transcriptomic Technologies

Transcriptome analysis is based on the detection and quantification of mRNA transcripts. The main advantage transcript profiling provides, relative to genomic approaches, is the ability to capture the *dynamic* response of a biological system under different conditions by measuring the expression profile of thousands of mRNA transcripts. There are approximately 25,000 human genes, yet only a small percentage (roughly 20%) is active at any given time. Transcriptome technology provides the researcher with a perspective closer to the functional response of the biological system. The technological platforms for transcript profiling are very similar to those used for genomic analysis, and they similarly can be subdivided into two categories: approaches that evaluate all mRNA without prior bias regarding the sequence, namely as a serial analysis of gene expression (SAGE), and analysis that is focused on a predefined set of genes, namely in DNA microarrays. Even though SAGE and DNA microarrays are based on different technologies, they have been demonstrated to correlate well in terms of mRNA quantitation, especially in the case of highly expressed transcripts [19]. Current technologies allow high density DNA microarrays to contain roughly 45,000 unique transcripts and genes that span the entire genome, with several commercial DNA microarrays now available at low to moderate cost (Affymetrix, Agilent, GE Healthcare, Applied Biosystems, etc.). Results from high-throughput transcript profiling approaches are frequently confirmed using lower throughput assays such as quantitative reverse transcript–polymerase chain reaction (qRT-PCR) or Northern blotting.

Similar to genomic approaches, transcriptomic technologies have facilitated the identification of putative targets and pathways, as well as provide predictions regarding drug efficacy and toxicity:

- Transcript analysis can identify mRNA transcripts that are strongly correlated with a disease (and indicate associated molecular pathways suitable for therapeutic intervention).
- Identification of on-target and off-target drug effects throughout the whole genome may influence drug efficacy and toxicity.
- Transcriptomic profiling of the biological mechanisms which are engaged in drug metabolism, distribution, and clearance.

For further information regarding current DNA microarray products and applications, the reader may refer to an excellent recent review on "Toxicogenomic Technologies to Predictive Toxicilogy" by the National Research Council of the National Academies [20]. In addition to genomic and transcriptomic profiling, several related areas of study show promise in furthering the understanding of drug efficacy but are beyond the scope of this chapter. These include technologies involved in detection of DNA methylation [21], microRNA technologies, and CpG microarrays [22].

2.1.3 Metabolomic Technologies

Metabolomics refers to the study of metabolites (i.e., products or small-molecule intermediates of the biological processes) as they exist in the cell, tissue, organ, or animal as a whole. Biological samples including cellular supernatants, blood, plasma, saliva, urine, and stool provide the source material that is typically analyzed using nuclear magnetic resonance (NMR) spectroscopy or mass spectrometry (MS). These technologies are capable of evaluating a wide range of metabolic components (e.g., disease-specific metabolome changes). Metabolites have also been used as biomarkers in order to quantify the toxic effects of drugs. For a complete review of metabolomic applications, the reader can refer to more focused reviews [23–25].

2.1.4 Proteomic and Protein Activity Technologies

Proteins are the ultimate executors of cellular function, and thus are directly responsible for a biological phenotype [26–30]. Proteomics is the study of the expression, modification, and activity of proteins in a biological system. In comparison to genomic or transcriptome approaches, proteomic profiling involves several unique challenges:

1. Screening of the entire proteome in a manner similar to whole genome or transcriptome is currently impossible and impractical.

2. The proteome cannot be defined using a constrained list of proteins (similar to genome approaches) because of the wide range of post-translational protein modifications, and these in turn can produce infinite combinations that are ultimately responsible for the phenotype.

3. Protein modifications such as phosphorylation, ubiquitination, methylation, sulfation and proteolytic cleavage (which are the main modulators of protein activity) cannot simultaneously be measured from a single assay [31].

4. Protein abundance from a single cell population can span more than six orders of magnitude, creating a bias toward high-abundance proteins.

5. Compared with DNA-based experiments, protein experiments lack a "protein-amplification" feature (similar to PCR for genes) that makes protein amount valuable.

6. The ability to broadly analyze protein binding affinity (the driving force in signal transduction) is not possible on a high-throughput scale.

As with the previously described genomic and transcriptomic techniques, protein analysis can be divided into two separate approaches: one that makes no a priori assumption about protein composition or structure (i.e., 2D-PAGE, capillary electrophoresis, and mass spectrometry [MS] technology), and another that is based on a predetermined set of target proteins (i.e., affinity-based approaches). In a 2D-PAGE approach, the control lysates are separated based on their physical properties (mass and charge). Diseased (or drug-treated lysates) are identically processed, and a comparative analysis is performed to evaluate protein expression between the two samples. The MS approach, which often complements 2D-PAGE, entails protein digestion to generate a mixture of peptides, which are then separated and analyzed using liquid-chromatography-coupled mass spectrometry (LC-MS). Depending on specific physical properties, each peptide generates a unique signature (i.e., MS-MS spectra) that can be identified by a semiautomated search against proteomic databases. This approach, known as shotgun proteomic analyses, enables the automated characterization of hundreds of proteins in a complex mixture. Both 2D-PAGE and MS approaches have the disadvantage of being biased toward high-abundance proteins and can only process a very low number of samples at a time.

Affinity-based assays utilize capture entities (antibody, peptide, nucleotides, etc.) to preferentially bind target proteins of interest. In contrast to the 2D-PAGE and MS approaches, affinity-based assays identify proteins that can be recognized and captured by high-affinity molecules. Thus a well-developed affinity assay provides a high degree of specificity. A critical feature of affinity-based approaches is the ability to quantitate both protein concentration and protein activity, information that is essential for computational models. Antibody-based detection approaches are among the most commonly

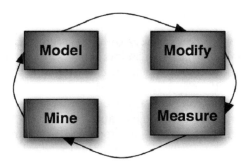

Figure 2.1 A systems biology approach for high-throughput protein-based datasets: The modify–measure–mine–model paradigm [32].

used for high-throughput protein analysis and therefore will be more thoroughly described later in this chapter.

High-throughput measurements of protein activity can capture the dynamic changes in intracellular signals, thus generating a large amount of data that encompasses high-quality protein-level information. These data carry valuable information regarding propagation of signals, a process known to be nonlinear and highly dynamic. Time-dependent and nonlinear processes have been well studied in many fields of engineering, a discipline known as dynamical systems. It is anticipated that similar methods can be utilized to extract valuable information from protein activity measurements to describe the biological phenotype. Thus the combination of high-throughput data under different conditions (perturbations) and mathematical modeling (see Figure 2.1) supported by bioinformatics tools is a paradigm in which a systems biology approach can have an impact on drug development, efficacy and toxicity [32,33].

2.2   EXPERIMENTAL PLATFORMS FOR PROTEIN ACTIVITY QUANTIFICATION

This section describes high-throughput and multiplexed protein activity-based measurements in cells. First, we introduce the basics for high-throughput protein measurements. Then, we focus on select platforms that are based on antibody detection and list their major advantages and limitations. This is not an exhaustive list of all proteomics platforms as the technology is constantly developing and new assays are continually emerging. We do not discuss single-cell based approaches (fluorescence-activated cell sorting—FACS— high content screening/microscopy) because they are extensively covered in other chapters of this book. Last, we introduce computational tools that can be used for the analysis of protein signaling datasets obtained by high-throughput approaches.

2.2.1 Affinity-Based Assays

Affinity-based assays utilize molecules with high affinity and specificity for the capture and detection of target protein(s). The most commonly used high-affinity molecules are antibodies, whose selectivity and affinity for the target protein are critical for the outcome of the assay. Despite the fact that antibody development and production is a mature industry, scientists should continually be aware that a significant percentage of antibodies often recognize more than one target and thus are not suitable or interchangeable for every assay. Assays are only as good as the antibodies available. In addition, when we discuss antibody-based measurements of "protein activity," we are generally referring to the phosphorylation state of the protein and not to the actual protein activity. This is especially relevant for kinase molecules, in which the phosphorylation state of a substrate is a good surrogate of kinase activity. However, discrepancies between kinase phosphorylation status and activity are to be expected under varied conditions [34].

There are three main characteristics of every affinity based assay (Figure 2.2):

1. An *identification (multiplexing) scheme* in which a *solid support* (individual wells, spots on glass, beads, etc.) obtains a unique identity required for multiplexing. A solid support not only contributes to the

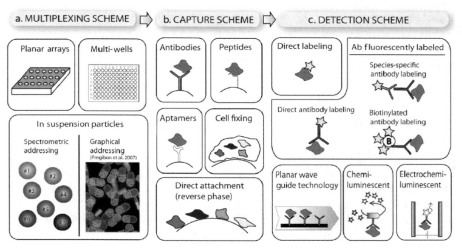

Figure 2.2 The three main characteristics of a high-throughput affinity based assay. (*a*) A multiplexing scheme in which solid supports (e.g., microparticles [35], beads, spots, or wells) obtain a unique identity. (*b*) A capture scheme immobilizes and/or isolates the protein of interest. (*c*) A detection scheme generates a readable output, which is linearly correlated to the amount of the immobilized protein of interest. (See color insert.)

multiplexability of the assay, it is essential for all steps in the assay, including washes, protein separation and coupling, and measurements. This unique identity can be obtained by either:

- *spatially distributed 2D arrangements*, whereby the individual coordinates on a 2D plane correspond to individual conditions, (such as well "B2" in a 96/384-well plates, spot with coordinates (n, m) on a printed glass slide, or combination of both (5th spot on the B2 well), or
- *microparticles in suspension* whereby each microparticle has a unique physical characteristic (i.e., emits a unique spectrometric signature, or carries a unique graphical signature; see Figure 2.2*a*).

2. A *capture scheme* that aims to immobilize the protein of interest to the uniquely addressed solid support. Three main approaches widely used for immobilization of a protein of interest are:

- a capture antibody, peptide, or aptamer attached to a solid substrate (plate, slide, bead);
- cell lysate directly spotted on a chemically derived glass slide (usually known as *reverse phase* approach); and
- cells that are directly fixed on a support (usually on a 96/384 well plate).

3. A *detection scheme* that aims to produce a signal that ideally is linearly proportional to the amount of the protein captured on the support. Depending on the multiplexing and capturing scheme there are at least four distinct categories of detection:

- *Fluorescent-labeled detection.* This can take one of three forms: (a) *direct labeling* whereby samples are chemically labeled with a fluorophore, as has successfully been applied to study cancer markers [36], but not widely adopted because it involves chemical modifications of the samples that may affect their biochemical properties; (b) *single-antibody labeling* whereby proteins that have been covalently immobilized on a substrate are recognized by a single antibody that is either directly labeled, biotinylated (for binding fluorescent Streptavidin) or recognized by a species-specific antibody (i.e., anti-goat fluorescent secondary antibody); or (c) *double-antibody labeling (or sandwich assay)* whereby the protein of interest is captured between an immobilized antibody and a secondary antibody that can be directly labeled, biotinylated, or recognized by a species-specific antibody.
- *Enzymatic labeled detection.* Typically a biotinylated secondary antibody is bound by a streptavidin-linked horseradish peroxidase that yields amplified chromogenic products.
- *Planar wave guide technology.* This technology, implemented by Zeptosens (www.zeptosens.com), uses a guided light that is passed over a thin film located below the detection antibody. The electromagnetic

field created by the propagation of the light can lead to measurements with a 50-fold increase in sensitivity compared to regular fluorescent schemes.

- *Electrochemiluminescent detection.* This technology, implemented by Meso Scale Discovery (MSD, www.meso-scale.com), is based on the electrical induction of an oxidation-reduction cycle resulting in emitted light. The technology is similar to that of planar wave guide technology, but only labels proximal to the captured antigen surface can be detected, resulting in minimal background signals.

A novel detection scheme recently reported is the proximity ligation procedure in which detection signals can be generated by a PCR-type reaction. This assay is based on pairs of primers that are separately coupled to individual antibodies that recognize closely related epitopes. Thus, when the antibodies bind their targets and come in close proximity, a PCR reaction can generate a DNA product that verifies the proximity and presence of the antibodies ([37–40]).

2.2.2 Specific Platforms for Protein Measurements

Protein Microarrays   Protein microarrays (or capture microarrays) employ a capture antibody (alternatively: peptide, nucleotide, etc.) that is covalently bound to a slide (or membrane) in an ordered manner; multiple distinct antibodies may be affixed at separate locations on the same slide. Their main advantage is the ability to measure dozens to hundreds of proteins in each sample although the total number of samples that can be processed is somewhat limited (Figure 2.3 and Table 2.1). Even spotting of the antibody is critical for proper interaction with analytes and subsequent reading of the slide. Following blocking of the free microarray surfaces to reduce nonspecific binding (and improve signal to background noise ratio), lysate bathes the entire slide. Detection and quantification of an interaction between the capture antibody and analyte can be achieved either by direct labeling or by sandwich assay, as mentioned above. The advantage of direct labeling is the simultaneous measurement of many analytes and a requirement for only a single antibody (the capture antibody). However, uneven labeling of all proteins and the chemical alteration of the labeled protein is a source of false-positive and high background signals. On the other hand, a sandwich assay employs two antibodies, a captured protein and a detection antibody. The detection antibody binds to a protein that is already immobilized to the surface via the capture antibody. Subsequently a fluorescent-labeled secondary antibody associates with the capture antibody, allowing for detection and quantification of the signal. The sandwich assay avoids labeling of the sample and ensures more accurate and specific detection of a positive signal. In turn, a limitation is the requirement for two high-quality antibodies. Identification of high-quality

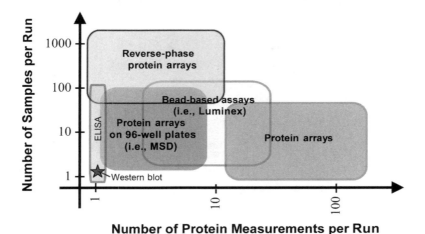

Figure 2.3   High-throughput proteomics platform comparison based on the number of samples and the number of analytes that can be processed.

antibodies is a common theme for all protein microarrays and poses a challenge beyond identifying antibodies suitable for Western blotting, which detects denatured proteins. In either case (direct labeling or sandwich assay), slides are analyzed using readers that are fairly common equipment in many laboratories today. An alternative to fluorescent detection is the planar wave guided technology by Zeptosens, which offers increased signal sensitivity and lower background. However, this methodology requires specialized instrumentation and the proprietary technology makes the assay more expensive.

Meso-scale Discovery   MSD is a multi-array technology that utilizes electro-chemiluminescent detection of antibody–analyte interactions. Its main advantage is the ability to measure a few proteins (up to 10) in a large number of samples (96 per plate) (Figure 2.3, Table 2.1). Capture antibodies are bound to the surface of the wells of a 96-well plate. Each well can accommodate up to 10 distinct antibodies at defined locations (multi-spot). Lysates and supernatants are incubated in each well, followed by the addition of a capture antibody containing a proprietary SULFO-Tag. Electrochemical stimulation is then initiated by carbon electrodes located in the base of the microplate. Activation of SULFO-Tags within close proximity to the electrode results in the emission of light which is read by the specialized MSD reader. The reader can process a plate in 1 to 3 minutes and does not involve any fluidics. One drawback is the reader's inability to re-read plates, if needed, as the signal is significantly reduced after the plate has been read. The assays are quite sensitive (to near 10 attamole for some analytes) and have a dynamic range of approximately 5 logs. However, because of the specialized nature of the MSD

TABLE 2.1 Some Commercial and Generic High-Throughput Assays for Protein-Based Measurements

Assay	Multiplexing Scheme	Capture Scheme	Detection Scheme	Size of Samples (per Run)	Size of Signals (per Run)
ELISA (i.e. R8.0)	Multi-wells (96 or 384)	Sandwich antibodies	Fluorescent or Enzymatic	100/plate	1 per well
In-cell Western *LICOR*	Multi-wells (usually 96)	Fixed cell and single antibody	Fluorescently labeled antibody	100/plate	1–2 per well
Protein arrays (e.g. Ray Bie)	Planar array slides/membranes	Sandwich antibodies	Fluorescently labeled antibody	1/slide	~100 per slide (Ab pair limited)
Protein arrays on multi-wells	Planar array slides/membranes on multi-wells (usually 96)	Sandwich antibodies and different sample per well	Fluorescently labeled antibody	100/plate	~10 spots/well (spot size limited)
Protein arrays reverse phase	Planar array slides/membranes	Spotting and single antibodies	Fluorescently labeled antibody	1000s/slide	Usually 1 per slide
Protein arrays reverse phase on multi-wells	Planar array slides/membranes on multi-wells (usually 96)	Spotting and single antibodies per well	Fluorescently labeled antibody	~10 spots/well	~100 per plate
Protein arrays meso-scale discovery	Planar array on multi-wells (usually 96)	Sandwich antibodies and different sample per well	Electrochemiluminescent labeled antibody	100/plate	~10 spots/well (spot size limited)
Protein arrays *Zeptosens*	Planar array on slides	Antibody or peptides	Antibody with planar wave technology	32/chip	Up to 6 per chip
Protein arrays reverse phase *Zeptosens*	Planar array on slides	Direct attachment (spotting)	Antibody with planar wave technology	200/chip but scalable 1000s/run	1 per chip
Bead-based (luminex or cytometric bead array)	In suspension bead particles on multi-wells (usually 96)	Sandwich antibodies	Fluorescently labeled antibody	100/plate	~30 per well (Ab pair limited)
Flow cytometry	Individual vials or wells	Fixed/live cell	Fluorescently labeled antibody	1 per vial or 100 per well	Up to 4 signals on 1000s of single cells

plates, customers are limited to targets available from the company, or alternatively must develop their own plates. The specialized MSD reader, plates, and reagents are commercially available at an appreciable cost.

xMAP Technology   xMAP technology developed by the Luminex Corporation (www.luminexcorp.com) is a bead-based assay that allows for the simultaneous analysis of up to 100 different analytes from a single well. Microspheres (5.6 μm polystyrene beads) are internally dyed to generate up to 100 distinct spectral signatures. Each uniquely identified bead can in turn be coupled to a different capture antibody (or enzyme substrate, DNA, receptors, antigens, etc.). The distinctly conjugated beads can then be mixed (multiplexed) and incubated with a single sample. A mixture of biotinylated detection antibodies is subsequently added to form a sandwich assay on the surface of the bead; a fluorescently labeled reporter molecule (StreptAvidin PhycoErythrin—SAPE) binds the detection antibody, allowing for detection and quantification. A flow cytometer-based instrument equipped with two lasers and associated optics excites the dyes and allows for quantification of the fluorescent signal representing each analyte. The red diode (635 nm) laser excites and identifies the bead as one of 100 distinct signatures. The green diode (532 nm) laser simultaneously excites the fluorescent reporter tag bound to the detection antibody, with the resultant amount of green fluorescence proportional to the amount of analyte captured in the assay.

The theoretical multiplex capabilities of xMAP technology are currently unparalleled; 100 proteins in each of 96 distinct samples can be measured (Figure 2.3, Table 2.1). In practice, however, there are several limitations with regard to the number of targets which simultaneously can be evaluated including antibody cross-reactivity, natural protein abundance, and antibody competition for protein complexes [41]. A further advantage in using bead suspensions (relative to planar microarrays) is the fast reaction kinetics and the high surface-to-volume ratio, which leads to better washes and homogeneous chemical reactions. As with other antibody-based assays, scientists are limited to commercially available targets or developing their own assays, although several vendors currently provide a growing list of analytes. The vacuum-based protocol and plate-reading time is moderately time-consuming and limits the number of plates that can be processed. However, advances including the use of magnetic bead technology and automated assay/readers promise to couple the tremendous amount of data per well with the ability to increase the plates throughput. The xMAP technology requires a specialized bead-reader, although a comparable technology has also been developed by Becton Dickinson and Company (Cytometric bead array) that utilizes a more typical FACS instrument.

Reverse Phase   Reverse phase assays also utilize an antibody-based approach, but in contrast to capture microarrays, the cell lysate itself is immobilized on a solid support (typically a chemically treated slide or membrane). A real strength of this approach is that multiple lysates (dozens to several hundreds) corresponding to different treatments or conditions can be arrayed and processed on a single slide (Figure 2.3, Table 2.1). The entire slide can be probed with a single antibody or alternatively, distinct individual primary antibodies can be compartmentalized at discrete locations. A labeled secondary antibody binds the capture antibody, allowing for detection and quantification. Reverse phase arrays only require a single antibody for detection, which is an advantage over the necessity to identify two reliable antibodies as is the case for sandwich assays. However, the signal that is generated by reverse phase represents the sum of specific and nonspecific antibody binding; thus it is very dependent on the quality of the antibodies being used (an issue avoided by Western blotting, in which individual proteins are separated). Thus, presence of all cellular proteins bound to a spot carries with it issues of specificity and decreased signal to noise ratio.

2.3   ORGANIZING AND ANALYZING DATA

The tremendous amount of data obtained using these high-throughput approaches necessitates an organized system of data storage and handling. Context specific information (conditions under which the data were obtained, protocols used, cell type, etc.) should accompany the experimental data. A popular approach to storing data (widely used in genomics) is relational database management systems (RDBMS). In a relational database, the subdivision of data and its storage follows a predefined schema which allows one to identify and maintain links between disparate pieces of information. However, this approach comes at the price of limited flexibility: it is difficult for a relational database to accommodate frequent changes in data formats and to incorporate unstructured information. Such changes and adaptations may be common during the experimental process and thus should be considered when deciding on a system for data storage. There are a number of RDBMS type databases adapted for proteomics data, such as SBEAMS (http://www.sbeams.org) or Bioinformatics Resource Manager [42]. In order to overcome the limitations of RDBMS, we have developed *DataRail*, a free and open-source (http://code.google.com/p/sbpipeline/) MATLAB (http://www.mathworks.com/) toolbox for data management which stores, processes, and visualizes experimental data. *DataRail* supports both scripting and GUI-based interaction, and incorporates a variety of data processing algorithms (normalization, scaling, etc.) and visualization routines. The information derived from a set of experiments is organized into a structure called a compendium, which consists of multiple *n*-dimensional data arrays. The algorithms and parameters used during data processing are stored with each array to maintain a record of the provenance of the data [43].

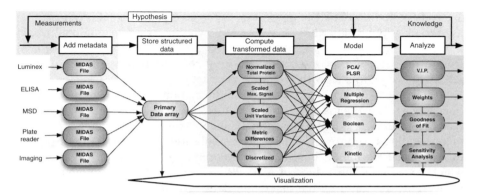

Figure 2.4 DataRail Workflow. DataRail helps to close the iterative loop between measurements, modeling and generation of hypothesis characteristic of systems biology (see Figure 2.3). Experimental measurements are first converted into a MIDAS format and then used to assemble a multidimensional primary data array. Different algorithms transform the data to create new data arrays (orange) that can then be modeled using internal (full-line boxes) or external routines (dashed boxes) [43].

Besides its flexibility, the strength of *DataRail* is its ability to link the data to mathematical models. Data are imported and exported using a MIDAS (minimal amount of information for data analysis in systems biology) format, a derivative of the MIACA (minimum information about a cellular assay, http://miaca.sourceforge.net/) format. In addition import of the data generated by disparate devices (Luminex reader, ELISA, etc.), as well as export to specific modeling tools (*CellNetAnalyzer* [44] and the differential-equation based modeling package *PottersWheel* (http://www.PottersWheel.de/)) are possible (see Figure 2.4).

High-throughput data sets are inherently difficult to interpret solely based on inspection and intuition. Thus mathematical analyses can help extract information that is not readily apparent. There are two main approaches: strictly studying the data in a hypothesis-free manner using "data-driven models" [45] or comparing the data to a priori biological knowledge encoded in a mathematical framework [32].

2.3.1 Data-Driven Models

Data-driven approaches to data analysis encompass several methods derived mainly from machine learning and statistics. Methods of machine learning follow one of two paradigms: supervised or unsupervised learning [46]. In supervised learning, such as the support vector machine (SVM) algorithm, a set of objects (e.g., drugs) with certain properties (e.g., their effect on intracellular signals) are assigned to different groups (e.g., toxic or nontoxic). Rules are constructed that link the properties to the groups. These rules can then be used to classify objects whose class is unknown. For example, one could train a classification system with information (e.g., based on intracellular signals) from drugs known to be either toxic or nontoxic, and then use this system to screen new compounds with unknown toxicity [47].

In unsupervised learning there is no information about which group each object (e.g., drug) belongs to, and therefore one tries to define such groups (called clusters) based on similarities. One application of clustering is to organize signaling responses based on their similarities [45]. Another method of unsupervised learning is based on the computation of principal components, which transforms the values of a single measurement into combinations of measurements capturing the maximum data variability. For example, instead of considering individual phosphorylation of particular proteins [48], one considers the combined phosphorylation of groups of proteins [45]. This approach has the additional feature that it reduces the dimension of the data. Principal component analysis (PCA) can be helpful to obtain biological insight. Using signaling profiles, PCA was employed to qualitatively discriminate apoptotic cell fates [45]. Partial least squares regression (PLSR) is another technique similar to PCA. However, in PLSR, the data are structured into independent and dependent variables (inputs and outputs), whereas in PCA there is only one set of data. PLSR reduces the inputs and outputs to their principal components and then identifies a linear solution that relates the former to the latter [45]. PLSR not only provides biological insight; it can also be used to predict the results of new experiments. Multiple linear regression (MLR) is a technique used to extract correlations between inputs and outputs and can be viewed as simplified PLSR. In MLR the linear solution is computed directly between the measured variables. It does not reduce the components as PLSR does. On the other hand, the resulting correlations are links between experimentally measured variables, and therefore the results are easier to interpret. For example, the results of MLR can be visualized as a pathway map that connects phosphoprotein activity to cytokine release [41]. Therefore MLR can be used as a means to reconstruct the network topology from the experimental data. There are also more sophisticated methods to construct pathways maps out of data that constitute a field known as reverse engineering [49]. Reverse engineering has been extensively applied to gene regulatory networks [49], and to a lesser extent to signaling networks [50,51].

In addition to *DataRail*, a number of tools are available to perform data-driven analyses, including the free open source systems R/Bioconductor [46] as well as commercial software such as MATLAB specific toolboxes.

2.3.2   Topology-Based Models

The methods described above make use of only the data, and in some cases a classification scheme (categorization of objects into classes in the case of supervised learning). Knowledge accumulated from decades of research and gathered in the form of thousands of scientific publications is not utilized. An in silico replica of the current knowledge of the signaling system under consideration may be generated to take advantage of this vast resource. This model can then be interrogated with respect to its ability to reproduce the experimental data in order to obtain mechanistic insight. There are several mathematical formalisms that can be used to describe signaling networks, varying in the level of detail they incorporate. An extensive review is outside the scope of this chapter, but we will describe the most popular approaches and refer to reviews for further reading.

Probably the simplest description of a signaling network is what is known in mathematics as a graph: each species (typically proteins) is represented as a node, and the nodes are linked with edges ("lines" representing the interactions). Using this simple description, one can unravel important structural properties of the network such as the presence of clusters of proteins (potentially involved in common biological functions), or to identify elements which are highly connected (known as hubs) representing central elements of a signaling network [52,53].

Directionality and sign (positive or negative) of the arrows (defining the effect between nodes) leads to interaction graphs that can capture the direct dependencies among species (see Figure 2.5). This description allows a useful analysis in terms of examining networks and data, that is, one can compute the paths from any species A to any other species B. Four possibilities exist: the paths are all positive, all negative, mixed positive and negative, or there is no path. Accordingly, the species A can be classified with respect to B as activator, inhibitor, ambiguous, or nonaffecting. By comparing the *possible* connections (positive, negative, ambiguous) between two proteins with the experimental data, one can identify consistencies and discrepancies, and thereby build a model that best represents the cellular system [54]. For example, in the case of an intervention in which a particular protein A is blocked (e.g., with an inhibitor), if the activity of a different protein B increases, A cannot have a direct positive effect on B.

In cellular networks, an interaction (edge) often represents a relationship among more than two species (nodes). In an interaction graph,

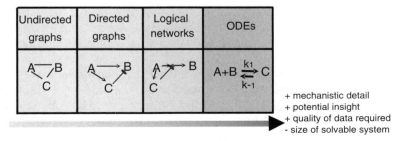

Figure 2.5 Different representations of pathway topology in mathematical terms.

the interpretation of such cases can be ambiguous: if two kinases both have a positive effect on a third C, does it mean that either of them can activate C, or rather that both together are required? The logical gates AND (for the latter case) and OR (for the former) can be used to distinguish the possibilities. Thus, by including some additional information about the logic of the signal propagation, one obtains a more accurate description. This type of refinement of interaction graphs is called interaction hypergraphs and is the framework for boolean (or logical) networks (see Figure 2.5), in which all states have a discrete value (in the simplest case, either ON or OFF) [54].

Within this framework it is possible to test the consistency between the network topology and experimental data across different cell types and conditions. Measurements of protein activation under different conditions can automatically be compared with the predictions of a model based on a certain topology. By comparing the models with data from different cell types, one can uncover significant differences in the signaling networks. Furthermore experimental data that cannot be reconciled with the a priori knowledge encoded in the maps suggests gaps in our current knowledge that point to potential new connections [41].

Additional insight can be unlocked by constructing and subsequently analyzing detailed, mechanistic, kinetic models. Here, one first considers the individual chemical processes underlying signaling events, and then defines the reactions consuming and producing species, leading to balanced concentrations. This procedure is typically encoded as a set of ordinary differential equations (ODEs) that describes the time-dependent concentration of the protein species as a function of kinetic parameters and initial concentration [32,64]. However, the large number of unknown parameter values and entities (enzymatic activities, binding constants, etc.) make modeling a very large network in a mechanistic manner an arduous task. If large amounts of data are available, one can try to calibrate the model by finding parameter values so that the model optimally describes the data. This is nevertheless a very challenging problem [55,56], so fully calibrated models are typically only available for small systems or subsets of systems.

A wide range of methods is suitable for the analysis of ODE models: analysis of nonlinear behavior (e.g., oscillations), calculation of sensitivities (the variations of the activation level of certain proteins upon changes in the model parameters, which reveal key parameters in the signaling network, have importance for drug discovery) or finite-time Lyapunov exponents (which discern how initial transients in a signaling network determine alternative cell fates) [32,56].

Many computational tools are now available that allow scientists to establish, simulate, and analyze models. A number of these tools are graph based (Cytoscape, visANT, etc.; see Aittokallio for reviews [52]), others analyze biochemical systems from a qualitative perspective (GNA:[57], GINsim:[58], CAN:[44]), and a still larger number are suitable for kinetic modeling ([59,60]). Most of these computational tools help with the setup and analysis of models through user interfaces and/or programming of scripts. The standard formats CellML and specially SBML ([61]) are widely used because they allow exchange of data between different programs. Information on how to set up specific models is readily available in the literature and also on the Web, where extensive discussion can be found on signaling pathways, interactions between molecules (binding, substrate/enzyme relationships, etc.) and cell-specific information. Tools that mine data are invaluable for facilitating the retrieval of such information.

2.4 CONCLUSION

Knowledge is power. Scientists have long sought to extract as much informa-tion as possible from their experiments in order to maximize understanding of the systems they study. This effort is demonstrated, for example, by the wide range of genomic screening approaches undertaken by academics and industry in the much celebrated Human Genome Project and in the ongoing International HapMap Project. Several computational tools have evolved around such datasets that seek a global view of biological systems.

When it comes to protein-based measurements, scientists have been reluc-tant to follow similar approaches. The main reason is the tremendous (if not impossible) task of generating large proteomic datasets using standard biologi-cal assays such as Western blots or ELISAs [62,63]. However, the recent high-throughput protein platforms such as the ones described in this chapter have provided scientists with the opportunity to use computational models to harvest the power of protein and phosphoprotein based measurements [41,47,48]. That said, despite the fact that current protein datasets lack the scope of whole genome sequencing, phosphoprotein measurements incorpo-rate knowledge much closer to a cell's biological function.

The pharmaceutical industry has a vested interest in applying a systems biology approach to the drug discovery process. For target identification, the interconnectivity of biological pathways can be incorporated into models to elucidate the optimal novel targets. Scientists can then evaluate whether a single-target approach is preferential to a multitargeted scheme that may be carried out either by co-dosing regimen or "nonspecific" inhibitors. For lead compound discovery, cell-based protein screens can complement chemical screens for understanding the effects of "on-target" inhibition on the rest of the cellular network. For toxicity studies, compounds can be classified as toxic or nontoxic based on their effect on the intracellular and extracellular protein space [47]. The contribution of such knowledge to the success or failure of a drug therapy is obvious.

As the sizes of protein-based datasets increase, computational tools will become increasingly necessary for understanding cellular biology. Nevertheless, combining mathematical models with protein datasets is not a trivial task, and certain limitations may need to be overcome prior to the implementation of a model or the generation of an expensive dataset. For example, correlation algorithms such as PCA, PLSR or MLR cannot handle time and space as efficiently as an ODE model. ODE models in turn cannot handle large topologies (because they are computationally expensive) and require time-dense, high-quality experimental data. Boolean models, on the other hand, can handle large topologies but with a limited description of the time domain. Other algorithms, such as SVM, can optimally handle classification problems (e.g., toxic or nontoxic drugs) but require a sizable dataset.

For a given proteomic platform, two of the main reasons that limit the size of protein datasets are bench time and cost. On the other hand, there are many requirements that increase the dataset size: time points, dosing concentrations, measured signals, stimuli selection, inhibitors (especially for compound screening), and the number of replicates. This is actually a multidimensional cost–benefit optimization problem where the several dimensions of the dataset (time, inhibitors, etc.) should be designed to work in harmony with the computational model. The complexity of both experimental approaches and computational algorithms also highlights the importance of interdisciplinary collaboration among scientists.

The pairing of high-throughput proteomic approaches with advanced computational models promises to vastly increase our understanding of biological systems and their behavior. It will be up to the pharmaceutical industry to use this knowledge to develop more efficient and effective drug strategies.

REFERENCES

1. Csermely P, Agoston V, Pongor S. The efficiency of multi-target drugs: the network approach might help drug design. *Trends Pharmacol Sci* 2005;26:178–82.
2. Araujo RP, Liotta LA, Petricoin EF. Proteins, drug targets and the mechanisms they control: the simple truth about complex networks. *Nat Rev Drug Discov* 2007;6:871–80.
3. Hanahan D, Weinberg RA. The hallmarks of cancer. *Cell* 2000;100:57–70.
4. Koch WH. Technology platforms for pharmacogenomic diagnostic assays. *Nat Rev Drug Discov* 2004;3:749–61.
5. Teufel A, Staib F, Kanzler S, Weinmann A, Schulze-Bergkamen H, Galle PR. Genetics of hepatocellular carcinoma. *World J Gastroenterol* 2007;13:2271–82.
6. Wilkens L, Bredt M, Flemming P, Klempnauer J, Heinrich Kreipe H. Differentiation of multicentric origin from intra-organ metastatic spread of hepatocellular carcinomas by comparative genomic hybridization. *J Pathol* 2000;192:43–51.
7. Bosch FX, Ribes J, Borras J. Epidemiology of primary liver cancer. *Semin Liver Dis* 1999;19:271–85.
8. Abou-Alfa GK. Hepatocellular carcinoma: molecular biology and therapy. *Semin Oncol* 2006;33:S79–83.

9. Thorgeirsson SS, Grisham JW. Molecular pathogenesis of human hepatocellular carcinoma. *Nat Genet* 2002;31:339–46.

10. Lynch TJ, Bell DW, Sordella R, Gurubhagavatula S, Okimoto RA, Brannigan BW, et al. Activating mutations in the epidermal growth factor receptor underlying responsiveness of non–small-cell lung cancer to gefitinib. *N Engl J Med* 2004; 350:2129–39. Epub 004 Apr 29.

11. Paez JG, Janne PA, Lee JC, Tracy S, Greulich H, Gabriel S, et al. EGFR mutations in lung cancer: correlation with clinical response to Gefitinib therapy. *Science* 2004;304:1497–500.

12. Ingelman-Sundberg M, Oscarson M, McLellan RA. Polymorphic human cytochrome P450 enzymes: an opportunity for individualized drug treatment. *Trends Pharmacol Sci* 1999;20:342–9.

13. Desta Z, Zhao X, Shin JG, Flockhart DA. Clinical significance of the cytochrome P450 2C19 genetic polymorphism. *Clin Pharmacokinet* 2002;41: 913–58.

14. Syvanen AC. Toward genome-wide SNP genotyping. *Nat Genet* 2005;37:S5–10.

15. Bumol TF, Watanabe AM. Genetic information, genomic technologies, and the future of drug discovery. *JAMA* 2001;285:551–5.

16. Evans WE, Relling MV. Pharmacogenomics: translating functional genomics into rational therapeutics. *Science* 1999;286:487–91.

17. Evans WE, McLeod HL. Pharmacogenomics—drug disposition, drug targets, and side effects. *N Engl J Med* 2003;348:538–49.

18. Phillips KA, Veenstra DL, Oren E, Lee JK, Sadee W. Potential role of pharmacogenomics in reducing adverse drug reactions: a systematic review. *JAMA* 2001;286:2270–9.

19. Kim HL. Comparison of oligonucleotide-microarray and serial analysis of gene expression (SAGE) in transcript profiling analysis of megakaryocytes derived from CD34+ cells. *Exp Mol Med* 2003;35:460–6.

20. Committee on Applications of Toxicogenomic Technologies to Predictive Toxicology and Risk Assessment NRC. *Applications of toxicogenomic technologies to predictive toxicology and risk assessment*. Washington, DC: National Academies Press, 2007.

21. Bibikova M, Lin Z, Zhou L, Chudin E, Garcia EW, Wu B, et al. High-throughput DNA methylation profiling using universal bead arrays. *Genome Res* 2006;16:383–93.

22. Jabbari K, Bernardi G. Cytosine methylation and CpG, TpG (CpA) and TpA frequencies. *Gene* 2004;333:143–9.

23. Raamsdonk LM, Teusink B, Broadhurst D, Zhang NS, Hayes A, Walsh MC, et al. A functional genomics strategy that uses metabolome data to reveal the phenotype of silent mutations. *Nat Biotechnol* 2001;19:45–50.

24. Goodacre R, Vaidyanathan S, Dunn WB, Harrigan GG, Kell DB. Metabolomics by numbers: acquiring and understanding global metabolite data. *Trends Biotechnol* 2004;22:245–52.

25. Haugen AC, Kelley R, Collins JB, Tucker CJ, Deng C, Afshari CA, et al. Integrating phenotypic and expression profiles to map arsenic-response networks. *Genome Biol* 2004;5:R95. Epub 2004 Nov 29.

26. Anderson NL, Anderson NG. The human plasma proteome—history, character, and diagnostic prospects. *Mol Cell Proteomics* 2002;1:845–67.

27. Aebersold R, Mann M. Mass spectrometry-based proteomics. *Nature* 2003;422: 198–207.

28. Ideker T, Thorsson V, Ranish JA, Christmas R, Buhler J, Eng JK, et al. Integrated genomic and proteomic analyses of a systematically perturbed metabolic network. *Science* 2001;292:929–34.

29. Pandey A, Mann M. Proteomics to study genes and genomes. *Nature* 2000;405: 837–46.

30. Gygi SP, Rist B, Gerber SA, Turecek F, Gelb MH, Aebersold R. Quantitative analysis of complex protein mixtures using isotope-coded affinity tags. *Nat Biotechnol* 1999;17:994–9.

31. Mann M, Jensen ON. Proteomic analysis of post-translational modifications. *Nat Biotechnol* 2003;21:255–61.

32. Aldridge BB, Burke JM, Lauffenburger DA, Sorger PK. Physicochemical modelling of cell signalling pathways. *Nat Cell Biol* 2006;8:1195–203.

33. Albeck JG, MacBeath G, White FM, Sorger PK, Lauffenburger DA, Gaudet S. Collecting and organizing systematic sets of protein data. *Nat Rev Mol Cell Biol* 2006;7:803–12.

34. Janes KA, Albeck JG, Peng LX, Sorger PK, Lauffenburger DA, Yaffe MB. A high-throughput quantitative multiplex kinase assay for monitoring information flow in signaling networks: application to sepsis-apoptosis. *Mol Cell Proteomics* 2003;2:463–73.

35. Pregibon DC, Toner M, Doyle PS. Multifunctional encoded particles for high-throughput biomolecule analysis. *Science* 2007;315:1393–6.

36. Knezevic V. Proteomic profiling of the cancer microenvironment by antibody arrays. *Proteomics* 2001;1:1271–8.

37. Fredriksson S, Gullberg M, Jarvius J, Olsson C, Pietras K, Gustafsdottir SM, et al. Protein detection using proximity-dependent DNA ligation assays. *Nat Biotech* 2002;20:473–7.

38. Gustafsdottir SM, Schlingemann J, Rada-Iglesias A, Schallmeiner E, Kamali-Moghaddam M, Wadelius C, et al. In vitro analysis of DNA-protein interactions by proximity ligation. *Proc Natl Acad Sci USA* 2007;104:3067–72.

39. Schallmeiner E, Oksanen E, Ericsson O, Spangberg L, Eriksson S, Stenman U-H, et al. Sensitive protein detection via triple-binder proximity ligation assays. *Nat Meth* 2007;4:135–7.

40. Soderberg O, Gullberg M, Jarvius M, Ridderstrale K, Leuchowius K-J, Jarvius J, et al. Direct observation of individual endogenous protein complexes in situ by proximity ligation. *Nat Meth* 2006;3:995–1000.

41. Alexopoulos LG, Saez-Rodriguez J, Cosgrove B, Lauffenburger DA, Sorger PK. Context sensitive pathway maps of primary and transformed human hepatocytes reveal profound alterations in NfkB signaling. *In preparation*, 2008.

42. Shah AR, Singhal M, Klicker KR, Stephan EG, Wiley HS, Waters KM. Enabling high-throughput data management for systems biology: the Bioinformatics Resource Manager. *Bioinformatics* 2007;23:906–9.

43. Saez-Rodriguez J, Goldsipe A, Muhlich J, Alexopoulos LG, Millard B, Lauffen-burger DA, et al. Flexible informatics for linking experimental data to mathemati-cal models via DataRail. *Bioinformatics* 2008;24:840–7.

44. Klamt S, Saez-Rodriguez J, Gilles E. Structural and functional analysis of cellular networks with CellNetAnalyzer. *BMC Sys Biol* 2007;1:2.

45. Janes KA, Yaffe MB. Data-driven modelling of signal-transduction networks. *Nat Rev Mol Cell Biol* 2006;7:820–8.

46. Tarca AL, Carey VJ, Chen XW, Romero R, Draghici S. Machine learning and its applications to biology. *PLoS Comput Biol* 2007;3:e116.

47. Alexopoulos LG, Saez-Rodriguez J, Lauffenburger DA, Sorger PK. Support vector machine approach for classification of drug toxicity based on their effects on the intracellular and extracellular signaling motifs. *In preparation*, 2008.

48. Espelin C, Goldsipe A, Sorger PK, Lauffenburger DA, de Graaf D, Hendriks BS. Multidimensional phosphoprotein and cytokine profiling reveals context-dependent behavior of kinase inhibitors in U937 macrophages. *In preparation*, 2008.

49. Cho KH, Choo SM, Jung SH, Kim JR, Choi HS, Kim J. Reverse engineering of gene regulatory networks. *Iet Sys Biol* 2007;1:149–63.

50. Sachs K, Perez O, Pe'er D, Lauffenburger DA, Nolan GP. Causal protein-signaling networks derived from multiparameter single-cell data. *Science* 2005;308:523–9.

51. Santos SDM, Verveer PJ, Bastiaens PIH. Growth factor-induced MAPK network topology shapes Erk response determining PC-12 cell fate. *Nat Cell Biol* 2007;9:324–30.

52. Aittokallio T, Schwikowski B. Graph-based methods for analysing networks in cell biology. *Brief Bioinform* 2006;7:243–55.

53. Barabasi A-L, Oltvai ZN. Network biology: understanding the cell's functional organization. *Nat Rev Genet* 2004;5:101–13.

54. Klamt S, Saez-Rodriguez J, Lindquist JA, Simeoni L, Gilles ED. A methodology for the structural and functional analysis of signaling and regulatory networks. *BMC Bioinform* 2006;7:56.

55. Jaqaman K, Danuser G. Linking data to models: data regression. *Nat Rev Mol Cell Biol* 2006;7:813–9.

56. Kremling A, Saez-Rodriguez J. Systems biology—an engineering perspective. *J Biotechnol* 2007;129:329–51.

57. de Jong H, Geiselmann J, Hernandez C, Page M. Genetic Network Analyzer: quali-tative simulation of genetic regulatory networks. *Bioinformatics* 2003;19:336–44.

58. Gonzalez AG, Naldi A, Sanchez L, Thieffry D, Chaouiya C. GINsim: a software suite for the qualitative modelling, simulation and analysis of regulatory networks. *Biosystems* 2006;84:91–100.

59. Vacheva I, Eils R. Computational systems biology platforms. *IT Info Technol* 2006;48:140–47.

60. Alves R, Antunes F, Salvador A. Tools for kinetic modeling of biochemical net-works. *Nat Biotech* 2006;24:667–72.

61. Hucka M, Finney A, Sauro HM, Bolouri H, Doyle JC, Kitano H, et al. The systems biology markup language (SBML): a medium for representation and exchange of biochemical network models. *Bioinformatics* 2003;19:524–31.

62. Gaudet S, Janes KA, Albeck JG, Pace EA, Lauffenburger DA, Sorger PK. A compendium of signals and responses triggered by prodeath and prosurvival cytokines. *Mol Cell Proteomics* 2005;4:1569–90.

63. Janes KA, Albeck JG, Gaudet S, Sorger PK, Lauffenburger DA, Yaffe MB. A systems model of signaling identifies a molecular basis set for cytokine-induced apoptosis. *Science* 2005;310:1646–53.

64. Hendriks BS, Hua F, Chabot JR. Analysis of mechanistic pathway models in drug discovery: p38 pathway. *Biotechnol Prog* 2008;24:96–109.

3

CELLULAR SYSTEMS BIOLOGY APPLIED TO PRECLINICAL SAFETY TESTING: A CASE STUDY OF CELLCIPHR™ PROFILING

Lawrence Vernetti, William Irwin, Kenneth A. Giuliano, Albert Gough, Kate Johnston, and D. Lansing Taylor

Contents

Drug Efficacy, Safety, and Biologics Discovery: Emerging Technologies and Tools,
Edited by Sean Ekins and Jinghai J. Xu
Copyright © 2009 by John Wiley & Sons, Inc.

3.1 INTRODUCTION

3.1.1 Challenge in the Pharmaceutical Industry

The goal of the pharmaceutical industry should be to create drugs that exhibit high efficacy, low toxicity, and high patient specificity. To reach this goal, there must be changes in the approaches applied in the continuum from early drug discovery, through drug development and clinical trials/diagnostics. This chapter addresses the application of Cellular Systems Biology (CSB)™ to safety testing at the interface between discovery and preclinical testing. CSB can be applied across the continuum from early drug discovery to clinical trials and diagnostics [1,2].

3.1.2 Cellular Systems Biology (CSB)™

Cellular Systems Biology (CSB)™ is the investigation of cells as integrated and interacting networks of genes, proteins, and metabolic processes that give rise to either normal or pathological conditions. Cells are the first level of biological organization that integrate the activities of constituents such as genes, proteins, and metabolites into a functioning system. Cells, of course, form the basis of higher order tissue and organ systems that in turn make up organisms. In addition to providing the basic functions required of tissues and organs, cells are involved in mediating their interactions.

Individual cells and combinations of cells are complex enough to yield important systems information and knowledge, but simple enough to manipulate and measure if we take advantage of the last few decades of reductionist exploration of isolated cellular constituents ("omics") to create moderate-throughput assays and profiles (Figure 3.1). The paradigm shift in applying CSB is that we can now look at individual cells and collections of cells as surrogate systems, not just "containers" of independent target molecules and specific pathways. The goal of CSB is to understand the systems response of cells to various chemical and biological challenges and the relationships between those responses and organ and organismal (dys)function. Analysis of the response profiles of a panel of target molecules and pathways allows the identification of characteristic patterns that can be used to reduce the complexity of CSB data to simpler mechanistic interpretations as well as an index value that can be used to make decisions.

CSB builds on the "omics" approaches by harnessing genomics, proteomics, and metabolomics analyses to guide the selection of panels of functional biomarkers. In addition the CSB approach takes advantage of the evolution of cell-based assays and instrumentation over the last 10 years from whole plate cell population averages to high content screening (HCS) methods [3]. CSB is the next generation of cell-based discovery, and it can be applied in basic

Cellular Systems

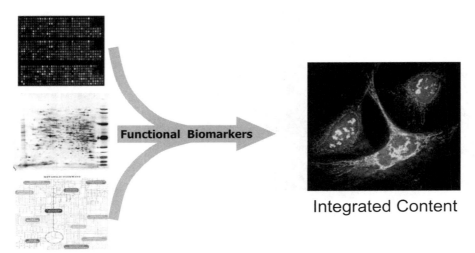

Integrated Content

Figure 3.1 Cellular systems biology is the study of the integrated and interacting network of genes, proteins, and metabolic processes that give rise to normal and abnormal conditions. The cell, as the simplest of complex biological systems, exhibits properties in response to external stimulus that are not always anticipated from detailed knowledge of its component parts, or component functions and can be measured and analyzed using panels of fluorescently labeled, functional biomarkers coupled with advanced informatics. (See color insert.)

biomedical research, drug discovery, drug development, and clinical trials, as well as, in diagnostics to create more powerful answers in less time and for lower cost.

3.1.3 Tools of CSB

The tools of CSB are designed to manipulate and to measure biomarkers of key processes and pathways in models of cellular and tissue functions [1]. Furthermore ideal tools provide precise spatial, temporal, and contextual information on the interrelationships between biomarker activities within the same cells. Currently CSB profiling data can be captured with high content imagers multiplexed across multiple wells of the same cell preparations. Final integration of CSB profiling data employs computational software to

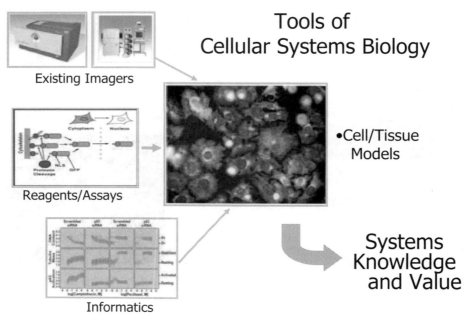

Figure 3.2   Tools of cellular systems biology. Cells or tissue models are plated in high density 384-well microtiter plates and exposed to treatments. At the end of exposure time the cells are evaluated for 10 or more measurements using panels of fluorescent-based reagents. The 384-well plates are scanned using existing high-content reader instruments with image analysis algorithms. Informatics tools extract contextual information from the multiplex of functional cell features. Databases containing large compound profiles sets can be mined for knowledge. (See color insert.)

interrogate, summarize, and transform CSB profiling information into new systems knowledge (Figure 3.2).

Cellular Systems Biology Assays   CSB assays utilize a panel (usually >6) of functional biomarkers to extract, a "cellular systemic response" to a treatment or condition in the form of a panel of "features" [1]. The assays are performed in a high-throughput format (384 well plates) often with an HCS reader. The assays can be fixed end point, where the cells are fixed and labeled with multiplexed, fluorescence-based reagents after treatment, or they can be live cell assays, where the treatment and readouts are performed directly on living cells.

CellCiphr™ Profiles   Automated, computational analyses of the data are derived from a set of cellular systems biology assays. The resulting summary index can help guide decisions.

3.2 PRECLINICAL SAFETY TESTING AS ONE KEY CHALLENGE

3.2.1 Improved Prioritization of Leads and Clinical Candidates

The pharmaceutical industry is under high pressure to reduce the overall failure rate in drug development while meeting tougher human regulatory standards. The cost to drive one drug successfully to approval is estimated at $897 million, of which approximately $200 million is spent during the preclinical phase of development, and the remainder for clinical testing [4]. However, if the cost of failed drugs is taken into account, the cost of developing a successful new drug has been estimated to be approximately $1 billion [5]. Attrition of compounds is evident at all levels of drug discovery and development. Out of 10,000 compounds synthesized only one will ever be marketed as a drug. Approximately 9000 have undesirable chemical properties such as solubility and reactive groups; another 750 fail due to overt toxicity, lack of efficacy, or IP protection issues. Of the remaining 250 compounds that could possibly move into preclinical testing, only 10 will eventually enter clinical trials with just one of those gaining approval.

Current human safety requirements still rely heavily on the in vivo animal toxicity testing protocols that have changed little in decades. Although animal testing will remain pivotal as the safety testing standard involved in the development and approval process of new drug applications for the foreseeable future, half of new drug applications failed since 1990 because of unpredicted toxicities that animal safety studies were not able to present [6]. Furthermore the industry has been subject to withdrawals of approved drugs due to safety concerns. Terfenadine, troglitazone, bromfenac, cisapride, and cerivastatin have been pulled from the market for toxicological issues, and many others have received use restriction labels [7]. The withdrawal of two high-profile drugs, valdecoxib (Bextra) in 2005 and rofecoxib (Vioxx) in 2004 heightened criticism of the regulatory agency and its current drug safety policies [8], which is expected to level additional safety burdens on the industry. Besides the pressure to foresee human drug risks that are not likely to present under existing animal toxicity safety protocols, the industry is faced with the need to reduce the failure rate and costs in developing drugs. The pharmaceutical industry must therefore find new protocols or technologies to improve the efficiency with which compounds enter the postdiscovery stage development. Among these considerations are higher throughput methods that can better prioritize compounds for animal testing and be more predictive of human toxicity.

Recently toxicogenomics, the study of how the genome responds to environmental stressors or toxicants, has been applied to whole animal toxicity testing to elucidate mechanisms of action (MOA) [9,10]. The full value of the toxicogenomics-based approach to pharmaceutical sciences is, however, limited by two critical deficits: (1) gene array information does not reflect functional effects, such as posttranslational modifications and molecular inter-actions in time and space, and (2) the protocols have as yet unresolved chal-lenges to interpretation and reproducibility of data. With regard to the "omics" revolution, in general, these deficits prompted Scott Gottlieb, deputy FDA commissioner for medical and scientific affairs, to observe in 2006 that pro-teomics, genomics, and microarrays have only added to the cost of discovery and development without making the process any faster or more certain. [6,11]. Nevertheless, the toxicogenomics data are useful in selecting panels of functional biomarkers for CSB profiling in specific-tissue and cell types.

3.2.2   Early Cytotoxicity Assays Were Too Simple

Healthy cells extract energy from the environment to build and maintain the intricate, energy-rich subcellular structures, pathways, and processes involved in a range of cellular functions including homeostasis, motility, and self-replication. Disease from infections, genetic defects, environmental stress, or xenobiotic insult impairs normal phenotypic responses. For example, insulin-resistant liver cells exhibit decreased glucose and small cell lung cancer cells grow uncontrollably as a result of eliminated cell cycle check points. However, if the insult or injury is of sufficient duration and intensity to push the extent of the injury beyond the cell's capacity for repair, regeneration, or re-adaptation, a series of cascading cellular events occur that are collectively called cytotoxicity [12].

Historically simple cytotoxicity assays depended on cell loss or decreases in cell health indicators such as MTT, Alamar Blue, ATP, or increased leakage of cytosolic enzymes to determine a cytotoxic response [13]. In 2000 the Scandinavian Society for Cell Toxicology published the results of a large study from an initiative began in 1988 as the MultiCenter Evaluation of In Vitro Cytotoxicity (MEIC) [14]. The study compared the results of 50 reference compounds screened by 39 laboratories using 67 single end-point in vitro assays conducted in a variety of 60 "test" systems of established or primary cell types from humans, animals, insects, or bacteria and found an 84% cor-relation of 4 assays to acute human lethality. The assays were as follows: (1) 24-hour protein content in Hep G2 cells, (2) 24-hour ATP levels in HL-60 cells, and (3) two morphology assessments in Chang liver cells. Despite the positive association of the in vitro assays to predict lethal doses in humans, these simple cell health indicators had limited value to predicting the sub-lethal toxicity with an overall accuracy below 50%.

3.2.3   Cytotoxicity Assays Still Not Optimal

Given the difficulty in generating, analyzing, and interpreting toxicogenomic data, the cytotoxicity assay that continues to dominate in many labs is a single measurement involving one component of a biological system, whether a phenotypic marker (cell death, decreased mitochondrial membrane potential, intracellular ATP) or change in one gene or protein (DNA repair gene, stress gene activation). But as determined in the MEIC study, these single measurements have not proved to be a reliable indicator of sub-lethal whole organ or animal toxicity. Early attempts to combine the single measurement assays together were useful, but the layered approach was still separated from the context of the function of the intact cellular system [15].

A crucial step in the generation of useful biological information is the choice of the cell type and method of measurement of cell activities. O'Brien et al. reported better than 80% correlation between the safety data and a five-parameter HCS assay using HepG2 cells as an indicator of human in vivo hepatotoxicity [16]. Although HepG2 cells are generally a well-regarded cell line for human liver studies when primary cells are inconvenient, or of questionable quality or unobtainable, HepG2 cells do not possess physiologic levels of the most abundant liver metabolizing enzyme CYP 3A4 [17]. Additional cell types may be necessary to identify drugs requiring metabolic activation through this enzyme. Nonetheless, some researchers regard HepG2 cells better as a indicator of general toxicity than as an indicator of specific hepatotoxin activity. Because hepatotoxicity is generally regarded as one of the major limiting factors in drug discovery [18,19], cytotoxicity panels using liver-based models would be predicted to decrease delays and expenses throughout the discovery and development process Hepatotoxicity is also often cited as a major reason for failure to gain approval for new drug applications, which can lead to expensive drug withdrawals and label restrictions [7]. Consequently there is a continued need for more powerful test systems to identify potential hepatotoxins. Primary hepatocytes have emerged as a relevant and dependable model test system. When isolated and handled appropriately, hepatocytes express a broad range of metabolizing enzyme activities, hepatic transporters, and other differentiated functions [20,21]. Furthermore numerous laboratories have reported correlations between the primary hepatocyte model and in vivo metabolic profile of drugs [22–25]. Taken together, the primary hepatocyte is well suited to assess hepatocellular liver injury or hepatotoxicity using a CSB approach. Given that animal liver cells can process drugs quite differently than human liver cells [26,27], that rats are the most often used animal species in drug safety studies [28], and the need for reliable screening tests at the decision-junctures between drug discovery and preclinical safety assessment, the primary rat hepatocyte becomes one good candidate for CSB profiling.

3.2.4 CSB as a New Approach to Preclinical Safety Testing

Cellular Systems Biology can be applied to toxicity testing and used to pull identification of problematic side effects forward into the interface between early drug discovery and drug development. CSB brings in the contextual information missing from the single end-point measures, adds cause and effect relational information missing from toxicogenomics, and importantly, offers tremendous advantages in the speed and number of compounds that can be tested earlier in the process to yield a safety index that can be used to make decisions to prioritize the compounds that move forward into preclinical testing. Better decisions will be made possible through application of CSB profiling in relevant cell types. Here is described the application of CSB to cytotoxicity profiling and a report on a case study of the performance of the first generation CellCiphr™ toxicity profiling tools.

3.3 APPLYING CELLULAR SYSTEMS BIOLOGY TO CYTOTOXICITY PROFILING

3.3.1 Case Study: 100 Compound CellCiphr™ Panel 1 Profile

CellCiphr™ cytotoxicity assays are designed to be used as stand-alone assays or in combination to provide a more detailed profile. The assays are performed in 384 well plates with extensive intra- and interplate quality controls using HCS readers. The images collected from each well of the dose–response series are processed using off-the-shelf software applications provided with the existing high-content instruments. The results are extracted as measurements from a dose series that is fit to a dose–response curve (Figure 3.3a) using a standard four-parameter logistics model. A set of QC metrics are used to automatically accept or reject curves based on the quality of the fit and the likelihood that the curve accurately represents a dose–response relationship. Cell feature responses can increase or decrease depending on the treatment, and these changes are monitored as appropriate by the slope of dose–response curve (Figure 3.3b, c). The concentration at which the population average response is 50% of the control activity range (AC_{50} value) is calculated from the curve and the collection of AC_{50} values over the entire cell feature set comprises the response profile. The profiles are then analyzed with proprietary visual and quantitative data mining tools including CellCiphr classifiers, correlation analysis and cluster analysis.

The CellCiphr™ cytotoxicity panel 1 uses the Hep G2 cell line derived from human liver hepatoma and panel 2 uses primary rat hepatocytes to profile the cellular responses to toxic challenges in a cell-specific set of fixed end-point assays (Table 3.1). The cell features are captured in time- and concentration-dependent responses to toxicants at 1, 24, and 72 hours in HepG2, at 1, 24, and 48 hours in rat hepatocytes, and in 10 concentration ranges from 0.003 to 100 μM for the two panels.

The performance of the CellCiphr™ panel 1 was assessed in a set of 136 compounds with preclinical safety reference data. A total of 100 of the compounds were blinded test compounds provided by a consortium of pharmaceutical companies, while the remaining 36 compounds were well-known compounds. Initially each compound was assigned to a categorical toxicity

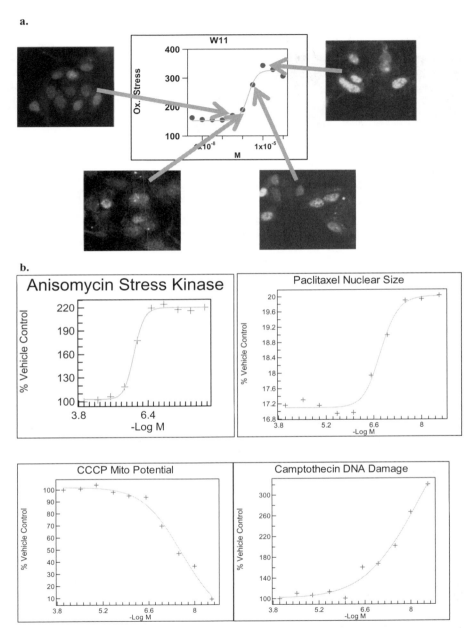

Figure 3.3 Example of CellCiphr™ panel 1 data processing. (*a*) Image analysis extracts cell features as numeric data forming a 10-point dose–response curve. (*b*) Representative control response curves from CellCiphr™ HepG2 assay.

c.

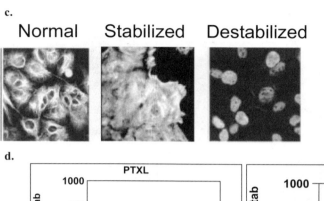

d.

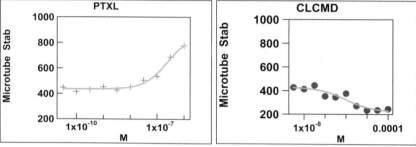

Figure 3.3 (*c*) Certain biomarkers can increase or decrease dependant on treatment. Images of microtubules showing normal, stabilized (increased staining intensity), and destabilized (decreased staining intensity) tubulin formation. (*d*) Dose–response curves of Paclitaxel-stabilized and colcemid-destabilized tubulin.

TABLE 3.1   CellCiphr™ Assays Used to Evaluate Compound Effects over a Broad Range of Indicators

CellCiphr™ Panel 1 HepG2	CellCiphr™ Panel 2 Rat Hepatocytes
Cell loss	Cell loss
DNA degradation	DNA degradation
Nuclear size	Nuclear size
Cytoskeletal disruption	DNA damage
DNA damage response	Phospholipidosis
Oxidative stress	Apoptosis
Mitosis marker	Mitochondria function
Stress kinase activation	Steatosis
Mitochondria function I	
Mitochondria function II	
Cell cycle arrest	

class based on a severity score derived from the analysis of drug safety studies by two separate toxicologists. This toxicity score along with the CellCiphr™ profiling results for approximately half of the unknown compounds was used as the training set to build the computational Classifier algorithm (Figure 3.4*a*, *b*). The classifier is an analysis method by which a two-stage regression model is applied to the cell feature data with the outcome being a categorical classification of the overall response as a function of the strength and frequency of the variables. Once created, classifier performance was then tested against the remainder of the unknown compounds (the test set) and an independent set of control compounds (Figure 3.4*c*).

Because CellCiphr™ profiling was developed to provide facilitated decision making from complex sets of response profile data, the results are presented in several forms. Each compound can be reported simply as a noncorrelated individual response profile or after computational analysis to reduce dose- and time-dependent data into a set of descriptors that are used to tease out cellular modes of toxicity, so as to provide a relative ranking score and safety index predictor (Figure 3.4*d*). Clustered heat maps are used to identify patterns of responses in large data sets (Figure 3.5). Statistical tools such as the Pearson's correlation coefficient are used to compare compound profiles for similarity, which can also be visually assessed in overlaid profile plots. The profile similarity plots are used to identify potential mechanisms of action by direct interpretation of functional responses as well as the mechanisms predicted by the correlations between the unknown test compounds and known control compounds (Figure 3.6) with known mechanisms of action. The relative toxicity of compounds in a series, such as a lead series or SAR, predicted by the CellCiphr™ classifier provides a rank order of toxicity that can be utilized to prioritize compounds for additional follow-on studies or for preclinical candidacy. This safety risk index has been demonstrated in the study presented here to reliably predict potential in vivo liabilities. Additional results, such as the earliest and the most potent cell feature response of a compound, can also be easily extracted from the data. These results may be useful to identify a single end-point assay for more extensive toxicity SAR campaigns, as well as mechanisms of action campaigns.

3.3.2   Performance of First-Generation CellCiphr™ in the Case Study

The first generation, two-stage classifier produces three output classifications: significant toxicity, moderate toxicity, and minimal toxicity. When applied to the 136 compounds in the HepG2 assay panel, if the unbiased automated CellCiphr™ classifier identified a compound as significantly toxic, it was indeed, in all cases toxic, giving an accuracy of 100%. (Table 3.2). The accuracy over the entire 136 compound set of unknowns to identify compounds with in vivo toxicity was 76%, a substantial improvement over the less than 50% accuracy found in the MEIC study. Although the performance accuracy for classifying minimal/negative toxins was low, it was improved

a.

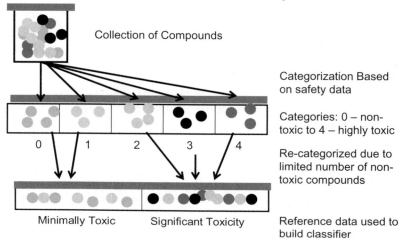

Building the Generation 1 Classifier for Compound Toxicity

Collection of Compounds

Categorization Based on safety data

Categories: 0 – non-toxic to 4 – highly toxic

Re-categorized due to limited number of non-toxic compounds

Minimally Toxic   Significant Toxicity

Reference data used to build classifier

Figure 3.4 Constructing the classifier. (*a*) Basic classifier construction method. The collection of compounds having categorical in vivo safety reference data are binned according to in vivo severity so that 0 are nontoxic, 1 minimally toxic, 2 and 3 moderately toxic, and 4 significantly toxic compounds. A limited number of nontoxic compounds existed in this initial set of compounds necessitating a combination of compounds scored 0 and 1 into minimally toxic and 2, 3, or 4 into significantly toxic bins. (*b*) A subset of each bin was randomly selected to use as a training set. Regression analysis using a two-stage approach was applied to the training set to identify patterns and changes between minimally toxic and significantly toxic profiles, creating an algorithm to simplify the profile to a single number called the toxicity score. The safety score algorithm was then applied to classification of the test set of compounds. (*c*) An independent set of control compounds with drug safety reference data was used to validate the findings of the classifier. (*d*) The results are tabulated according to the simple binning and ranked according to the calculated toxicity score. (See color insert.)

compared to the single end-point assay method, with the advantage that the accuracy can be refined with addition of larger sets of compounds in the database additional cell types and additional assay panels targeted to other toxicity mechanisms.

Several of the control compounds used in the large study are currently marketed or market-withdrawn drugs. Table 3.3 compares the results of two drugs still on the market against one marketed with a warning label for hepatotoxicity and four that were market-withdrawals due to safety issues. The classifier performed very well in identifying correctly the compounds with safety issues. These drugs would have failed the CellCiphr™ "filter" early in

b.

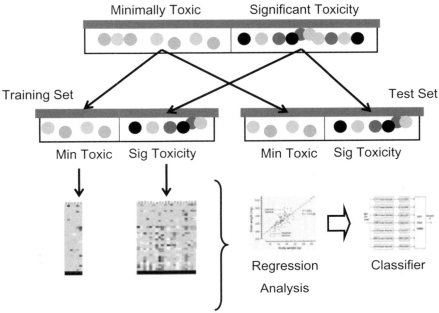

Building the Gen 1 Classifier

Minimally Toxic   Significant Toxicity

Training Set   Test Set

Min Toxic   Sig Toxicity   Min Toxic   Sig Toxicity

Regression   Classifier

Analysis

c.

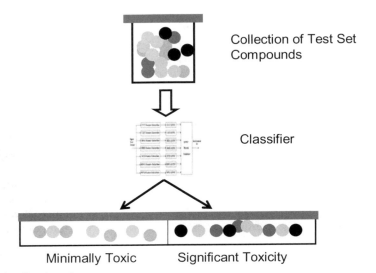

Using the Generation 1 Classifier

Collection of Test Set
Compounds

Classifier

Minimally Toxic   Significant Toxicity

Figure 3.4   *Continued*

d.

Classifier output of training and test set of compounds building the algorithm

Cmpd	Score	Sig Toxic	Min Toxic	Cmpd	Score	Sig Toxic	Min Toxic	Cmpd	Score	Sig Toxic	Min Toxic
W11	1.00	•		A29	0.53	•		H85	0.50	•	•
Y30	0.85	•		W91	0.53		•	C67	0.49	•	
O3	0.82	•		Y50	0.53	•		T72	0.48	•	
F84	0.78	•		X49	0.53	•		M26	0.48	•	
R90	0.76	•		R50	0.53	•		E72	0.47	•	
T42	0.74	•		R40	0.53		•	J27	0.46	•	
A55	0.73	•		O53	0.53		•	K32	0.45	•	
A85	0.71	•		Z22	0.53	•		M36	0.45		•
U28	0.71	•		D61	0.53	•		X39	0.44	•	
E7	0.70	•		G1	0.53		•	I98	0.44		•
C77	0.69	•		H35	0.53		•	F44	0.44		•
N6	0.69	•		D11	0.53	•		F94	0.44		•
L38	0.67	•		B54	0.53	•		T52	0.43		•
Z12	0.67	•		D51	0.53	•		B24	0.43	•	
N16	0.67	•		E62	0.53	•		X69	0.43		•
I78	0.65	•		S63	0.53	•		L15	0.43	•	
S23	0.63	•		Z82	0.53	•		J37	0.43	•	
B4	0.63	•		P70	0.53	•		H25	0.43		•
W61	0.61	•		D71	0.53	•		U68	0.43	•	
T63	0.60	•		G61	0.53	•		U58	0.42	•	
O45	0.60	•		B64	0.53	•		D19	0.42	•	
L75	0.60	•		W81	0.53	•		G18	0.42	•	
V27	0.60		•	T2	0.53	•		I17	0.41		•
L65	0.60	•		Z42	0.53	•		Z62	0.41	•	
S13	0.60	•		O93	0.51		•	Y60	0.41	•	
B74	0.60	•		K59	0.51	•		S73	0.40	•	
Y10	0.58	•		A75	0.51	•		P20	0.40		•
F34	0.57	•		H27	0.50		•				

Figure 3.4 *Continued*

their development phase, if applied. This would have given the investigators key information to help make decisions and could have saved a large amount of time and money. In comparison, the single end-point cell viability assessment would prioritize Tacrine and Troglitazone ahead of Lovastatin, Haloperidol, Astemizole, and Cerivastatin simply on cell loss AC_{50} values of $115, 26, 14, 25, 10$, and $0.2 \mu M$, respectively. CSB assay data linked to classification proved to be a powerful tool that could be used to confidently prioritize unknown compounds early in drug discovery process prior to preclinical safety assessment.

In the set of unknown compounds, approximately 7% of them produced profiles that have a correlation coefficient with known control compounds of greater than 0.8, while an additional 10% showed a correlation of at least 0.7 when compared with known controls. The unknown set of compounds produced an average of 9 cell feature responses, while the control compounds averaged 11 cell feature responses. As expected, nearly all features show increased frequency and decreased AC_{50} with exposure time. All cell feature assays showed activity for at least one compound. DNA degradation was the least frequent while changes to nuclear size and cell loss were the features affected most frequently. Nearly a third of the compounds caused significant cell loss (>20%) at 1 hour and 80% showed measurable cell loss at the chronic

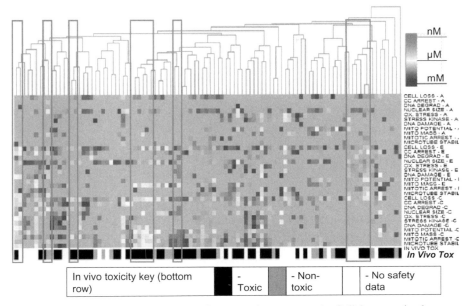

In vivo toxicity key (bottom row)	■ - Toxic	▨ - Non-toxic	□ - No safety data

Figure 3.5 Hierarchical clustering of case study compounds. Cell features in the profiles are color coded by AC_{50} value so that red is nM, yellow is µM, and blue is mM concentrations. In vivo results are shown on the bottom axis. Blue rectangles indicate compounds with high degree of in vitro similarity, thus with a high likelihood that they will produce similar responses in vivo. Heat maps are used to identify patterns in response profiles between compounds in large data sets. (See color insert.)

time point (72 h). Overall the selectivity (frequency of features responding) correlated better to in vivo toxicity than sensitivity (mean AC_{50} of the responses).

3.3.3 Combining Multiple CellCiphr™ Panels

Detailed analysis of the compounds that exhibited toxicity, but were not classified as toxic by the first-generation classifier, indicates that the toxic mechanisms involved were not expected to be active in the HepG2 panel. Mechanisms including immune-mediated toxicity, neuropathies, cardiac, renal, and respiratory toxicities highlight the need for development of additional assay panels. To address this need, and to further optimize detection in rats, a primary rat hepatocyte panel has been developed. Although the two panels were designed with different functional endpoints and only the HepG2 panel results are reported here, preliminary results from the rat hepatocyte panel show that the different cell types produce results consistent and unique to the cellular biology. Diclofenac is a NSAID compound that requires CYP3A4 metabolic

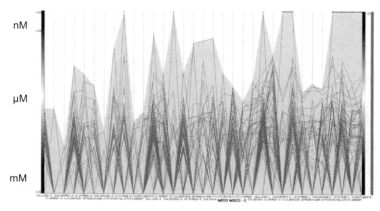

Unknowns I17 (blue) and I98 (gray) with high similarity to Terfenadine (red)

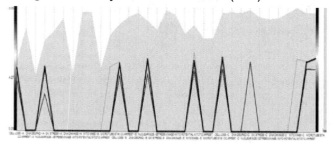

Unknown H25 with high similarity to Etoposide

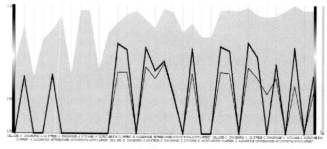

Figure 3.6 Application of Pearson's correlation plot similarity analysis. (*a*) The universe of all compounds plotted as cell features against magnitude of the response. The lines represent individual compounds, with the gray background showing the maximum value of feature responses for all compounds in the first-generation database. (*b*) Test compounds I98 and I17 have high similarity to Terfenadine (QT prolongation) while H25 has a nearly identical profile to Etoposide (myleotoxicity). Correlations such as these are used as mechanistic indicators for follow-up investigative toxicology studies. (See color insert.)

TABLE 3.2 Accuracy of CellCiphr Classifier 1

In Vivo Toxicity[a]	n	Accuracy CellCiphr Classifier
Significant	33	100%
Moderate	65	80%
Min	38	41%

[a]Includes 136 unknown and control compounds for which CellCiphr™ and drug safety data were available.

TABLE 3.3 Comparison of Two Examples of Currently Marketed Drugs and Five Failed or Warning Labeled Drugs Run in CellCiphr™ Classifier

Drug	Status	CellCiphr™ Safety Index
Lovastatin	Currently marketed	Low risk
Haloperidol	Currently marketed	Low risk
Tacrine	Label warning to monitor hepatotoxicity	High risk
Troglitazone	Withdrawn for hepatotoxicity	High risk
Cerivastatin	Withdrawn for rhabdomyolysis	High risk
Astemizole	Withdrawn for drug–drug interactions	High risk

activation to produce a toxic intermediate [29]. Cell responses to diclofenac were evident in rat hepatocytes but not in HepG2 cells (Figure 3.7a). Primary rat hepatocytes, but not HepG2 cells, maintain measureable levels of CYP 3A activity in short-term culture [17], so the results between the two panels are consistent with a metabolism-driven mode of toxicity. Another example of differential response to a compound from the test set is a compound which exhibited toxicity consistent with a toxic proliferation inhibitor. In vivo the compound presented bone marrow depletion, reduced blood counts, and thrombocytopenia, but minimal effect on liver cells. As demonstrated in the two CellCiphr™ panels, no measureable responses were evident in the rat hepatocyte panel, but significant number of features responded in HepG2 cells (Figure 3.7b). These results are consistent with an in vivo profile of a compound effect on cycling Hep G2 cells but no effect on noncycling cells such as primary hepatocytes. The two selected examples serve to show that multiple cell types or panels are required to cover the broad range of in vivo toxicity mechanisms.

3.4 CONCLUSION

The principles of CSB were used to address the problems arising during the drug development process by developing a reliable, new in vitro solution for identifying toxic compounds in an automated process. The first-generation CellCiphr™ cytotoxicity profiling system offers a rapid, inexpensive, cell-

a.

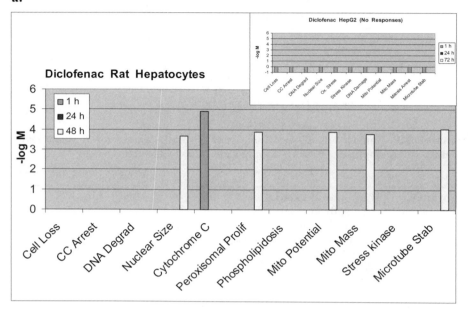

b.

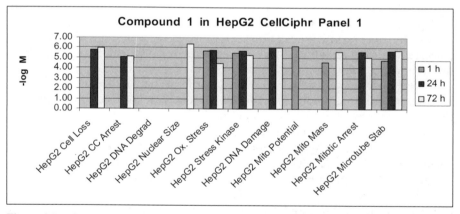

Figure 3.7 Comparison of CellCiphr™ profile responses of an in vivo hepatotoxic and myleotoxic compound in CellCiphr™ panels in Hep G2 and rat hepatocytes. (*a*) The NSAID compound diclofenac requires metabolic activation to a toxic intermediate to produce a liver-specific cytotoxicity. HepG2 have limited metabolic capacity to activate the toxic intermediate as evidenced by the lack of responses (insert). However, the primary rat hepatocytes contain a full complement of metabolic function depict early activation of apoptosis with time-dependent effects on mitochondrial mass and other cell features. Therefore the best system will probably include multiple cell types. (*b*) The test compound W11 was found to be a potent myleotoxic, nonhepatotoxic compound in drug safety studies; it produced numerous cell feature responses in cycling HepG2 cells but none in noncycling primary rat hepatocytes (not shown).

based method capable of accurate and sensitive identification of compounds associated with severe in vivo toxicity with the additional benefit of no occurrence of false-positives. The CellCiphr™ cytotox panels are designed to filter compounds for toxicity and would be employed anywhere that compound ranking for efficacy or preclinical safety assessment is useful. Further the multiplexed image-based data captured by the CellCiphr™ cytotoxicity profile tools offers advantages over single end point well-based assays by providing deeper insight into potential mechanisms of action.

The CellCiphr™ HepG2 panel presented here is the first in a series of panels to be developed aimed at applying Cellular Systems Biology to in vitro toxicity assessment. Preliminary results from the CellCiphr™ primary rat hepatocyte panel, including some additional mechanistic insights resulting from the use of the two panels, were discussed. New panels making use of cells from other organs and additional measurements, coupled with a growing library of reference compound profiles will continue to improve the reliability of the classification, as well as add significantly to the mechanistic insights provided by the feature measurements and the correlations with the reference compounds in the database.

ACKNOWLEDGMENTS

The authors would like to thank Cambridge Healthtech Associates (CHA) and a consortium of pharmaceutical companies for their involvement in the project. In addition the Millipore Corporation, and in particular, Dennis Harris, Matthew Hsu, Andrew Ball, Rick Ryan, and Stella Redpath who collaborated with Cellumen in the production of the HepG2 panel as a panel kit co-marketed through Millipore. Finally, thanks to Carrie Langer and Seia Comsa for their valuable technical support.

REFERENCES

1. Giuliano KA, Premkumar D, Strock CJ, Johnston PA, Taylor DL. Cellular systems biology profiling applied to cellular models of disease. In: Tang F, Xu J, eds. *Combinatorial chemistry and high throughput screening*. In press, 2008.

2. Critchley-Thorne RJ, Lingle WL, Miller SM, Taylor DL. Applications of cellular systems biology in breast cancer patient stratification and diagnostics. In: Tang F, Xu J, eds. *Combinatorial chemistry and high throughput screening*, 2008, in press.

3. Taylor DL. Insights into high content screening: past, present and future. In: D. Lansing Taylor, Jeffrey R. Haskins, Kenneth A. Giuliano, eds. *High content screening: a powerful approach to systems cell biology and drug discovery*. Totowa, NJ: Humana Press, 2006, 3–18.

4. Tufts Center for Study of Drug Development. News Release. May 13, 2003. http://csdd.tufts.edu/NewsEvents/RecentNews.asp?newsid=29

5. Frank RG. New estimates of drug development costs. *J Health Econ* 2003;22:325–30.

6. Calfee JE. Playing catch up. *FDA, Science and Drug Regulation. Health Policy Outlook*. Mar 28, 2006. www.aei.org/publications/pubID.24130/pub_detail.asp

7. Meadows M. Why drugs get pulled off the market. *FDA Consumer Magazine*. Jan–Feb 2002. www.fda.gov/fdac/features/2002/102_drug.html

8. Avorn J. FDA standards—good enough for government work? *N Engl J Med* 2005;353(10):969–72.

9. Yang Y, Bloome EA, Waring JF. Toxicogenomics in drug discovery: from preclinical studies to clinical trials. *Chem Biol Interact*. 2004;150(1):71–85.

10. Baken KA, vandebriel RJ, Pennings JLA, Kleinjans JC, Van Loveren H. Toxicogenomics in the assessment of immunotoxicity. *Methods* 2007;41:132–41.

11. Gottlieb S. Modernizing development science to unlock new treatments. Remarks to the American Enterprise Institute, Washington, DC, Feb 7, 2006.

12. Trump BF, Berezesky IK. Calcium-mediated cell injury and cell death. *FASEB J.* 1995;9(2):219–28.

13. Barile FA. In: *In vitro cytotoxicity: mechanisms and methods*. Boca Raton, FL: CRC Press, 1994. p. 47–57.

14. Multicenter Evaluation on In vitro Cytotoxicity. Pt 1. MEIC evaluation of acute systemic toxicity: part VII. Clemedson C, et al. *ATLA* 2000;28:161–200. Pt 2. MEIC evaluation of acute systemic toxicity: part VIII. Ekwall B, et al. ATLA 2000;28:201–34.

15. Perlman ZE, Slack MD, Feng Y, Mitchison TJ, et al. Mulidimensional drug profiling by automated microscopy. *Science* 2004;306(12):1194–8.

16. O'Brien PJ, Iwin W, Diaz D, Howard-Cofield E, Kresja CM, Slaughter MR, et al. High concordance of drug-induced human hepatotoxicity with in vitro cytotoxicity measured in a novel cell-based model using high content screening. *Arch Toxicol* 2006;80(9):580–604.

17. Wilkening S, Stahl F, Bader A. Comparison of primary human hepatocytes and hepatoma cell line HepG2 with regard to their biotransformation properties. *Drug Metab Dispos* 2003;31(8):1035–42.

18. Willis RC. Learning about liver toxicity. *Drug Discov News* 2007(Oct). www.drugdiscoverynews.com/index.php?newsarticle=1238

19. Dambach DM, Andres BA, Moulin F. New technologies and screening strategies for hepatotoxicity: use of in vitro models. *Toxicol Pathol* 2005;33(1):17–26.

20. Farkas D, Tannenbaum SR. In vitro methods to study chemically-induced hepatotoxicity: a literature review. *Curr Drug Metab* 2005;6(2):111–25.

21. Guillouzo A. Liver cell models in in vitro toxicology. *Envir on Health Perspec* 1998;106:S2.

22. Hewitt NJ, Burhins KU, Dasenbrock J, Haunschild J, Ladstetter B, Utesch D, Studies comparing in vivo:in vitro metabolism of three pharmaceutical compounds in rat, dog, monkey, and human using cryopreserved hepatocytes, microsomes, and collagen gel immobilized hepatocyte cultures. *Drug Metab Dispos* 2001;29(7): 1042–50.

23. Salonen JS, Nyman L, Boobis AR, Edwards RJ, Watts P, Lake BG, et al. Comparative studies on the cytochrome p450-associated metabolism and interaction

potential of selegiline between human liver-derived in vitro systems. *Drug Metab Dispos* 2003;31(9):1093–102.

24. Bort R, Ponsoda X, Carrasco E, Gomez-Lechon MJ, Castell JV. Comparative metabolism of the nonsteroidal anti-inflammatory drug, aceclofenac, in the rat, monkey, and human. *Drug Metab Dispos* 1996;24(9):969–75.

25. Ponsida X, Pareja E, Gomez-Lechon MJ, Fabra R, Carrasco E, Trullenque R, et al. Drug biotransformation by human hepatocytes: in vitro/in vivo metabolism by cells from the same donor. *J Hepatol* 2001;34(1):19–25.

26. Martelli A, Mattioli F, Angiola M, Reiman R, Brambilla G. Species, sex and inter-individual differences in DNA repair induced by nine sex steroids in primary cultures of rat and human hepatocytes. *Mutat Res* 2003;536(1–2):69–78.

27. Brambilla G, Martelli A. Human hepatocyte primary cultures in toxicity assessment. *Cytotechnology* 1993;11(suppl1):S6–8.

28. Tatsuji N. Concept for establishment of rat outbred global standard strains. In: *Proc US/Japan conf microbial standards and genetic evaluation of mice and men*. International Committee of the Institute for Laboratory Animal Research. National Academy Press, Washington, D.C., 2000.

29. Park KB, Kitteringham NR, Maggs JL, Pirmohamed MY, et al. The role of metabolic activation in drug-induced hepatotoxicity. *Ann Rev Pharmacol Toxicol* 2005;45:177–202.

4

SYSTEMS PHARMACOLOGY, BIOMARKERS, AND BIOMOLECULAR NETWORKS

Aram S. Adourian, Thomas N. Plasterer,
Raji Balasubramanian, Ezra G. Jennings,
Shunguang Wang, Stephen Martin, Jan van der Greef,
Robert N. McBurney, Pieter Muntendam,
and Noubar B. Afeyan

Contents

Drug Efficacy, Safety, and Biologics Discovery: Emerging Technologies and Tools,
Edited by Sean Ekins and Jinghai J. Xu
Copyright © 2009 by John Wiley & Sons, Inc.

4.1　INTRODUCTION

Recent decades have witnessed a robust increase in both the volume and diversity of information derived from measurements of biological systems. Steady progress in analytical measurement technologies and advances in data analysis techniques have provided the ability to measure orders of magnitude more components of biological systems than previously possible. Concurrently the life sciences community has broadly come to the realization that to the extent biological systems are not characterized in their inherent complexity, the completeness and accuracy of our understanding of health, disease, and pharmacological intervention are significantly compromised. Recent advances in analytical measurement technologies have been seen in areas such as biological mass spectrometry, gene expression measurement, nucleic acid sequencing, nuclear magnetic resonance measurement, multiplexed protein assay platforms, and a multitude of other techniques that are often collectively referred to as "molecular profiling technologies [1]. In addition a wide variety of in vivo biological imaging modalities such as PET, CT, and MRI have made significant advances in the last decades; these imaging technologies are, however, beyond the scope of this chapter. Generally situated under the rubrics of "proteomics," "metabolomics," "transcriptomics," "genomics," and the like, these molecular profiling technologies, tools, and approaches collectively measure, characterize, and quantify an increasingly diverse and expansive set of components in a given biological system. Reviews of the applications of molecular profiling approaches have been published on transcriptomics [2], metabolomics [3,4], and proteomics [5,6], for example. As these tools continue to advance in capability and become increasingly adopted by the life sciences community, they promise to have significant consequences for drug discovery and development. The purpose of this chapter is to explore these implications, summarize the current applications for which they are being exploited, and extrapolate the possible consequences of the increasing integration of these technologies into the research and development process.

4.1.1　Systems Pharmacology and Molecular Biomarkers in Pharmaceutical Development

The paradigm of target-centric drug discovery as traditionally practiced by the pharmaceutical industry has recently come under scrutiny, particularly in light of decreasing productivity, dramatically increasing research, and development costs, and well-publicized safety and efficacy concerns [7]. Many have proposed that advanced molecular measurement technologies and their application to the life sciences herald and enable "systems-level" analyses spanning functions from target validation to lead optimization to efficacy and safety evaluation, providing important decision support tools in drug discovery and development as well as in clinical patient management [8–14]. A fundamental definitional aspect of "systems-level" approaches is: What exactly is the "system" under question? In the literature the biological "system" can range from a relatively minimal one, such as an isolated enzyme–substrate complex, to an intact organism, or to even an entire ecosystem. For the purposes of this chapter, the word "system" is understood to refer to a specific single or multiple biomolecular attribute(s) within a unicellular or multicellular organism in a particular condition (healthy, diseased, perturbed with a pharmacological agent, etc.). For example, biochemical signaling pathways and their constituent components related to inflammation in dendritic cells underlying a particular disease in a mammalian species would be considered to constitute a "system"; the human endocrine system comprising the brain, thyroid, heart, striated muscle, adipose, liver, kidney, and other organs would similarly be considered a "system" in the present context.

A fundamental principle of systems-level analyses is that biological systems do not merely comprise a collection of independent components—be they genes, proteins, biochemical pathways, or cells—but that inherent degrees of "connectivity" between and among components lead to various levels of organizational complexity and emergent properties [15,16]. The premise of systems pharmacology is that it is the response of these organizational units to pharmacological intervention that must be evaluated in order to assess more fully the effects of a perturbation to the system such as the efficacy of a drug compound [17,18]. Indeed the concept that biology and medicine are suited to a systems-level approach is not a new one. The works of von Bertalanffy in the midtwentieth century on the application of systems theory to complex biological organisms are perhaps among the early ventures into systems-level perspectives in the life sciences [19].

What has proved challenging is matching systems-level approaches and capabilities to real problems in modern drug discovery and development. Recently, however, the number of studies, initiatives, and large-scale public and private research and development programs that explicitly invoke systems-level approaches and molecular profiling methodologies has dramatically increased [20–29]. The terms "systems pharmacology" and "systems pathology" have recently been coined, the former referring to the application of systems-level approaches for understanding the effects of therapeutic interventions in complex systems, and the latter having to do with better understanding disease etiology and subsequent pathological processes [9,30].

Broadly considered, systems pharmacology, systems pathology and molecular profiling can be considered to be of particular relevance to two general objectives of the contemporary drug discovery and development community. The first of these is a more comprehensive understanding of the on-target, off-target, and systemwide effects induced by pharmaceutical compounds and their metabolites, both in preclinical models and in humans. In this context, studies have been reported in the literature on the use of molecular profiling and systems-level analysis to investigate the perturbative effects of different compounds on systems [31,32], for target discovery and validation [33], and for the selection of appropriate preclinical models for translational purposes

[34,35]. More recently, proteomic, metabolomic, and other molecular profiling tools have been applied to complement genomic and transcriptomic (gene expression) approaches for the analysis of samples ranging from in vitro cell lines to clinical samples from treated patients. In such studies, objectives include better understanding the mode of action of a compound [36], assessing the efficacy of a compound [37], evaluating the toxicity and sources of toxicity of a compound [38–40], reducing or eliminating adverse drug effects (often by informing subsequent cycles of pharmaceutical chemistry) [41], exploring dose-dependent effects [42,43], and investigating combinations of distinct agents as therapeutics [44].

The second general area of relevance of systems-level analysis to drug discovery and development is in the area of biological markers, or "biomarkers." The term "biomarker" has been used in the life sciences community with often differing meanings. The definition we adopt here is one developed by the National Institute of Health Biomarkers Definition Working Group, namely that a biomarker is a characteristic that is objectively measured and evaluated as an indicator of (1) normal biologic processes, (2) pathogenic processes, or (3) pharmacologic responses to a therapeutic intervention [45]. A biomarker can be a characteristic, such as an analyte or set of analytes, that is derived from a broader systems-level analysis; as such, molecular biomarkers often comprise selected subsets of results from a larger molecular profiling study. In order for a biomarker to be meaningful in drug discovery and development and, further, in the clinical setting, it often must advance to the criteria of providing a "surrogate end point." Generally, a surrogate end point is an expression level of biomarker that is intended to serve as a substitute for a clinical end point, and such equivalency is assumed to be based on epidemiologic, pathophysiologic or other established scientific evidence. A useful biomarker is also generally considered one that can be relatively accessible for measurement through minimally invasive procedures in living organisms, for example, derived from biological matrices such as peripheral blood, urine, other bodily fluids, or biopsy material. Indeed, regulatory agencies such as the Food and Drug Administration have expounded on the use of biomarkers in a variety of framework, guideline, and guidance documents [46,47]. Biomarkers of efficacy, toxicity, response, and other aspects have become increasingly important elements in the modern drug discovery and development process [48,49].

Molecular biomarker discovery often proceeds from molecular profiling, systems pharmacology, and systems pathology studies. These studies are necessary but not sufficient elements in yielding a successful biomarker for drug discovery and development purposes, as will be discussed in subsequent sections of this chapter. In drug discovery and development, biomarkers as defined above assume roles throughout the process from target discovery to compound optimization to clinical trials, both as decision support tools and potentially as companion diagnostics for approved therapeutic compounds. Indeed certain biomarkers have already proved useful in increasing the efficiency of the drug discovery and development process. In particular, biomarkers derived from molecular profiling studies have had impact on target validation, drug safety and efficacy evaluation, and patient selection for clinical trials and as companion diagnostics. Widely reported are studies for discovering and validating novel biomarkers relevant to drug discovery and development, to date primarily of transcriptomic and genomic origin but increasingly incorporating other molecular profiling technologies as well [50–54].

4.1.2 Challenges of Systems Pharmacology Approaches

The challenges inherent in systems pharmacology and related biomarker studies can be generally categorized as (1) challenges involving measurement and (2) challenges involving data analysis and interpretation. Challenges involving measurement are present in activities from experimental design to instrumentation and process control. As with any experiment in pharmaceutical research and development, a study must comprise a sufficient number of distinct samples available for analysis in order to achieve an acceptable level of statistical power. Systems-level studies typically measure many hundreds or thousands of individual analytes or features, while the number of available distinct samples in preclinical or early-stage clinical studies is often on the order of 10 or 100. This inequality is the opposite of that typically encountered in, for example, traditional late-stage clinical trials, where often one or a few outcome measures or surrogate end points are tested in a population of hundreds or thousands of individuals. While a number of strategies have been proposed and are used to address this statistical regime, the implications are often insufficiently considered, leading to inconclusive or misleading results [55].

Systems pharmacology studies also place extremely stringent demands on measurement technologies, instrumentation, and laboratory practices. Inherent in systems pharmacology and molecular profiling is the objective of measuring, characterizing, and quantifying as many biomolecular components of a system as possible. The diversity and often incompatibility of techniques to extract and detect different types of analytes from biological matrices, ranging from peptides, proteins, nucleic acids, to endogenous metabolites such as lipids necessitate a diverse set of distinct bioanalytical platforms and sample preparation protocols. Because of the often limited volumes of starting material available for study, and a lack of amplification techniques analogous to polymerase chain reaction for analyte types other than nucleic acids, minimizing sample consumption across each bioanalytical platform is of paramount importance; this is a particularly important consideration in preclinical small animal experiments. Mass spectrometric techniques, for example, are favored for proteomic and metabolomic studies in part due to their relatively small sample volume consumption. The large range in concentration of many endogenous analytes of all classes presents a measurement challenge as well, and the consequence is often a balance between extensive sample preparation and analytical repeatability.

Another challenge involving measurement in systems pharmacology approaches is the required stringency of analytical consistency, reproducibility, repeatability, and accuracy. The demands of measuring tens or hundreds of samples using bioanalytical platforms such as mass spectrometry or oligonucleotide microarrays are dramatically different than those for protocols to measure one or a few specimens. Internal and external standards, elaborate analysis order randomization schemes, and other analytical protocols and practices are broadly used in molecular profiling and systems pharmacology experiments [56–59]. The driving imperative is to ensure that for as many analytes as possible, the measurement variability not overwhelm the inherent biological variability across distinct samples that the experiment is designed to measure. This imperative is complicated by the sheer numbers of analytes that are simultaneously, or within a short time span, being measured, and the differing natural biological variability of each analyte.

Challenges involving data analysis and interpretation are similarly varied, and their successful management is fundamental to successful systems pharmacology experiments. While systems-level experiments generate large volumes of data, this is most often not the most daunting challenge. Rather, the heterogeneity and diversity of data sets derived from different bioanalytical platforms poses challenges that are significant. Innovative approaches to normalizing and integrating disparate data sets, which often differ in size, format and number of measured features have recently emerged in systems-level analyses. Indeed the inequality in the number of analytes measured by any two given bioanalytical platforms presents a data analysis challenge in itself. For example, an experiment seeking to integrate genomewide expression profiles using oligonucleotide arrays that may contain tens of thousands of probe sets with a metabolomics data set that measures and quantifies on the order of 100 analytes represents a purely quantitative imbalance; if not addressed, this may result in a skewing of results to the overwhelmingly larger data set. When incorporating public or third-party data sets in systems pharmacology analyses, a lack of accessibility of both data collection and analysis methods can also pose a significant challenge. Although uniform reporting standards are emerging for various bioanalytical measurement technologies, their adoption by the community at large often remains incomplete [60–64].

As important, with the ability to detect and quantify hundreds or thousands of analytes in a single experiment, interpretation of results becomes a fundamental challenge. The "list paradigm" in which analyte concentrations, "mean-fold changes," standard deviations, and probability values are accumulated, ranked, and "listed" is ill-suited to molecular profiling experiments. This approach inherently ignores the relationships between and among discrete biological components, as well as fundamental levels of biological organizational complexity. Indeed the most relevant observed effects due to pharmacological intervention or disease are often the more subtle changes observed.

In subsequent sections of this chapter, methodologies will be reviewed that implement top-down, bottom-up, and hybrid approaches to providing a context to molecular profiling measurements and observations. The objective of these endeavors is to take fuller advantage of systems pharmacology and biomarker data sets and to move beyond the "list paradigm," ultimately to enable the use of such studies as key decision-making tools in drug discovery and development.

4.2   A SYSTEMS-BASED VIEW OF MOLECULAR PROFILING AND BIOMARKERS

4.2.1   Biological Systems and Networks

In contemporary systems-based studies in the life sciences, frameworks of analysis based on "networks" have become prominent. The field of network analysis has its roots in information science, and borrows many of its fundamental elements from applied mathematics, physics, and graph theory. Ever since Euler pioneered network theory in the late eighteenth century, network analyses have been exploited to investigate the properties of complex systems in disciplines such as sociology, economics, computer science, and transportation. In the context of biology these approaches have been applied to metabolic networks [65,66], neuronal networks [67], gene regulatory networks [68–71], protein interaction networks [72–74], and drug-target networks [75–78], among others. Generically and simply defined, a network is an interconnected system of components. By the terminology adopted from applied mathematics, each component of a network is referred to as a "node," and each connection between a pair of nodes a "link" or "edge." In working with biological systems, these expressions have largely been preserved. For example, in a biological network a node may refer to an analyte such as a protein, while an edge or link may indicate a known protein–protein interaction (see Table 4.1); there are a few exceptions in which a complementary representation is used where nodes represent reactions and edges represent enzymes [79]. Biochemical pathways as traditionally defined can be considered to comprise such networks. Biological networks can be constructed from experimental data and evidence, for example, from yeast two-hybrid experiments for protein–protein interactions, or from dynamic mathematical modeling approaches using techniques such as systems of coupled differential equations [80–82]. The current chapter focuses primarily on the former, evidence-based type of network construction.

Understanding biological networks and using them in practice is a primary challenge in systems pharmacology. The increasing capabilities and availability of data from broad molecular profiling approaches, together with data from focused sources such as protein–protein interaction, localization, and regulation studies, generally provide pairwise evidence of biological relationships

TABLE 4.1 Types of Relationships in Biological Networks

Relationship	Reference
Protein–protein interaction	[83,84]
Metabolic process	[65,66]
Cell-signaling process	[85,86]
Transcriptional regulation	[87,88]
Drug–target interaction	[76,77]
Drug–drug interaction	[89,90]
Literature co-occurrence	[91,92]
Ontology	[93,94]
Linear statistical association	[95,96]
Nonlinear statistical association	[97,98]
Mathematically modeled reaction	[81,99]

between various analytes. Cellular processes, however, involve higher order relationships among genes, proteins, metabolite, exogenous compounds, and other analytes that act together in specific concerted, coordinated ways to carry out various biological processes. Biological network analysis is a means to investigate such multiparametric systems and their behavior under different conditions. The relationships among analytes in a given network can be quite varied, and can be based on empirically based observations (e.g., those derived from molecular profiling or other experiments), or on a priori knowledge or hypotheses of network properties. Further, for example, observed associations among components involved in metabolic processes may be defined by strict stoichiometric constraints, while relationships among constituents in signaling pathways may be less uniquely determined. Table 4.1 lists some of the types of relationships that can be captured in biological networks.

Importantly, network approaches inherently transcend the so-called list paradigm, and therefore represent an important element in systems pharmacology. By considering biological networks, and considering experimental observations within such frameworks, the unit of analysis is extended from individual analyte properties to the properties of multiple related components that together often form modules of functional or other similarity. Further biological networks, as other networks, exhibit dramatic hierarchical structural properties characterized by distinct levels of organization, information storage and processing [100]. For example, cellular components such as proteins, metabolites, and nucleic acids can be considered as fundamental building blocks of biological networks; regulatory motifs and metabolic pathways represent a higher level of organization and interconnectivity; and functional modules define yet larger scale cellular organization and processes [15].

As in other fields that utilize network analysis, biological networks are often visualized in a two-dimensional plane, with nodes and edges represented graphically. The types and interpretations of various network layouts and topologies can differ based on the information that has been used to derive and arrange the visualization [101,102]. Figure 4.1 shows a biological network that integrates and relates multiple types of data. In this figure experimental transcriptomic and proteomic data are associated with the cellular component hierarchy as defined by gene ontology [103]. Within the network shapes of nodes indicate the data source, and the color of the node indicates whether the measured abundance of the analyte was greater or less than a baseline level in this particular experiment. Further the two types of edges in the network indicate whether the shown association is derived from gene ontology or on known sequence-based association between gene transcripts and proteins. As such, the edges in this network are all based on a priori annotated biological knowledge, and the experimental (transcriptomic and proteomic) results, represented as the square and hexagonal nodes, are fitted within this scaffold. In the graphical representation of the network in Figure 4.1, there is no meaning to the length of the edges between the nodes; the algorithm for organizing nodes arranges both nodes and edges for maximal clarity in this case.

Figure 4.2 shows a network which is relatively more complex than that of Figure 4.1. The network of this figure comprises five distinct types of nodes and two types of edges, and was constructed in an unsupervised manner from experimental data and from accessible biological data sources. Nodes and edges that denote a priori defined biological knowledge are those that represent co-occurrence of analyte nomenclature terms in PubMed abstracts (document icons), and associations with disorders as annotated in the Online Mendelian Inheritance in Man (OMIM) database (crosses) [104]. In contrast with the network of Figure 4.1, the network in Figure 4.2 further integrates experimental results from this particular study. For example, the blue edges between pairs of proteomic, metabolomic or transcriptomic nodes represent statistical correlation, as observed in this specific experiment, among analytes. The color shading of the nodes representing analytes denotes the statistical abundance changes of each analyte observed within this study. The topological layout of the network in Figure 4.2 is such that clusters of nodes that appear in close topologic proximity are connected by a higher density of edges than nodes that are spatially farther removed from such clusters. Note that not every analyte node (protein, transcript, or metabolite) is associated with a PubMed abstract or OMIM node. Indeed a minority of the experimental nodes are so connected. This reflects generally the relatively incomplete annotation and curation of measurable molecular analytes into existing knowledge bases, a topic that is discussed in subsequent sections of this chapter.

Use of a network-based approach is relevant to drug discovery and development, as it is motivated by the goal of capturing both biological complexity and pharmaceutical chemistry. The inherent complexity and connectivity characterizing biological systems implies that even a hypothetical drug of perfect selectivity and specificity addressing a known target will have effects of modulating an intact system beyond the putative target. Similarly

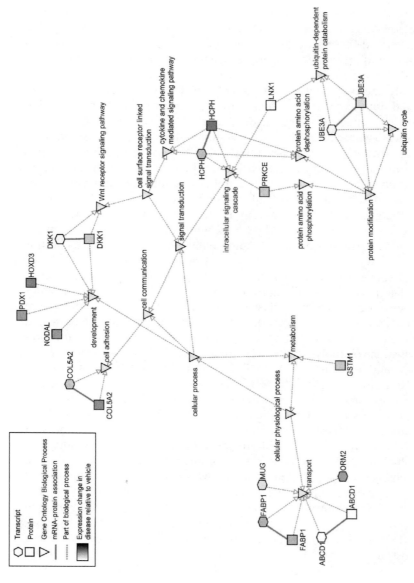

Figure 4.1 Biological network integrating experimental data from a preclinical study with Gene Ontology data [97]. Nodes and edges are as described in the legend. The biological process hierarchy of Gene Ontology is shown. The shades of gene transcript nodes (hexagon icons) and protein nodes (square icons) indicate changes in abundance of these analytes: Dark (light) shades indicat increase (decrease) relative to a baseline state. Gene and protein annotations follow HUGO nomenclature.

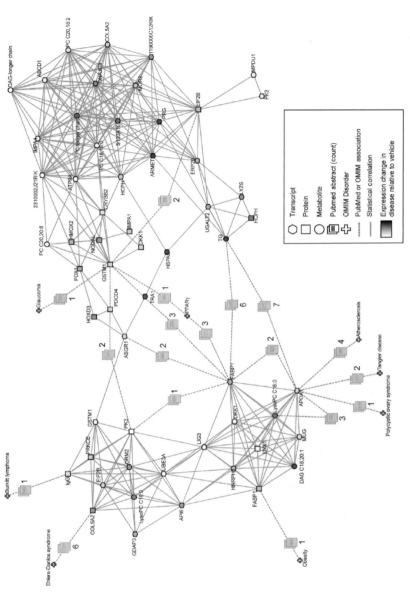

Figure 4.2 Biological network integrating experimental data from a preclinical study with literature co-occurrence data using PubMed and the Online Mendelian Inheritance in Man (OMIM) resource [97]. Nodes and edges are as described in the legend. The number of distinct PubMed abstracts connecting pairs of nodes is indicated below each document icon. Statistical correlations are based on a kernel PCA metric as described in Clish et al. [105]. The shades of gene transcript and protein nodes indicate changes in abundance of these analytes: dark or light shades indicate increase or decrease, respectively relative to a baseline state. Gene and protein annotations follow HUGO nomenclature.

exogenous drugs that affect multiple components in a biological system or, for example, yield bioactive metabolites will similarly perturb a highly connected system in a complex manner.

Figure 4.3 illustrates this phenomena. In contrast to the networks presented thus far, the components, nodes, and edges in Figure 4.3 are solely empirically derived, based on Pearson product-moment correlations; such correlation networks are discussed further in Section 4.3.4. As with analyte abundance changes, correlations among analytes can be tested statistically, and confidence metrics such as p-values assigned and adjusted for multiple hypothesis testing [106]. In Figure 4.3 the broad effects of a single drug compound administered in vivo on a biological network that centers on cholesterol and HDL and spans serum and adipose tissue in a rodent model are shown. Three networks are illustrated: one for normal phenotype animals (network a), one for disease phenotype animals (network b), and a corresponding network for disease phenotype animals administered a therapeutic compound for the disease (network c). These networks are graphical representations of the covariance matrices across all animals in each group. Apart from the imposed criterion that adipose analytes must be either one or two correlation links away from either serum cholesterol or serum HDL, these networks are derived in an entirely unsupervised manner. The colors of the edges represent the strength and sign of the statistical correlation, and the analyte node colors represent the concentration changes in each analyte relative to the normal phenotype state.

As can be seen in Figure 4.3, administration of the drug to diseased animals has dramatic and widespread effects not only on analyte concentrations (represented by node colors) but also in the measured correlations among analytes. None of the analytes shown in this figure were the putative target of the drug under study. While the drug is seen to reduce levels of serum cholesterol and serum HDL in the disease phenotype (as denoted by the coloring of the nodes representing these two analytes), drug administration is also seen to induce positive correlations among three gene transcripts that are not correlated in either the normal or disease phenotype (the circumscribed area labeled c' in Figure 4.3). This drug-induced effect may be the consequence of unintended modulation of reactions or pathways in adipose tissue in this disease model. This type of observation may well merit further investigation to determine whether such coordinated drug-induced changes among these particular analytes are detrimental, inconsequential, or perhaps beneficial and protective in terms of the properties of this particular compound. Another set of correlated analytes in tissue that is of interest is the area labeled c'' in Figure 4.3. These three analytes are seen to be correlated only in the disease phenotype, and the correlations are broken upon administration of the drug. These three analytes reflect a common pathophysiologic process in this disease state, and changes observed in their network relationship indicate that the drug compound reverts their coordinated behavior to that of the normal phenotype. Such an observation is a significant one in terms of assessing drug efficacy that

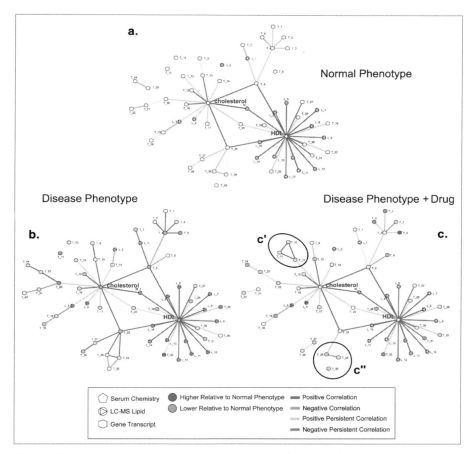

Figure 4.3 Cross-compartment subnetwork constructed from observed changes in a rodent model due to disease and drug administration. The top network (*a*) is the correlation network generated using data from normal phenotype animals. The left network (*b*) is the corresponding network for the disease phenotype group. The right network (*c*) is the corresponding network for a disease phenotype group administered the therapeutic compound. Node positions are fixed to compare identical analytes in the three treatment groups. Apart from imposing inclusion criteria that analytes be either one or two correlation links away from either serum cholesterol or serum HDL, each network was generated in an unsupervised manner. Except for the two serum clinical chemistry nodes, cholesterol and HDL, all nodes represent analytes in adipose tissue. Node colors in networks *b* and *c* reflect concentration levels relative to the baseline normal phenotype state (*a*). "Persistent correlations," (edges colored gold or blue) are unchanged across these three states. Highlighted in network *c* are two areas of interest, namely c″, a group of three analytes among which the disease induces correlations that are in turn reverted by drug administration, and c′, a group of another three analytes among which the drug induces correlations that were not observed in either the normal phenotype or the disease phenotype. All correlations shown are based on Pearson product–moment correlation metrics. Analytes have been de-identified except for serum cholesterol and serum HDL. (See color insert.)

goes significantly beyond evaluating analyte concentration levels on an analyte-by-analyte basis.

4.2.2 Biological Networks and Molecular Biomarkers

A recent but increasingly active area of investigation in biological networks involves their potential use for the discovery of more robust, sensitive, and specific biomarkers. A motivation once again can be traced to the shortcomings associated with the list paradigm, in which measurements that exhibit large changes between or among groups are often prioritized as putative biomarkers. In contrast, systems-based network approaches have been shown to highlight analytes that, while exhibiting perhaps more subtle changes in expression or abundance, are nonetheless more fundamental to a specific biological process compared to downstream effectors that exhibit larger magnitudes (and variability) of change.

These hypotheses have led a number of groups to investigate networks of biomolecules, or "network biomarkers," comprising analytes within, for example, a common canonical biological pathway or metabolic process as better biomarkers of the outcome of interest [107–112]. Such approaches often face the challenge that a majority of genes and proteins in higher species have not yet been assigned to definitive pathways. However, the use, for example, of protein–protein interaction data (e.g., derived from the literature, yeast two-hybrid experiments, transcriptional interaction screens, or mass spectrometry measurements) expands the inclusion criteria for such network biomarkers by effectively expanding the network to include associations that are more empirical in nature (such as protein-protein interaction measurements) than a priori defined biological pathways (e.g., from a database of biochemical pathways). An extension of this approach is the generation of yet more complex biomarkers comprising multiple distinct subnetworks, with each subnetwork in turn comprising discrete functional pathways or complexes. Because network-based biomarkers comprise multiple analytes, a quantitative scoring metric is often devised for validation and implementation in subsequent studies [110]. Ultimately, because network-based biomarkers are composed of multiple analytes that are presumably functionally related, they in effect sample more of the "biological space" within a biological system and hold the promise to be more robust to variability within any single constituent component, in addition to being more specific to the particular pathologic or drug-induced processes of interest.

Related to the concept of network biomarkers described above are unsupervised correlation networks used to identify molecular biomarkers. In contrast to other types of biological networks, the construction of networks such as correlation networks begins with a strictly empirical, mathematical and unsupervised data analysis approach. As such, correlation networks as defined here do not at the outset use a priori determined associations among analytes, such as known regulatory pathways or protein–protein interactions. Because the starting point for correlation network construction is a mathematical computation, for example, yielding a covariance matrix, the network itself is a visualization of underlying empirical relationships within the data. Correlation network construction is discussed in additional detail in Section 4.3.4.

As with network biomarkers described previously, correlation networks can also be used to construct subnetworks as multiparametric biomarkers that are more robust than single analyte biomarkers. An example is shown in Figure 4.4 (network c), which illustrates a correlation subnetwork comprising tissue lipids that were found to be conserved across species in this disease model. Lipids and other endogenous metabolites are attractive in cross-species studies, in part, because of their invariance across species. The networks are arranged in this visualization such that the spatial coordinates of the nodes (which have been de-identified) are aligned between the human and rodent networks.

Note that although the individual analyte concentrations in the disease state relative to nondisease normal phenotypes match quite well across species (i.e., the node colors across networks a and b in Figure 4.4), the empirical correlation structure is significantly different between the rodent disease model and the human disease condition. An approach to identifying a correlation network-based biomarker is to filter for those correlations the respective human and rodent networks that are common to both. The underlying hypothesis in doing so is that empirical correlations among analytes are a result of common metabolic pathways and processes. In choosing the intersection set of the two networks from human and animal, one captures those pathophysiologic biological processes that are common across species. As such, these common subnetworks serve as candidate cross-species network-based biomarkers that inherently capture important biological processes common to both species. These types of complex biomarkers hold the promise of more accurate assessment measures in evaluating drug efficacy or drug safety in translational studies.

4.3 TOP-DOWN APPROACHES: PATHWAY, REACTION, AND INTERACTION MAPPING

Contextualization, or biological contextualization, is the process of mapping experimental results onto known and defined bioinformatics data sources. The goal of this exercise is to gain an understanding of the relationships between experimental measurements that support or refute biological hypotheses. Top-down approaches most often involve overlaying experimental findings, as often embodied in a "list paradigm"—namely collections of analyte identities and respective changes in concentration, structure, location, and the like, onto a priori defined frameworks of biomolecular pathways, reactions, interactions, or other processes. These defined information sources often represent biological knowledge in a graphical construction, where nodes or vertices represent molecular analytes and edges or links represent a known biological

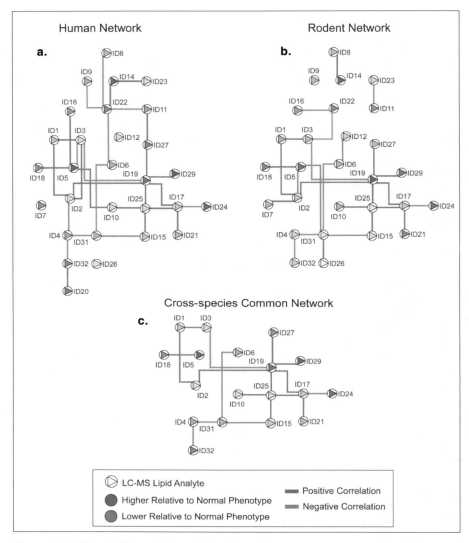

Figure 4.4 Correlation subnetworks constructed from molecular profiling measurements in a rodent model of disease and the human disease condition. Network *a* represents the correlation network in the human disease, and network *b* represents the correlation network in the rodent model. Network *c* is the intersection of networks *a* and *b*; it is a candidate network biomarker of disease common to both species. The spatial coordinates of all nodes are fixed across networks for clarity. Each node is a distinct lipid as measured by liquid chromatography and mass spectrometry (LC-MS). Node colors represent analyte concentration relative to the normal healthy phenotype of each species (normal phenotype networks not shown). Each network was generated in an unsupervised manner solely from the LC-MS lipid molecular profiling data. All network edges represent correlations based on Pearson product–moment correlation metrics. Analytes have been de-identified. (See color insert.)

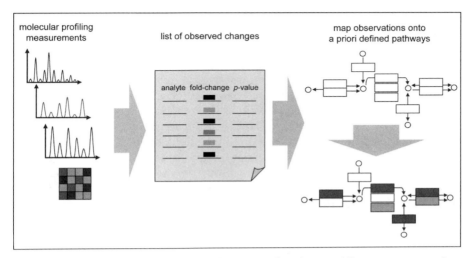

molecular profiling
measurements

list of observed changes

map observations onto
a priori defined pathways

analyte fold-change p-value

Figure 4.5 Schematic view of the top-down paradigm for providing context to molecular measurements. Results of molecular profiling experiments (*left*) are analyzed to generate lists of analytes and associated statistics (*middle*); this is referred to in the text as the list paradigm. Subsequently analytes are placed in the context of a priori defined biochemical relationships (*right*) for further interpretation.

or biochemical relationship between pairs of analytes. After mapping experimental analytes such as sets of gene transcripts, proteins, and metabolites onto such a graph structure, bioinformaticists and domain experts set out to infer the behavior of the system. This is referred to here as a "top-down" (knowledge on top of data) approach (Figure 4.5).

Bioinformatics data sources are derived broadly from three types of curated knowledge bases: pathway databases, ontologies, and literature. Other sources may include drug–protein interactions, disease databases, and sequence databases, which may annotate relationships with other genes or proteins. In practice, particularly in drug discovery and development, a combination of all three sources is used. Implementation often entails a collection of commercial, academic and "home-grown" bioinformatics sources and applications. The bioinformatics data source may be coupled directly to visualization schemes or may be decoupled, requiring distinct mapping and visualization steps. Some applications are able to offer near "one-stop shopping" but may entail a trade-off in terms of either breadth of coverage or insufficient fit to the experiment and data under study.

4.3.1 Pathway, Ontology, and Literature Mapping Approaches

Of the three primary bioinformatics data sources, pathway sources are among the most specialized. They differ depending on the types of relationships of interest to their curators. For example, some specialize in metabolic reactions, signal transduction reactions, gene regulatory events, or protein–protein interactions. A thorough resource of current pathway data sources is maintained by the Pathguide Web site (www.pathguide.org, [113]).

An overview of just some bioinformatics sources is presented here. The *Kyoto Encyclopedia of Genes and Genomes* (KEGG) [114], Ligand and Enzyme databases, are extensive sources for metabolic networks across multiple species. KEGG and EcoCyc [115], an *Escherichia coli* derived metabolic pathway database, were among the first in the field, dating to 1995 for KEGG and 1992 for EcoCyc. Many subsequent metabolic network data sources have leveraged KEGG directly or indirectly. Both *Nature* (The Signaling Gateway, [116]) and *Science* (Signal Transduction Knowledge Environment, STKE, [117]) host Web sites that act as both signal-transduction focused journals as well as signal transduction databases. *Nature*'s Signaling Gateway is part of the Alliance for Cell Signaling [118]. Biobase's Proteome Knowledge Base (PKB, [119]) and TRANSPATH database [120] also capture signal transduction relationships. Biobase's TRANSFAC [121] database focuses on gene regulatory relationships. It captures transcription factors, binding sites, regulated genes and other genetic elements. The Mammalian Promoters Database (MPromDB, [122]) focuses on mammalian promoters, cis-regulatory elements, and chromatin immunoprecipitation (including ChIP-chip) results. The Biomolecular Interactions Network Database (BIND, [123], and its successor the Biomolecular Object Network Databank), the Database of Interacting Proteins (DIP, [124]), IntAct [125], and many other databases focus on protein–protein interactions, with a mix of experimentally derived and computationally predicted interactions. Protein–protein interactions included in such data sources may be derived from reported experimental results of yeast two-hybrid systems, affinity purification and mass spectrometry, phage display, gene co-expression studies, fluorescence resonance energy transfer, among others [126,127].

Specialized applications such as Gene Map Annotator and Pathway Profiler (GenMAPP, [128]) provide environments for mapping experimental measurements onto one or more bioinformatics pathway data sources. VisAnt [129] and MEGU [130] are visualization programs built on top of KEGG's Ligand database. Cytoscape [131] was originally designed to visualize protein–protein interactions but has been subsequently expanded by an ambitious user group. Cell Designer [132] also allows pathway visualization along with more complex systems modeling. A number of commercial packages, such as Ingenuity Pathway Analysis (IPA, [133]) and GeneGo's Meta-Core [134] provide environments to integrate bioinformatics information as well. IPA has coupled visualization with the database source, displaying canonical pathways for analysis and interaction. Reactome [135] is an ambitious pathway and process knowledge base whose underlying data model aggregates metabolic, signal transduction, and gene regulatory content into a single unified model.

The use of ontologies in the life sciences, identified here as structured and controlled vocabularies relating scientific concepts, has been pursued by, among others, Michael Ashburner and colleagues at the Gene Ontology (GO) consortium, initially while members of Flybase, the Mouse Genome Database (MGD), and the Saccharomyces Genome Database (SGD), as a way to categorize and structure sequence-derived biological knowledge [103]. Most ontological mapping today is accomplished by fitting analytes into the three branches of the Gene Ontology [136] hierarchy. Because this ontology was constructed to capture relationships within analytes both at low and high levels of hierarchy, it is not analogous to pathway mapping and can be exploited for complementary purposes. The GO Biological Process hierarchy can provide indications of what cellular processes are affected in an experiment, while the GO Cellular Component hierarchy delineates cellular locations that may be relevant. Mapping to the Molecular Function hierarchy can elucidate what classes of related enzymes may be affected in a particular study. As with other mapping approaches, multiple viewers and mapping programs, such as Gene Ontology's browser AmiGO, GO TermFinder [137], and GO Miner [138], exist to place analytes graphically within the GO hierarchies.

Curated literature sources arise from the application of either manual or automated text mining. A number of commercial products such as Ingenuity Pathway Analysis (IPA) and GeneGo's MetaCore build their biological networks and network visualization primarily on top of such curated literature. Users submit lists of analytes for mapping, which are placed into the context of a background network constructed from curations. Ariadne Genomics' Medscan [139], for example, allows users to create their own networks from their own libraries and literature as well. An extensive description of text-mining approaches in biology is beyond the scope of this work; Ananiadou and Spasic [140,141] provide a review of these approaches in the context of systems biology.

4.3.2 Advantages and Limitations of Available Knowledge

The top-down approach is a de facto standard in the systems pharmacology and systems pathology communities in drug discovery and development. It is relatively easy to implement, especially for Web-based commercial applications, and can map many analyte identifiers from different molecular profiling platforms. Most of these tools were built to support microarray experiments, and as such, they do a comparatively better job of placing gene transcripts into biological context. Mapping protein identifiers is also fairly straightforward, but again, context can be challenging. A relatively few approaches such as KEGG Ligand, IPA and MetaCore are able to map endogenous metabolites. No approach currently enables lipid contextualization specifically, although the Lipid Maps initiative [142] has been established to resolve this shortcoming.

The first, and perhaps obvious, challenge with a top-down approach is determining what data sources and visualization methods are appropriate for a given experiment. Many are highly specialized to either a particular biological process or a small number of biological species. Using an inappropriate approach can both give very few matches to your experimental data and can potentially place results in an unsuitable context. Some of the more comprehensive commercial packages perform well in terms of depth of coverage, but often at the expense of a loss of contextual information that would make a more relevant "fit" to a particular data set. Even among commercial efforts, with teams of researchers curating literature and adding links, there remains a high level of incompleteness. For example, only a small fraction of all genes that are able to be currently measured have been mapped to canonical pathways or processes. This reflects the biological community's inevitable focus on a minority of genes in the genome, which is consequently manifest in biological literature and related sources. One is also often encountered with a problem of consistency in mapping onto predefined information structures. For example, if a set of genes are measured and identified as belonging to a canonical pathway, what is to be interpreted if a subset of those genes are up-regulated while others are down-regulated? Is the pathway or process deemed to be up- or down-regulated? Indeed a challenge remains to capture the complexity, redundancy, and interconnectedness within biomolecular systems in contemporary representations of biological function.

From the computational perspective the plethora of biological data sources has inspired innovative approaches for integration and contextualization. Many larger pharmaceutical, biotechnology, and research organizations have devoted significant resources of staff, software, and hardware to parsing, integrating, maintaining, and updating public and private bioinformatics data sources to develop in-house biological "knowledge bases," often building search and visualization tools on top of these infrastructures. Semantic layers are often constructed for traversing different data sources using both unified data source queries and a visualization modality. There are a number of parallel public efforts at standardizing data source formats, such as BioPAX [143] and the Systems Biology Markup Language (SBML [144]) as well as larger efforts governed by biological ontologies under the Semantic Web Health Care and Life Sciences Interest Group with its prototype application called BioDash [145].

The history of biological data sources is also of key importance in terms of their utility. Historically, biological data sources have been constructed to support the key biological initiatives of the last few decades, and as a consequence often reflect the designs at the time of conception. During the pursuit to sequence the first free-living organism, for example, involving Craig Venter's group at the Institute for Genomic Research (TIGR, sequencing *Haemophilus influenzae*) and Fred Blattner *E. coli* Consortium centered at the University of Wisconsin (sequencing *Escherichia coli* strain K-12), databases were constructed to support these efforts including EcoCyc [146] and what has grown into the Comprehensive Microbial Resource [147], among others. These databases were annotated primarily by sequencing groups, with help from the scientific community. These particular bacterial genomes were from species streamlined for rapid reproduction and, for the most part, comprise genes for coding regions of single-domain proteins. This annotation foundation was carried over onto the annotation of other, more complex, eukaryotic genomes where multidomain proteins are common and a bewildering set of splice variants are possible. This leads to the challenge of "annotation transitivity" where functions for an incorrect protein domain can be assigned on the basis of high-scoring sequence alignments [148,149]. The multidomain annotation transitivity issue is confounded by so-called moonlighting proteins; that is, enzymes with a well-known canonical function that often have other functions as well [150,151]. Enolase is a classic moonlighting protein; canonically it converts 2-phosphoglycerate to phosphoenolpyruvate during glycolysis, but it can also function as a heat shock protein, an eye-lens crystallin, a DNA-binding protein, and a plasminogen receptor [152]. Relatively few bioinformatics data sources capture all of the known relationships regarding such moonlighting proteins.

Context is also a key aspect of biological interpretation that represents a challenge for the broader bioinformatics community. For example, consider an experiment evaluating human protein biomarkers of liver toxicity in plasma. After verifying protein identities, a scientist may begin the contextualization process with a set of identifiers, typically from Uniprot [153] or the International Protein Index (IPI, [154]). Subsequently a set of identifiers may be submitted to a mapping tool. Are the networks returned by the program known to be valid in plasma? Are they valid in humans? Does the mapping account for posttranslational processing of proteins in the network? Is the mapping from the protein sequence identifier to the pathway element an exact match or a more generalized class representation? While this example is deliberately focused on a particularly complex issue, relatively few contextualization methods address comparatively simpler contextual discrepancies such as that between gene transcripts and inferred protein product behavior. The distinction between transcript protein product is as of yet often undeveloped. Reactome and aMAZE [155] are examples of data sources that explicitly model transcripts and proteins as separate entities, and the broader community is maturing toward increasing levels of content refinement.

4.3.3   Bottom-up Approaches: Empirical Relationships and Network Construction

As a complement to the top-down approaches outlined in the previous section, other methodologies have been advanced to further the analysis and understanding of complex molecular profiling datasets. One such unsupervised approach mentioned earlier in this chapter is the correlation network construct, in which empirical relationships between and among analytes are determined and mined. This type of bottom-up unsupervised analysis, followed by subsequent top-down bioinformatics-based interpretation, can be summarized by the maxim "unsupervised discovery, supervised interpretation." Figure 4.6 is a schematic illustrating the general concept.

Networks in which the links between nodes are derived empirically and in an unsupervised manner from a molecular profiling data set are of particular interest as starting points for understanding behavior of a system to disease or drug intervention. The family of network-based approaches in which network nodes represent analytes and links reflect a measure of pairwise association between analytes is quite broad. These associations can be mathematical correlations [96,97,156,157], measures of pairwise entropy and mutual information [98,158,159], and Bayesian constructs [160–162] among others [163–165].

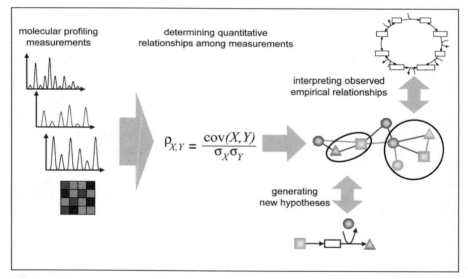

Figure 4.6 Schematic view of the bottom-up paradigm for providing context to molecular measurements. Results of molecular profiling experiments (*left*) are analyzed not only to generate lists of analytes and associated statistics but also for empirical associations and relationships between and among measured analytes (*middle*; the equation, related to Pearson's product–moment correlation coefficient, is only for illustration). In coupling bottom-up and top-down approaches, network structures that result from bottom-up analyses (*right*) can be subsequently compared to a priori defined biochemical frameworks (*right, top*), which may explain observed network structures, or can be exploited as evidence to suggest novel hypotheses (*right, bottom*).

4.3.4 Correlation Network Approaches

In the case of Pearson's product–moment correlations as the association measure, the network graphs are in essence visualizations of covariance matrices of the experimental molecular profiling data sets. Such correlation networks are particularly useful for integrating large and diverse molecular profiling data because, as mathematical constructs derived from the data, they are agnostic to the class of analyte; indeed among the most interesting correlations are those measured across different analyte types. Further, because covariance matrices are independent of absolute concentration measurements for analyte abundances and rely on relative quantitation measures, such network constructs are very useful for molecular profiling data sets in which absolute analyte concentrations are not typically determined. Correlation networks exploit the subtle but intrinsic biological variability across study subjects, and as such are often thought of as orthogonal to the "list paradigm" in which variability within a nominally homogeneous group is detrimental to statistical power and in which analyte concentrations within an a priori defined group are averaged or otherwise combined. Although data integration by correlation analysis requires extremely stringent tolerances on bioanalytical platforms, namely that the measurement variance be consistently less than the individual-to-individual biological variability, the additional information is essential in detecting subtle and early modulations of biochemical pathways and mechanisms [97,105,156,166,167]. The networks shown in Figure 4.3 and Figure 4.4, for example, are correlation networks.

Correlation networks that span biological compartments are particularly useful in selecting and prioritizing biomarker candidates from in vivo models. Because calculation of correlation metrics such as covariance matrices is agnostic to both the type of analyte and its biological compartment, correlation networks spanning multiple compartments such as plasma and tissue have recently been reported [95]. With an unsupervised approach, analyte data from molecular profiling sources are first well-qualified based on instrument and other experimental criteria, and then selected based on statistical metrics. True to its definition, unsupervised data mining typically does not involve any prior filtering or selection of analytes based on existing biological hypotheses.

From the set of all analytes, correlations can be determined both within and across platforms, within and across tissues or compartments, and within treatment groups. These correlations are qualified using conventional statistical confidence values [168,169], often correcting for multiple hypothesis testing consequences inherent to large data sets [170,171]. From this background matrix of correlations, subnetworks may be selected that best match the experimental objectives. These subnetworks may be further refined for particular relationships in the data. For example, analytes may be selected only if they are individually different in concentration between experimental groups of interest, that is, of statistical significance with some biological plausibility, within the experiment.

Correlation edges can also be compared across treatment groups to determine relationships that differ or persist. For example, a correlation edge can be tested to see if a correlation is significantly different between a vehicle-treated normal group, a vehicle-treated diseased group and a drug-treated diseased group. Correlation patterns can be evaluated for relationships that exist in the normal group, are altered by disease, and are restored with drug treatment, or the complementary case. Relationships may exist only in the diseased state, possibly indicative of a systemic response to disease. Relationships may also exist only in drug-treated states, indicative of potential off-target effects. Perhaps not as intuitive, relationships that persist across all treatment groups are of interest as well. Such a scenario may indicate that either the system cannot tolerate perturbations to these relationships and compensates, or that the disease and drug do not affect these relationships. Examples of these types of correlation network behavior are shown in Figures 4.2, 4.3, and 4.4.

4.3.5 Emergent Properties of Biomolecular Networks

Focusing on correlations in analysis has important implications during interpretation. It moves the systems biologist out of the "list paradigm" and into systems frameworks. No longer is the focus on explaining a fold-change or p-value of a particular analyte, but rather on the empirical relationships between and among larger sets of analytes. In drug discovery and development, this enters the realm of systems pharmacology [8]. When considering the behavior of a given analyte, it cannot be realistically divorced from its local and global context. Where is it located? With whom does it interact? What factors determine its transcription and translation? What factors make it active? What recycles it?

It is possible to investigate these associations by examining correlations between and among analytes. For example, one might predict that the expression of proteins participating in a macromolecular complex forms a strongly correlated set. In the absence of sufficient and matching expression of the components of a molecular machine, it would be unlikely to properly assemble. Figure 4.7 illustrates such results from a recent experiment in which the expression of both subunits of the eukaryotic ribosome were observed. In a liver tissue from a group of rodents, 37 distinct ribosomal proteins were measured and identified that gave rise to 478 correlations links among them, the observed Pearson's correlation values ranging from +0.80 to +0.99. The measurements of the proteins in this case involved mass spectrometric proteomic analysis of liver tissue. In the network comprising these proteins, shown on the left in Figure 4.7, node density is particularly striking (Figure 4.7, right); the majority of subunits have between 24 and 34 correlations to other subunits while a small subset has between 1 and 6, strongly supporting

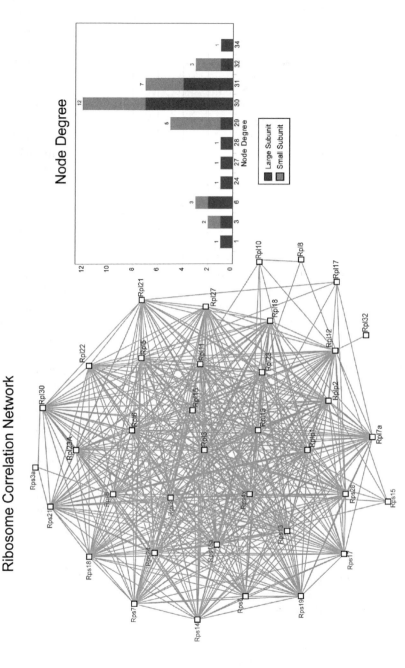

Figure 4.7 Correlations observed among rodent liver ribosomal proteins as measured by mass spectrometry. Small subunit proteins begin with "Rps" while large unit proteins begin with "Rpl". Most subunits have a high node degree (N_k), defined as the number of connections a given node has to its neighbors.

the concept of co-expression for this particular molecular machine in this experiment.

While strong correlations often exist for proteins that are components of a common molecular machine, this finding does not imply that these correlations necessarily exist at the mRNA message level. Likewise relationships within a metabolic pathway need not be correlated. Morgenthal et al. have shown strong correlations between the metabolic neighbors glucose 6-phosphate and fructose 6-phosphate, substrates and products of phosphoglucoisomerase in the Calvin cycle; however, other substrate/product relationships are uncorrelated or even anti-correlated, while longer distance correlations, such as that between sucrose and triose phosphate in the same pathway, are observed [167].

In addition, techniques adopted from network graph theory may also be used to characterize and select subnetworks from larger networks. These include approaches to analyzing the structure and topology of networks in order to discern potentially important subnetworks representing, for example, regulatory motifs or other functional subunits. Correlation networks are directionless graphs and, as such, can be characterized using simple metrics from graph theory. One method is to filter networks using node degree, a simple count of the number of edges. This will select "hubs" in a network, recognized as a key property for regulators in protein–protein interaction networks, signaling networks, and metabolic networks [15,100,172]. Other graph properties, such as analysis of cliques, or maximally connected subgraphs, can be used to find functional units such as the ribosome described above [15,173,174]. An example of graph theoretic properties of correlation networks based upon molecular profiling exercises is shown in Figure 4.8. While there are insufficient data to evaluate the scale-free properties of this network, the general distribution of analyte nodes and correlated edges, particularly at high correlation thresholds, is as expected based on other studies of biological networks; most analytes have relatively few connections to others (low node degree), while considerably fewer analytes exhibit properties of "hubs" that are characterized by a high number of connections to other analytes within the network (high node degree).

4.4   SYNTHESIS OF TOP-DOWN AND BOTTOM-UP APPROACHES

4.4.1   Convergence of Pathway Mapping and Unsupervised Network Construction

Correlation networks are very useful at determining relationships among analytes that may not have been previously recognized. The next step is determining what underlying biochemical processes give rise to the observed relationships. This is where supervised interpretation is implemented. After a network has been qualified based on statistical criteria, experimental objec-

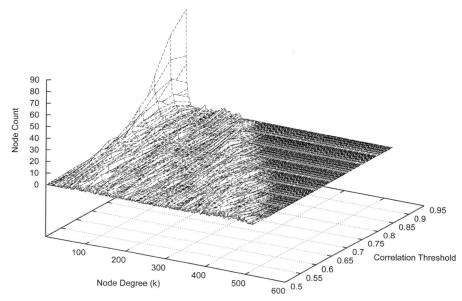

Figure 4.8 Plot of the count of nodes as a function of node degree and correlation threshold in a correlation network derived from a molecular profiling experiment in a rodent model of disease.

tives and graph theory approaches, the next step is to layer knowledge from bioinformatics data sources on top of the network, often as additional edges in the network. Figure 4.2 is an example where literature data from PubMed and OMIM edges are added to a molecular correlation network structure.

Building on top of the common industrial model of a data warehouse for public and private bioinformatics data sources, one can model all relationships among analytes—whether experimental or from existing bioinformatics database sources—as edges, and build a system to query the resulting graph structure for particular relationship types. Such a system uses both direct and indirect semantic typing of nodes to achieve this goal. A typical use case would be to determine all protein–protein interactions from a network of gene transcripts. While there is no direct interaction between transcripts, a goal of this database traversal is to find interactions among their protein products. The rule for such a relationship begins with the set of Affymetrix identifiers from the gene transcript network as an input data set, maps them into Unigene, then Entrez Gene, then into UniProt protein identifiers, and then the system determines interacting partners from the IntAct table within the UniProt record. Figure 4.9 shows such a traversal. Any transcript pair satisfying this rule would then be annotated with an interaction edge. Other bioinformatics data sources and routes through the data warehouse can subsequently be

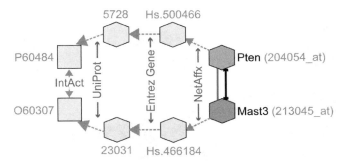

Figure 4.9 Database traversal layered upon empirical correlation. Two gene transcripts, Pten and Mast3, were observed to be positively correlated empirically in an experiment (*solid edge*). The data sources NetAffx, Entrez Gene, and Uniprot were used to map identifiers from Affymetrix, Unigene, Entrez Gene, Uniprot, and the IntAct database. The traversal yields a multiple reported interactions involving IntAct between Pten and Mast3. After the traversal is completed an interaction edge is added (double arrow) to the network.

traversed by the query and added to the graphical network representation. In the example illustrated in Figure 4.9, a mathematical correlation was observed between the gene transcripts Pten and Mast3. Subsequently the NetAffx, Entrez Gene, and Uniprot databases were automatically traversed to submit a query using appropriate identifiers to the IntAct database. The IntAct database returned evidence, based on multiple publications, of physical interaction between and phosphorylation involving Pten and Mast3. Given the IntAct database evidence, as well as the observed experimental correlation between these two analytes, a supplemental, confirmatory interaction edge (dark in Figure 4.9) is added to the network. Indeed many vendors encourage interaction with their data sources either through the use of programming interfaces, such as Ingenuity's IPA-Integration Module, or by providing their data model and schema directly, such as Biobase's Proteome Knowledge Base.

4.4.2 A Case Study in the Synthesis of Approaches

Fenofibrate is among the more commonly prescribed drugs used to treat dyslipidemia and metabolic key risk factors in cardiovascular disease and type 2 diabetes mellitus [175]. It targets and activates peroxisome proliferator activated receptor alpha (PPAR-alpha), which then activates a set of genes involved in lipid transport, lipid catabolism and energy utilization, predominantly in the liver and type I muscle fibers. Common side effects of fenofibrate and other fibrate drugs in this class are muscle pain, weakness, and rhabdomyolysis. We used a synthesis of the bottom-up and top-down approaches to compare shared properties of fenofibrate and a novel PPAR-alpha activating

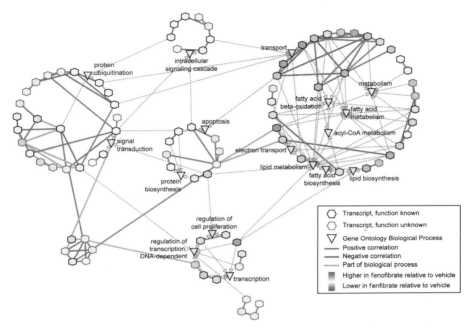

Figure 4.10 Gene Ontology Biological process database traversal on top of a rat skeletal muscle correlation network. Red and green edges denote correlations shared between fenofibrate and a novel PPARα agonist. Dotted lines denote inclusion in a particular biological process node (triangle), and node color indicates direction of transcript abundance change between fenofibrate and a vehicle group. Transcripts that are either unidentified or poorly characterized have a blue border. (See color insert.)

compound in rat skeletal muscle both to see that the treatments generated expected biological behavior and to see if any novel gene expression patterns could be detected with this approach. Under this approach, all common, significant correlation in skeletal muscle were generated and analytes were placed in the context of the Biological Process branch of the Gene Ontology hierarchy (Figure 4.10). By this approach, expected GO enrichment in fatty acid metabolism, fatty-acid beta oxidation, lipid metabolism, and fatty acid biosynthesis were demonstrated (gray triangles). Enrichment in protein biosynthesis, apoptosis, transcription, and signal transduction is also evident. However, there were many poorly characterized or unidentified transcripts that were also brought into this network on the basis of strong correlations to well-characterized genes (blue-bordered hexagons). These unidentified transcripts represent potential novel targets of PPAR-alpha or potential off-target effects. By bringing together the expert-guided interpretive power of the top-down approach with the mathematically guided power of the bottom-up approach, one is able indeed to gain insight at a much broader and extensive level than with either approach alone.

REFERENCES

1. Stoughton RB, Friend SH. How molecular profiling could revolutionize drug discovery. *Nat Rev Drug Discov* 2005;4:345–50.

2. Stoughton RB. Applications of DNA microarrays in biology. *Ann Rev Biochem* 2005;74:53–82.

3. van der Greef J, Davidov E, Verheij E, Vogels J, Van Der Heijden R, Adourian A, et al. The role of metabolomics in systems biology: a new vision for drug discovery and development. In: Harrigan GG and Goodacre R, eds. *Metabolic profiling: its role in biomarker discovery and gene function analysis*. Berlin: Springer, 2003. p. 170–98.

4. Lindon JC, Holmes E, Bollard ME, Stanley EG, Nicholson JK. Metabonomics technologies and their applications in physiological monitoring, drug safety assessment and disease diagnosis. *Biomarkers* 2004;9:1–31.

5. de Hoog CL, Mann M. Proteomics. *Ann Rev Genomics Hum Genet* 2004;5: 267–93.

6. Aebersold R, Mann M. Mass spectrometry-based proteomics. *Nature* 2003;422: 198–207.

7. Woosley RL, Cossman J. Drug development and the FDA's Critical Path Initiative. *Clin Pharmacol Ther* 2007;81:129–33.

8. van der Greef J, Martin S, Juhasz P, Adourian A, Plasterer T, Verheij ER, et al. The art and practice of systems biology in medicine: mapping patterns of relationships. *J Proteome Res* 2007;6:1540–59.

9. van der Greef J, McBurney RN. Innovation: Rescuing drug discovery: in vivo systems pathology and systems pharmacology. *Nat Rev Drug Discov* 2005;4: 961–67.

10. Loscalzo J, Kohane I, Barabasi AL. Human disease classification in the postgenomic era: a complex systems approach to human pathobiology. *Mol Syst Biol* 2007;3:124.

11. Butcher EC, Berg EL, Kunkel EJ. Systems biology in drug discovery. *Nat Biotechnol* 2004;22:1253–59.

12. Hood L, Perlmutter RM. The impact of systems approaches on biological problems in drug discovery. *Nat Biotechnol* 2004;22:1215–17.

13. Walgren JL, Thompson DC. Application of proteomic technologies in the drug development process. *Toxicol Lett* 2004;149:377–85.

14. Kitano H. Systems biology: a brief overview. *Science* 2002;295:1662–4.

15. Barabasi AL, Oltvai ZN. Network biology: understanding the cell's functional organization. *Nat Rev Genet* 2004;5:101–13.

16. Hartwell LH, Hopfield JJ, Leibler S, Murray AW. From molecular to modular cell biology. *Nature* 1999;402:C47–52.

17. Fishman MC, Porter JA. Pharmaceuticals: a new grammar for drug discovery. *Nature* 2005;437:491–93.

18. Hughes TR, Marton MJ, Jones AR, Roberts CJ, Stoughton R, Armour CD, et al. Functional discovery via a compendium of expression profiles. *Cell* 2000;102:109–26.

19. von Bertalanffy L. *General systems theory: foundations, development, application.* New York: Braziller, 1968.

20. Biological Network Modeling Center at the California Institute of Technology; 2007. http://bnmc.caltech.edu

21. Center for Cancer Systems Biology, 2007. http://ccsb.dfci.harvard.edu

22. MIT Computational and Systems Biology, 2007. http://csbi.mit.edu

23. Harvard Medical School Department of Systems Biology, 2007. http://sysbio.med.harvard.edu

24. Simons Center for Systems Biology at the Institute for Advanced Study, 2007. http://www.csb.ias.edu

25. Lewis-Sigler Institute for Integrative Genomics at Princeton University, 2007. http://www.genomics.princeton.edu

26. Netherlands Institute for Systems Biology, 2007. http://www.sysbio.nl

27. Pacific Northwest National Laboratory Biomolecular Sciences Initiative, 2007. http://www.sysbio.org

28. Institute for Systems Biology, 2007. http://www.systemsbiology.org

29. The Systems Biology Institute, 2007. http://www.systems-biology.org

30. Alizadeh AA, Ross DT, Perou CM, van De Rijn M. Towards a novel classification of human malignancies based on gene expression patterns. *J Pathol* 2001;195: 41–52.

31. Lamb J, Crawford ED, Peck D, Modell JW, Blat IC, Wrobel MJ, et al. The Connectivity Map: using gene-expression signatures to connect small molecules, genes, and disease. *Science* 2006;313:1929–35.

32. Lehar J, Zimmermann GR, Krueger AS, Molnar RA, Ledell JT, Heilbut AM, et al. Chemical combination effects predict connectivity in biological systems. *Mol Syst Biol* 2007;3:80.

33. Lindsay MA. Target discovery. *Nat Rev Drug Discov* 2003;2:831–8.

34. van der Greef J, Adourian A, Muntendam P, McBurney RN. Lost in translation? role of metabolomics in solving translational problems in drug discovery and development. *Drug Discov Today Technol* 2006;3:205–11.

35. Swanson KS, Mazur MJ, Vashisht K, Rund LA, Beever JE, Counter CM, et al. Genomics and clinical medicine: rationale for creating and effectively evaluating animal models. *Exp Biol Med (Maywood)* 2004;229:866–75.

36. Hojer-Pedersen J, Smedsgaard J, Nielsen J. Elucidating the mode-of-action of compounds from metabolite profiling studies. *Prog Drug Res* 2007;64:103–29.

37. Gunther EC, Stone DJ, Gerwien RW, Bento P, Heyes MP. Prediction of clinical drug efficacy by classification of drug-induced genomic expression profiles in vitro. *Proc Natl Acad Sci USA* 2003;100:9608–13.

38. Slikker W, Jr, Paule MG, Wright LK, Patterson TA, Wang C. Systems biology approaches for toxicology. *J Appl Toxicol* 2007;27:201–17.

39. Waring JF, Gum R, Morfitt D, Jolly RA, Ciurlionis R, Heindel M, et al. Identifying toxic mechanisms using DNA microarrays: evidence that an experimental inhibitor of cell adhesion molecule expression signals through the aryl hydrocarbon nuclear receptor. *Toxicology* 2002;181–2:537–50.

40. Waring JF, Jolly RA, Ciurlionis R, Lum PY, Praestgaard JT, Morfitt DC, et al. Clustering of hepatotoxins based on mechanism of toxicity using gene expression profiles. *Toxicol Appl Pharmacol* 2001;175:28–42.

41. Guerreiro N, Staedtler F, Grenet O, Kehren J, Chibout SD. Toxicogenomics in drug development. *Toxicol Pathol* 2003;31:471–9.

42. Yengi LG. Systems biology in drug safety and metabolism: integration of microarray, real-time PCR and enzyme approaches. *Pharmacogenomics* 2005;6: 185–92.

43. Nicholson JK. Global systems biology, personalized medicine and molecular epidemiology. *Mol Syst Biol* 2006;2:52.

44. Keith CT, Borisy AA, Stockwell BR. Multicomponent therapeutics for networked systems. *Nat Rev Drug Discov* 2005;4:71–8.

45. Biomarker_Definitions_Working_Group. Biomarkers and surrogate endpoints: preferred definitions and conceptual framework. *Clin Pharmacol Ther* 2001;69: 89–95.

46. Goodsaid F, Frueh FW. Implementing the U.S. FDA guidance on pharmacogenomic data submissions. *Environ Mol Mutagen* 2007;48:354–58.

47. Frueh FW, Rudman A, Simon K, Gutman S, Reed C, Dorner AJ. Experience with voluntary and required genomic data submissions to the FDA: summary report from track 1 of the third FDA-DIA-PWG-PhRMA-BIO pharmacogenomics workshop. *Pharmacogenomics J* 2006;6:296–300.

48. Williams SA, Slavin DE, Wagner JA, Webster CJ. A cost-effectiveness approach to the qualification and acceptance of biomarkers. *Nat Rev Drug Discov* 2006;5:897–902.

49. Phillips KA, Van Bebber S, Issa AM. Diagnostics and biomarker development: priming the pipeline. *Nat Rev Drug Discov* 2006;5:463–69.

50. Roses AD, Saunders AM, Huang Y, Strum J, Weisgraber KH, Mahley RW. Complex disease-associated pharmacogenetics: drug efficacy, drug safety, and confirmation of a pathogenetic hypothesis (Alzheimer's disease). *Pharmacogenomics J* 2007;7:10–28.

51. Hanke JH, Webster KR, Ronco LV. Protein biomarkers and drug design for cancer treatments. *Eur J Cancer Prev* 2004;13:297–305.

52. Papadopoulos N, Kinzler KW, Vogelstein B. The role of companion diagnostics in the development and use of mutation-targeted cancer therapies. *Nat Biotechnol* 2006;24:985–95.

53. Colburn WA. Biomarkers in drug discovery and development: from target identification through drug marketing. *J Clin Pharmacol* 2003;43:329–41.

54. Lacana E, Amur S, Mummanneni P, Zhao H, Frueh FW. The emerging role of pharmacogenomics in biologics. *Clin Pharmacol Ther* 2007;82:466–71.

55. Farcomeni A. A review of modern multiple hypothesis testing, with particular attention to the false discovery proportion. *Stat Meth Med Res* 2008;17:347–88.

56. Yauk CL, Williams A, Boucher S, Berndt LM, Zhou G, Zheng JL, et al. Novel design and controls for focused DNA microarrays: applications in quality assurance/control and normalization for the Health Canada ToxArray. *BMC Genom* 2006;7:266.

57. Bucknall M, Fung KY, Duncan MW. Practical quantitative biomedical applications of MALDI-TOF mass spectrometry. *J Am Soc Mass Spectrom* 2002;13: 1015–27.

58. Ross PL, Huang YN, Marchese JN, Williamson B, Parker K, Hattan S, et al. Multiplexed protein quantitation in Saccharomyces cerevisiae using amine-reactive isobaric tagging reagents. *Mol Cell Proteomics* 2004;3:1154–69.

59. Hsu JC, Chang J, Wang T, Steingrimsson E, Magnusson MK, Bergsteinsdottir K. Statistically designing microarrays and microarray experiments to enhance sensitivity and specificity. *Brief Bioinform* 2007;8:22–31.

60. Lindon JC, Nicholson JK, Holmes E, Keun HC, Craig A, Pearce JT, et al. Summary recommendations for standardization and reporting of metabolic analyses. *Nat Biotechnol* 2005;23:833–8.

61. Orchard S, Salwinski L, Kerrien S, Montecchi-Palazzi L, Oesterheld M, Stumpflen V, et al. The minimum information required for reporting a molecular interaction experiment (MIMIx). *Nat Biotechnol* 2007;25:894–8.

62. Taylor CF, Paton NW, Lilley KS, Binz PA, Julian RK, Jr, Jones AR, et al. The minimum information about a proteomics experiment (MIAPE). *Nat Biotechnol* 2007;25:887–93.

63. Whetzel PL, Parkinson H, Causton HC, Fan L, Fostel J, Fragoso G, et al. The MGED Ontology: a resource for semantics-based description of microarray experiments. *Bioinformatics* 2006;22:866–73.

64. Brazma A, Hingamp P, Quackenbush J, Sherlock G, Spellman P, Stoeckert C, et al. Minimum information about a microarray experiment (MIAME)—toward standards for microarray data. *Nat Genet* 2001;29:365–71.

65. Ideker T, Thorsson V, Ranish JA, Christmas R, Buhler J, Eng JK, et al. Integrated genomic and proteomic analyses of a systematically perturbed metabolic network. *Science* 2001;292:929–34.

66. Herrgard MJ, Fong SS, Palsson BO. Identification of genome-scale metabolic network models using experimentally measured flux profiles. *PLoS Comput Biol* 2006;2:e72.

67. Herzog ED. Neurons and networks in daily rhythms. *Nat Rev Neurosci* 2007;8:790–802.

68. Stathopoulos A, Levine M. Genomic regulatory networks and animal development. *Dev Cell* 2005;9:449–62.

69. Pe'er D, Regev A, Tanay A. Minreg: inferring an active regulator set. *Bioinformatics* 2002;18(suppl 1):S258–67.

70. Hartemink AJ, Gifford DK, Jaakkola TS, Young RA. Using graphical models and genomic expression data to statistically validate models of genetic regulatory networks. *Pac Symp Biocomput* 2001:422–33.

71. Tavazoie S, Hughes JD, Campbell MJ, Cho RJ, Church GM. Systematic determination of genetic network architecture. *Nat Genet* 1999;22:281–85.

72. Stumpf MP, Kelly WP, Thorne T, Wiuf C. Evolution at the system level: the natural history of protein interaction networks. *Trends Ecol Evol* 2007;22: 366–73.

73. Rual JF, Venkatesan K, Hao T, Hirozane-Kishikawa T, Dricot A, Li N, et al. Towards a proteome-scale map of the human protein-protein interaction network. *Nature* 2005;437:1173–78.

74. Tucker CL, Gera JF, Uetz P. Towards an understanding of complex protein networks. *Trends Cell Biol* 2001;11:102–6.

75. Araujo RP, Liotta LA, Petricoin EF. Proteins, drug targets and the mechanisms they control: the simple truth about complex networks. *Nat Rev Drug Discov* 2007;6:871–80.

76. Strong M, Eisenberg D. The protein network as a tool for finding novel drug targets. In: Boshoff HI, Barry CE, eds. Systems Biological Approaches in Infectious Diseases. Basel: Birkhäuser Verlag; 2007. p. 191-215. *Prog Drug Res* 64:191,93–215.

77. Yildirim MA, Goh KI, Cusick ME, Barabasi AL, Vidal M. Drug-target network. *Nat Biotechnol* 2007;25:1119–26.

78. Ma'ayan A, Jenkins SL, Goldfarb J, Iyengar R. Network analysis of FDA approved drugs and their targets. *Mt Sinai J Med* 2007;74:27–32.

79. Nacher JC, Ueda N, Yamada T, Kanehisa M, Akutsu T. Clustering under the line graph transformation: application to reaction network. *BMC Bioinform* 2004; 5:207.

80. Kitano H. Computational systems biology. *Nature* 2002;420:206–10.

81. Chen T, He HL, Church GM. Modeling gene expression with differential equations. *Pac Symp Biocomput* 1999;29–40.

82. Szallasi Z, Stelling J, Periwal V. *System modeling in cellular biology*. Cambridge: MIT Press, 2006.

83. Giot L, Bader JS, Brouwer C, Chaudhuri A, Kuang B, Li Y, et al. A protein interaction map of Drosophila melanogaster. *Science* 2003;302:1727–36.

84. Li S, Armstrong CM, Bertin N, Ge H, Milstein S, Boxem M, et al. A map of the interactome network of the metazoan C. elegans. *Science* 2004;303: 540–43.

85. Tekirian TL, Thomas SN, Yang A. Advancing signaling networks through proteomics. *Expert Rev Proteomics* 2007;4:573–83.

86. Stagljar I. Finding partners: emerging protein interaction technologies applied to signaling networks. *Sci STKE* 2003:pe56.

87. Segal E, Shapira M, Regev A, Pe'er D, Botstein D, Koller D, et al. Module networks: identifying regulatory modules and their condition-specific regulators from gene expression data. *Nat Genet* 2003;34:166–76.

88. Tong AH, Lesage G, Bader GD, Ding H, Xu H, Xin X, et al. Global mapping of the yeast genetic interaction network. *Science* 2004;303:808–13.

89. Paolini GV, Shapland RH, van Hoorn WP, Mason JS, Hopkins AL. Global mapping of pharmacological space. *Nat Biotechnol* 2006;24:805–15.

90. Wishart DS, Knox C, Guo AC, Cheng D, Shrivastava S, Tzur D, et al. DrugBank: a knowledgebase for drugs, drug actions and drug targets. *Nucleic Acids Res* 2007;35:D521–26.

91. Cohen AM, Hersh WR. A survey of current work in biomedical text mining. *Brief Bioinform* 2005;6:57–71.

92. Jenssen TK, Laegreid A, Komorowski J, Hovig E. A literature network of human genes for high-throughput analysis of gene expression. *Nat Genet* 2001;28: 21–28.

93. Tao Y, Sam L, Li J, Friedman C, Lussier YA. Information theory applied to the sparse gene ontology annotation network to predict novel gene function. *Bioinformatics* 2007;23:i529–38.

94. Wang JZ, Du Z, Payattakool R, Yu PS, Chen CF. A new method to measure the semantic similarity of GO terms. *Bioinformatics* 2007;23:1274–81.

95. Adourian A, Jennings E, Balasubramanian R, Hines W, Damian D, Plasterer T, et al. Correlation network analysis for data integration and biomarker selection. *Mol Biosys* 2008;4:249–59.

96. Weckwerth W, Loureiro ME, Wenzel K, Fiehn O. Differential metabolic networks unravel the effects of silent plant phenotypes. *Proc Natl Acad Sci USA* 2004;101:7809–14.

97. Oresic M, Clish CB, Davidov EJ, Verheij E, Vogels J, Havekes LM, et al. Phenotype characterisation using integrated gene transcript, protein and metabolite profiling. *Appl Bioinforms* 2004;3:205–17.

98. Butte AJ, Kohane IS. Mutual information relevance networks: functional genomic clustering using pairwise entropy measurements. *Pac Symp Biocomput* 2000:418–29.

99. Vo TD, Greenberg HJ, Palsson BO. Reconstruction and functional characterization of the human mitochondrial metabolic network based on proteomic and biochemical data. *J Biol Chem* 2004;279:39532–40.

100. Jeong H, Tombor B, Albert R, Oltvai ZN, Barabasi AL. The large-scale organization of metabolic networks. *Nature* 2000;407:651–4.

101. Nikiforova VJ, Willmitzer L. Network visualization and network analysis. *Exs* 2007;97:245–75.

102. Bornholdt S, Schuster HG. *Handbook of graphs and networks: from the genome to the Internet*. New York: Wiley, 2003.

103. Ashburner M, Ball CA, Blake JA, Botstein D, Butler H, Cherry JM, et al. Gene ontology: tool for the unification of biology. Gene Ontology Consortium. *Nat Genet* 2000;25:25–9.

104. *OMIM Online Mendelian inheritance in man*. McKusick-Nathans Institute of Genetic Medicine, Johns Hopkins University and National Center for Biotechnology Information, National Library of Medicine, 2007.

105. Clish CB, Davidov E, Oresic M, Plasterer TN, Lavine G, Londo T, et al. Integrative biological analysis of the APOE*3-leiden transgenic mouse. *Omics* 2004;8:3–13.

106. Dudoit S, van der Laan MJ. *Multiple testing procedures with applications to genomics*. Berlin: Springer, 2007.

107. Rapaport F, Zinovyev A, Dutreix M, Barillot E, Vert JP. Classification of microarray data using gene networks. *BMC Bioinform* 2007;8:35.

108. Tian L, Greenberg SA, Kong SW, Altschuler J, Kohane IS, Park PJ. Discovering statistically significant pathways in expression profiling studies. *Proc Natl Acad Sci USA* 2005;102:13544–9.

109. Doniger SW, Salomonis N, Dahlquist KD, Vranizan K, Lawlor SC, Conklin BR. MAPPFinder: using Gene Ontology and GenMAPP to create a global gene-expression profile from microarray data. *Genome Biol* 2003;4:R7.

110. Chuang HY, Lee E, Liu YT, Lee D, Ideker T. Network-based classification of breast cancer metastasis. *Mol Syst Biol* 2007;3:140.

111. Subramanian A, Tamayo P, Mootha VK, Mukherjee S, Ebert BL, Gillette MA, et al. Gene set enrichment analysis: a knowledge-based approach for interpreting genome-wide expression profiles. *Proc Natl Acad Sci USA* 2005;102:15545–50.

112. Paik S, Shak S, Tang G, Kim C, Baker J, Cronin M, et al. A multigene assay to predict recurrence of tamoxifen-treated, node-negative breast cancer. *N Engl J Med* 2004;351:2817–26.

113. Bader GD, Cary MP, Sander C. Pathguide: a pathway resource list. *Nucleic Acids Res* 2006;34:D504–6.

114. Kanehisa M, Goto S, Kawashima S, Okuno Y, Hattori M. The KEGG resource for deciphering the genome. *Nucleic Acids Res* 2004;32:D277–80.

115. Karp PD, Keseler IM, Shearer A, Latendresse M, Krummenacker M, Paley SM, et al. Multidimensional annotation of the Escherichia coli K-12 genome. *Nucleic Acids Res* 2007;35:7577–90.

116. Saunders B, Lyon S, Day M, Riley B, Chenette E, Subramaniam S. The Molecule Pages database. *Nucleic Acids Res* 2007;36:D700–06.

117. Gough NR. Science's signal transduction knowledge environment: the connections maps database. *Ann NY Acad Sci* 2002;971:585–7.

118. Gilman AG, Simon MI, Bourne HR, Harris BA, Long R, Ross EM, et al. Overview of the Alliance for Cellular Signaling. *Nature* 2002;420:703–6.

119. Hodges PE, Carrico PM, Hogan JD, O'Neill KE, Owen JJ, Mangan M, et al. Annotating the human proteome: the Human Proteome Survey Database (HumanPSD) and an in-depth target database for G protein-coupled receptors (GPCR-PD) from Incyte Genomics. *Nucleic Acids Res* 2002;30:137–41.

120. Krull M, Pistor S, Voss N, Kel A, Reuter I, Kronenberg D, et al. TRANSPATH: an information resource for storing and visualizing signaling pathways and their pathological aberrations. *Nucleic Acids Res* 2006;34:D546–51.

121. Matys V, Kel-Margoulis OV, Fricke E, Liebich I, Land S, Barre-Dirrie A, et al. TRANSFAC and its module TRANSCompel: transcriptional gene regulation in eukaryotes. *Nucleic Acids Res* 2006;34:D108–10.

122. Sun H, Palaniswamy SK, Pohar TT, Jin VX, Huang TH, Davuluri RV. MPromDb: an integrated resource for annotation and visualization of mammalian gene promoters and ChIP-chip experimental data. *Nucleic Acids Res* 2006;34:D98–103.

123. Bader GD, Betel D, Hogue CW. BIND: the Biomolecular Interaction Network Database. *Nucleic Acids Res* 2003;31:248–50.

124. Salwinski L, Miller CS, Smith AJ, Pettit FK, Bowie JU, Eisenberg D. The Database of Interacting Proteins: 2004 update. *Nucleic Acids Res* 2004;32:D449–51.

125. Hermjakob H, Montecchi-Palazzi L, Lewington C, Mudali S, Kerrien S, Orchard S, et al. IntAct: an open source molecular interaction database. *Nucleic Acids Res* 2004;32:D452–5.

126. Shoemaker BA, Panchenko AR. Deciphering protein-protein interactions. Part I. Experimental techniques and databases. *PLoS Comput Biol* 2007;3:e42.

127. Saghatelian A, Cravatt BF. Assignment of protein function in the postgenomic era. *Nat Chem Biol* 2005;1:130–42.

128. Salomonis N, Hanspers K, Zambon AC, Vranizan K, Lawlor SC, Dahlquist KD, et al. GenMAPP 2: new features and resources for pathway analysis. *BMC Bioinform* 2007;8:217.

129. Hu Z, Ng DM, Yamada T, Chen C, Kawashima S, Mellor J, et al. VisANT 3.0: new modules for pathway visualization, editing, prediction and construction. *Nucleic Acids Res* 2007;35:W625–32.

130. Kono N, Arakawa K, Tomita M. MEGU: pathway mapping web-service based on KEGG and SVG. *In silico Biol* 2006;6:621–5.

131. Shannon P, Markiel A, Ozier O, Baliga NS, Wang JT, Ramage D, et al. Cytoscape: a software environment for integrated models of biomolecular interaction networks. *Genome Res* 2003;13:2498–504.

132. Funahashi A, Morohashi M, Kitano H. CellDesigner: a process diagram editor for gene-regulatory and biochemical networks. *Biosilico* 2003;1:159–62.

133. Ingenuity Pathways Analysis; 2007. http://www.ingenuity.com

134. Ekins S, Nikolsky Y, Bugrim A, Kirillov E, Nikolskaya T. Pathway mapping tools for analysis of high content data. *Meth Mol Biol* 2007;356:319–50.

135. Vastrik I, D'Eustachio P, Schmidt E, Joshi-Tope G, Gopinath G, Croft D, et al. Reactome: a knowledge base of biologic pathways and processes. *Genome Biol* 2007;8:R39.

136. Harris MA, Clark J, Ireland A, Lomax J, Ashburner M, Foulger R, et al. The Gene Ontology (GO) database and informatics resource. *Nucleic Acids Res* 2004;32:D258–61.

137. Boyle EI, Weng S, Gollub J, Jin H, Botstein D, Cherry JM, et al. GO: TermFinder—open source software for accessing Gene Ontology information and finding significantly enriched Gene Ontology terms associated with a list of genes. *Bioinformatics* 2004;20:3710–15.

138. Zeeberg BR, Feng W, Wang G, Wang MD, Fojo AT, Sunshine M, et al. GoMiner: a resource for biological interpretation of genomic and proteomic data. *Genome Biol* 2003;4:R28.

139. Novichkova S, Egorov S, Daraselia N. MedScan, a natural language processing engine for MEDLINE abstracts. *Bioinformatics* 2003;19:1699–1706.

140. Ananiadou S, Kell DB, Tsujii J. Text mining and its potential applications in systems biology. *Trends Biotechnol* 2006;24:571–9.

141. Spasic I, Ananiadou S, McNaught J, Kumar A. Text mining and ontologies in biomedicine: making sense of raw text. *Brief Bioinform* 2005;6:239–51.

142. Fahy E, Cotter D, Byrnes R, Sud M, Maer A, Li J, et al. Bioinformatics for lipidomics. *Meth Enzymol* 2007;432:247–73.

143. Luciano JS, Stevens RD. e-Science and biological pathway semantics. *BMC Bioinform* 2007;8(suppl3):S3.

144. Bornstein S, Doyle J, Finney B, Hucka M, Keating B, Kitano H, et al. Evolving a lingua franca and associated software infrastructure for computational systems biology: the Systems Biology Markup Language (SBML) project. *Syst Biol* 2004;1:41–53.

145. Quan D. Improving life sciences information retrieval using semantic Web technology. *Brief Bioinform* 2007;8:172–82.

146. Karp PD, Riley M, Paley SM, Pelligrini-Toole A. EcoCyc: an encyclopedia of *Escherichia coli* genes and metabolism. *Nucleic Acids Res* 1996;24:32–9.

147. Peterson JD, Umayam LA, Dickinson T, Hickey EK, White O. The Comprehensive Microbial Resource. *Nucleic Acids Res* 2001;29:123–5.

148. Smith TF, Zhang X. The challenges of genome sequence annotation or "the devil is in the details." *Nat Biotechnol* 1997;15:1222–23.

149. Zhang X, Smith TF. Yeast "operons." *Microb Comp Genomics* 1998;3:133–40.

150. Jeffery CJ. Moonlighting proteins. *Trends Biochem Sci* 1999;24:8–11.

151. Jeffery CJ. Molecular mechanisms for multitasking: recent crystal structures of moonlighting proteins. *Curr Opin Struct Biol* 2004;14:663–8.

152. Sriram G, Martinez JA, McCabe ER, Liao JC, Dipple KM. Single-gene disorders: what role could moonlighting enzymes play? *Am J Hum Genet* 2005;76:911–24.

153. Consortium U. The Universal Protein Resource (UniProt). *Nucleic Acids Res* 2007;35:D193–97.

154. Kersey PJ, Duarte J, Williams A, Karavidopoulou Y, Birney E, Apweiler R. The International Protein Index: an integrated database for proteomics experiments. *Proteomics* 2004;4:1985–88.

155. van Helden J, Naim A, Mancuso R, Eldridge M, Wernisch L, Gilbert D, et al. Representing and analysing molecular and cellular function using the computer. *Biol Chem* 2000;381:921–35.

156. Steuer R, Kurths J, Fiehn O, Weckwerth W. Observing and interpreting correlations in metabolomic networks. *Bioinformatics* 2003;19:1019–26.

157. Cohen J, Cohen P, West SG, Aiken LS. *Applied multiple regression/correlation analysis for the behavioral sciences*. Mahwah, N.J.: Lawrence Erlbaum, 2002.

158. Butte AJ, Tamayo P, Slonim D, Golub TR, Kohane IS. Discovering functional relationships between RNA expression and chemotherapeutic susceptibility using relevance networks. *Proc Natl Acad Sci USA* 2000;97:12182–6.

159. Steuer R, Kurths J, Daub CO, Weise J, Selbig J. The mutual information: detecting and evaluating dependencies between variables. *Bioinformatics* 2002;18 (suppl2):S231–40.

160. Schafer J, Strimmer K. An empirical Bayes approach to inferring large-scale gene association networks. *Bioinformatics* 2005;21:754–64.

161. Friedman N, Linial M, Nachman I, Pe'er D. Using Bayesian networks to analyze expression data. *J Comput Biol* 2000;7:601–20.

162. Yu J, Smith VA, Wang PP, Hartemink AJ, Jarvis ED. Advances to Bayesian network inference for generating causal networks from observational biological data. *Bioinformatics* 2004;20:3594–603.

163. Ucar D, Neuhaus I, Ross-MacDonald P, Tilford C, Parthasarathy S, Siemers N, et al. Construction of a reference gene association network from multiple profiling data: application to data analysis. *Bioinformatics* 2007;23:2716–24.

164. Janes KA, Lauffenburger DA. A biological approach to computational models of proteomic networks. *Curr Opin Chem Biol* 2006;10:73–80.

165. Xia Y, Yu H, Jansen R, Seringhaus M, Baxter S, Greenbaum D, et al. Analyzing cellular biochemistry in terms of molecular networks. *Ann Rev Biochem* 2004;73:1051–87.

166. Davidov E, Clish CB, Oresic M, Meys M, Stochaj W, Snell P, et al. Methods for the differential integrative omic analysis of plasma from a transgenic disease animal model. *Omics* 2004;8:267–88.

167. Morgenthal K, Weckwerth W, Steuer R. Metabolomic networks in plants: transitions from pattern recognition to biological interpretation. *Biosystems* 2006;83: 108–17.

168. Best DJ, Roberts DE. Algorithm AS 89: The upper tail probabilities of Spearman's rho. *Appl Stat* 1975;24:377–9.

169. Hollander M, Wolfe DA. *Nonparametric statistical inference*. New York: Wiley, 1973.

170. Storey JD. A direct approach to false discovery rates. *J Roy Stat Soc* 2002;64: 479–98.

171. Benjamini Y, Hochberg Y. Controlling the false discovery rate: a practical and powerful approach to multiple testing. *J Roy Stat Soc B* 1995;57:289–300.

172. Dobrin R, Beg QK, Barabasi AL, Oltvai ZN. Aggregation of topological motifs in the Escherichia coli transcriptional regulatory network. *BMC Bioinform* 2004;5:10.

173. Strogatz SH. Exploring complex networks. *Nature* 2001;410:268–76.

174. Milo R, Shen-Orr S, Itzkovitz S, Kashtan N, Chklovskii D, Alon U. Network motifs: simple building blocks of complex networks. *Science* 2002;298:824–7.

175. Keating GM, Croom KF. Fenofibrate: a review of its use in primary dyslipidaemia, the metabolic syndrome and type 2 diabetes mellitus. *Drugs* 2007;67: 121–53.

5

ZEBRAFISH MODELS FOR HUMAN DISEASES AND DRUG DISCOVERY

HANBING ZHONG, NING-AI LIU, AND SHUO LIN

Contents

Drug Efficacy, Safety, and Biologics Discovery: Emerging Technologies and Tools,
Edited by Sean Ekins and Jinghai J. Xu
Copyright © 2009 by John Wiley & Sons, Inc.

5.1 INTRODUCTION

The zebrafish is a small freshwater fish. It was given this name because there are five horizontal pigmented stripes on each side of its body. Native zebrafish live in the warm regions south of the Himalayas, including India, Pakistan, Bangladesh, Nepal, and Myanmar. Before it was recognized as a genetic model organism, the zebrafish was a popular pet fish for beginner aquariums.

The zebrafish was first taxonomically named *Cyprinus rerio* by Hamilton–Buchanan in 1822 in a book describing fish in the Ganges river area [1]. In 1981 Shrestha proposed that the taxonomic name of zebrafish should be *Danio rerio* [2]. Although there have been additional taxonomic names used, *Danio rerio* is now officially accepted.

5.1.1 Basic Biology

The adult zebrafish is approximately 4 cm long. The abdomens of females are normally bigger than those of males. The mating behavior is controlled by the light cycle. Under a 14-hour light and 10-hour dark cycle, one female zebrafish can often lay several hundred embryos per clutch. The fertilized zygotes develop quickly, and all organ rudiments of this vertebrate species become visible within 24 hours of development. By 5 days postfertilization, zebrafish embryos hatch out of the chorion and become free swimmers. Up to this point, the body is still transparent, allowing easy visualization of organs and tissues that are already fully functional. Under standard laboratory conditions, it takes approximately three months for a zebrafish to become sexually mature [3]. Zebrafish are genetically diploid, containing 25 pairs of chromosomes [4]. The haploid zebrafish genome contains about 1.7×10^9 bases of DNA [5], which is approximately half the size of the human and mouse genomes.

5.1.2 Establishment as a Model Animal

Because of its small size, fast external development, transparency of embryos, short generation times, and amenability to genetic analysis, zebrafish has become an ideal vertebrate animal model. Initially zebrafish were considered a useful animal model for monitoring water pollutants, for instance, mutagens, teratogens, and toxicants [6]. In 1981 George Streisinger first introduced zebrafish into the developmental genetics field through his pioneering work published in *Nature* [7]. His work demonstrated that zebrafish had the potential to combine the technologies of genetics, embryology, and molecular biology in a single organism. Since then the scientific community began to recognize that the zebrafish is a promising vertebrate animal model that bridges the gap between invertebrate models and mammals. To date, hundreds of research laboratories worldwide have adopted zebrafish as their animal model of choice.

In 1996 *Development*, the premier journal of developmental biology, devoted an entire issue (Vol. 123) to the zebrafish, publishing 37 papers that described zebrafish mutations affecting nearly every aspect of its development [8–10]. The work was accomplished by the laboratories led by Nusslein–Volhard of the Max Planck Institute in Tubingen, Germany, and by Driever and Fishman of Massachusetts General Hospital/Harvard Medical School in Boston. This was the first large-scale systemic genetic screening performed in a vertebrate species.

In 2001, the Sanger Institute, in collaboration with the zebrafish community, launched the Zebrafish Genome Project. The latest release on the Ensembl Web site is the zebrafish assembly version 7 (Zv7), based on integrating physical maps and whole genome shotgun sequences. In this version there are 17,330 known protein-coding genes, 2467 novel protein-coding genes, and 4162 RNA genes (http://www.ensembl.org/Danio_rerio/index.html). Most of these genes have conserved human homologs. The progress of the Zebrafish Genome Project has remarkably promoted and facilitated the research of zebrafish.

In addition to developmental biology studies, zebrafish have now been widely used in genetics analysis, behavioral studies, human disease modeling, and drug discovery. This chapter focuses on the use of zebrafish in studies of human diseases and drug discovery.

5.2 ZEBRAFISH TECHNOLOGIES

As the zebrafish became an established animal model, a good number of techniques have been developed for the zebrafish system. Several of the frequently used techniques are discussed here.

5.2.1 Mutagenesis

The zebrafish is a suitable vertebrate model to perform genetic screens. Several strategies of forward genetic screening have been established [11–13]. Here we focus on chemical mutagenesis with ENU (*N*-ethyl-*N*-nitrosourea) and insertional mutagenesis with a retrovirus.

N-ethyl-*N*-nitrosourea (ENU) is a potent alkylating mutagen that transfers its ethyl group to bases of DNA. ENU efficiently produces random point mutations in zebrafish germline cells [14–16]. The estimated frequency of independent mutations per locus per gamete is approximately 1.0×10^{-3} [16]. Two large-scale genetic screens using ENU yielded over 1700 mutants [9,10], which affected various developmental processes. Recently a number of individual laboratories have performed additional ENU genetics screens, in which investigators looked for specific phenotypes using in situ hybridization, behavioral analysis, or tissue-specific transgenic lines [12,17].

The ENU-mutated gene can be identified by positional cloning [18,19]. The first positional cloning of a zebrafish mutant was done by Zhang et al. in 1998 [20]. A novel gene, *oep* (one-eyed pinhead), related to epidermal growth factor (EGF) was isolated. In 2007 a group of international scientists finished a rough mapping of 319 zebrafish mutants using positional cloning [21].

TILLING (Targeting Induced Local Lesions IN Genomes) was developed to induce mutations in specific zebrafish gene loci by ENU treatment followed by identification of mutations by sequencing. The first TILLING cloning of a zebrafish mutant was done by Wienholds et al. in 2002 [22]. The TILLING method for zebrafish has been further developed by Wienholds et al. [23] and Draper et al. [24]. More recently lesions in specific zebrafish genes were induced by zinc finger nucleases (ZFNs) designed to cut DNA at specific DNA sequences (Scot Wolfe, personal communication). This is an exciting technology for zebrafish research as zinc finger proteins can be designed to specifically target virtually any gene sequence of choice.

Although ENU-mediated chemical mutagenesis is effective, both positional cloning and TILLING are time-consuming and laborious, which is the major disadvantage of chemical mutagenesis. Insertional mutagenesis is an alternative approach, in which foreign DNA is inserted into chromosomes as a mutagen and also serves as a tag to clone the mutated genes quickly. The pseudotyped retrovirus has been effectively used as an insertional mutagen, which is a modified Moloney Murine Leukemia Virus (MoMLV) genome packaged in an envelope containing glycoprotein of vesicular somatitis virus (VSV) [25]. Injection of MoMLV(VSV) into blastula stage zebrafish embryos creates mosaic founders, in which individual cells have integrated the retrovirus at multiple sites on chromosomes. When integrated into germline cells, provirus is transmitted to offspring in a Mendelian fashion. By inbreeding, mutations will be recovered in F2 progeny. Genomic DNA fragments adjacent to the retrovirus insertion site can be isolated by molecular biological means, for instance, linker-mediated PCR or inverse PCR. Using the sequence of adjacent genomic DNA to do an alignment search in databases, the insertion loci can be found rapidly [26]. Large-scale forward genetic screens with this strategy have been conducted successfully [27–29]. In the insertional screen performed by Amsterdam et al., 525 mutants were found. Among them, 315 mutated genes were identified [28]. Recently insertional mutagenesis with retroviruses has been further improved in a way that all genes in the zebrafish genome can be efficiently tagged and mutations can be stored in retrievable databases and resources. These resources will be extremely useful for studying disease genes, since many of them only show phenotypes in adults.

5.2.2 RNA Whole Mount In situ Hybridization

RNA in situ hybridization (ISH) is a technique that detects gene expression by combining molecular biological methods and histological methods. Labeled nucleotide probes are used to hybridize with the complementary target RNA sequences at their original sites within whole mount tissue or tissue section samples to reveal the expression level of gene transcripts. Since its invention in the 1960s [30], ISH has been developed into many variations and become a widely used tool in biomedical research [31]. The employment of digoxigenin-labeled antisense RNA probes, antibody-alkaline phosphatase conjugate, and BCIP/NBT staining makes ISH even easier and faster.

Because of the small size of the zebrafish embryo, ISH can be carried out in whole mount zebrafish embryo precluding the need for sectioning [32]. The whole mount in situ hybridization is a powerful tool to reveal temporal-spatial gene expression patterns in zebrafish embryos, providing extremely valuable information about functional and regulatory mechanisms of genes. Additionally tissue-specific genes can be used as molecular markers for studying biological processes before any tissues or organs become visually recognizable [33].

5.2.3 Gene Knockdown by Antisense Morpholino Oligos

Morpholino oligos are a type of antisense oligonucleotides in which the deoxyribose rings are replaced with morpholine rings and the phosphates are replaced with phosphorodiamidate to link the morpholine rings. These modifications make morpholino oligos highly stable in cells because they are unrecognizable and degradable by nucleases [34]. In zebrafish, morpholino oligos are injected into embryos at the 1 to 2 cell stage by a microinjection apparatus. Each morpholino oligo diffuses freely within a cell and distributes evenly among subsequent daughter cells. A trained researcher can inject hundreds of embryos in several hours.

A typical morpholino oligo is 25 bases in length. It binds to RNA by complementary nucleic acid base pairing and prevents other molecules from interacting with the target sequences. For protein-coding genes, morpholino oligos either bind to the region of the mRNA start codon to block protein translation in the cytoplasm or bind to the exon-intron junction of pre-mRNA to interfere the correct splicing within the nucleus. As a result morpholino oligos decrease the expression level of the targeted gene. The efficiency of a specific morpholino can be determined by Western blot for protein levels or RT-PCR for mature mRNA levels from splicing. Morpholino oligos mediated knockdown of gene expression in zebrafish provides a method to rapidly reveal gene function in vivo [35] and have been widely used since its initial introduction into zebrafish.

5.2.4 Transgenic Technologies

The first stable transgenic zebrafish exhibiting tissue-specific expression of a transgene that recapitulated the endogenous gene expression pattern was reported in 1998. In this first study, a DNA construct containing the putative zebrafish promoter sequence of GATA-1, an erythroid specific transcription factor, and the green fluorescent protein (GFP) reporter gene was microinjected into single-cell zebrafish embryos. The resulting transgenic zebrafish had GFP expression patterns that were reflective of the pattern of GATA-1 mRNA expression detected by RNA in situ hybridization. Since then additional technologies, including BAC (bacterial artificial chromosome) and transposon-mediated transgenesis, have been developed. Applications of these technologies produced a great number of stable tissue-specific transgenic lines, covering a wide range of tissues and organs, including neurons, blood cells, blood vessels (Figure 5.1C), pancreas (Figure 5.1A) [36], pituitary (Figure 5.1B) [37], thymus, muscle, germ cells, and so on [38]. These transgenic lines have been used as great tools in investigating developmental biology questions. Below we describe applications in gene regulation studies.

Gene expression is largely controlled by regulated interactions between DNA *cis*-elements and corresponding transcription factors. Here different fragments of regulatory genomic sequences of a gene are linked to GFP and the resulting constructs are injected into zebrafish embryos. Then the temporal and spatial expression pattern of GFP is quickly analyzed in the live transparent embryos to identify essential *cis*-elements required for tissue-specific expression of this gene. This approach was first employed by Meng et al. to identify regulatory regions of GATA-2 required for its tissue-specific expression [39]. Since then, this method has been successfully used to analyze the *cis*-elements of other zebrafish genes. It appears that genes expressed as

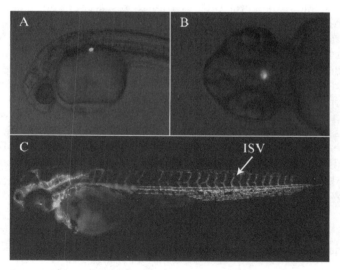

Figure 5.1 Representative transgenic zebrafish lines. (*A*) Insulin:gfp transgenic line, 30 hpf; (*B*) pomc:gfp and prol:rfp double transgenic line, 36 hpf (the pituitary is labeled with both GFP and RFP); (*C*) flk1:gfp transgenic line, 48 hpf. The white arrow points an ISV. (See color insert.)

terminally differentiated markers have shorter promoters and nearby enhancers, whereas the developmental regulatory genes have longer promoters and distal enhancers. For example, *islet1*, a transcription factor expressed in many types of neurons and endocrine cells, has an enhancer necessary for cranial motor neurons that is located about 62 kb upstream from the start codon [40]. Since it is not practical to clone DNA fragments larger than 10 kb into a conventional plasmid vector, BAC transgenesis is used to analyze distal enhancers (reviewed by Yang et al. [41]). BAC is a type of cloning vector that is capable of accommodating large DNA inserts (up to 300 kb). Transgenes can be inserted into BAC clones precisely at desired positions through homologous recombination. Modified zebrafish genomic BAC constructs have now been widely used to faithfully recapitulate endogenous gene expression patterns that require distal enhancers.

5.3 ZEBRAFISH MODELS OF HUMAN DISEASES

Animal models of human diseases are highly valuable tools that enable detailed investigation of molecular mechanisms that cannot be achieved in humans. Modern biomedical research therefore needs as many animal models as possible. Zebrafish resemble humans on multiple levels, including genomic sequence, molecular pathway, organ development, and physiology. This was first demonstrated by the fact that some mutants identified in the large-scale genetic screens phenocopied human diseases with mutations in the same genes. With the effort of the zebrafish community, a long list of zebrafish disease models has been established, covering neural system, cardiovascular system, blood, kidney, digestive system, behavior, and cancer [42–44]. Here we outline zebrafish disease models of blood cells, blood vessels, diabetes, and cancer.

5.3.1 Blood Cells and Blood Vessels

Blood cells and blood vessels develop together during embryogenesis, likely through a common progenitor called the hemagioblast. Similar to mammals, zebrafish blood cell development consists of two consecutive waves, primitive (embryonic) hematopoiesis and definitive (adult) hematopoiesis [45]. Although the anatomical locations of hematopoiesis are different, zebrafish and mammals share the same set of functionally critical genes. Those functionally important genes that were previously identified from mammals, such as *c-myb, gata-1*, and *scl*, are highly conserved in zebrafish [46]. Through large-scale mutagenesis screens, more than 50 mutants defective in hematopoiesis were identified [47,48]. Some of these zebrafish mutants are phenocopies of human homological diseases of hypochromic anemia, congenital sideroblastic anemia, anemia due to the defective iron transporter, porphyrias, and hemolytic anemia [42].

Blood vessel formation of vertebrates also occurs in two different and closely related ways, vasculogenesis and angiogenesis [49,50]. Vasculogenesis is the process of de novo blood vessel formation in which endothelial precursors are derived from the mesoderm. Angiogenesis is the process of new blood vessel formation based on preexisting vessels in which endothelial cells sprout from the existing vessels, migrate, and finally connect to each other to form new vessels. In development and growth, most blood vessels are formed by angiogenesis. Angiogenesis is involved in many pathological processes. For example, tumor growth and metastasis are angiogenesis dependent [50]. Without formation of new blood vessels, tumors are starved of oxygen and nutrients, thus cannot grow and metastasize. Studies have shown that normal development and pathological processes share almost the same angiogenic regulatory mechanisms.

Vascular development of zebrafish embryos has been well characterized [51,52]. The large axial vessels (dorsal aorta and caudal vein) and caudal plexus are formed by vasculogenesis while other vessels are formed by angiogenesis. This process is quite rapid in zebrafish. By 24 hours postfertilization the heart starts to beat regularly and the blood cells circulate in the dorsal aorta and caudal vein. In the trunk region the intersegmental vessels (ISVs) are explicit and thus ideal for angiogenic assays because their pattern is very stereotyped (Figure 5.1C). Unlike mammals, zebrafish embryos can survive and develop for one week without any blood circulation owing to its small body, readily accessible for the diffusion of oxygen and nutrients [53]. This ability offers a great chance to examine angiogenic defects that usually cause lethality in mammals. In addition several endothelial cell-specific GFP transgenic zebrafish have been generated with VEGFR2/KDR/flk1 and Fli1 promoters, which render easy, fast, and continuous observation of blood vessel development under the fluorescent microscope [54]. With the advantages above, zebrafish is an ideal animal model of angiogenesis. Using zebrafish as a model, mutations mimicking human vascular diseases have been identified. *Gridlock* is a recessive mutation in which blood flow to the tail is blocked by due to arterial-venous shunts [55]. The *gridlock* defect resembles coarctation of the aorta, a human congenital cardiovascular malformation of unknown etiology. Zebrafish studies suggest that notch signaling is involved in this pathway.

5.3.2 Diabetes

The development of the pancreas is well studied in zebrafish. As in mammals, the zebrafish pancreas is composed of both endocrine and exocrine glands. While there are differences in morphology, the molecular mechanisms including transcription networks and signaling pathways involved in pancreatic development and diseases are highly conserved between mammals and zebrafish [56,57]. Transgenic zebrafish lines expressing GFP in endocrine and exocrine pancreas have been created under the control of *pdx1, insulin* and elastase promoters [36]. In addition zebrafish mutants associated with human pancreatic diseases have been recovered.

Pancreatic disease MODY5 (maturity-onset diabetes of the young, type V) and familial GCKD (glomerulocystic kidney disease) are linked with mutations in homeobox gene *vhnf1* (variant hepatic nuclear factor 1). In mouse, lack of *vhnf1* leads to pancreatic agenesis by embryonic day 13.5. Zebrafish *vhnf1* mutants isolated by several groups also have defects in the pancreas, liver, and kidney, serving as a useful model for studying mechanisms of MODY5 and familial GCKD [58,59]. In the *vhnf1* mutant key pancreatic patterning genes *pdx1* and *shh* lose their proper expression pattern in endoderm. Further investigation showed that *Bmp, Fgf*, and retinoic acid (RA) signals converge upon *vhnf1* to control pancreas development.

Another pancreatic disease, neonatal diabetes mellitus, is affiliated with mutations in *ptf1a* (pancreas transcription factor 1 alpha) [60]. Mouse *ptf1a* null mutant exhibits a complete absence of exocrine pancreatic tissues, while the endocrine pancreatic tissue appears relatively normal until embryonic day 16 and then becomes scattered near then spleen [61]. Similarly knockdown of *ptf1a* with morpholino oligos in zebrafish results in an undifferentiated exocrine pancreas, but does not disrupt the normal differentiation and organization of the principal islet [62].

5.3.3 Cancer

Zebrafish cancer models are normally generated by chemical carcinogenesis, genetic mutations, and transgenic approaches [63,64].

Early in the 1960s, a chemical carcinogen diethylnitrosamine was shown to cause hepatic degeneration and neoplasia in treated zebrafish [65]. More recently Beckwith et al. described the cellular lesions of skin tumors caused by ENU treatment [66]. Angiogenesis was observed in papillomas larger than 1 mm. In 2006, comparative analysis of microarray data by Lam et al. showed that the molecular events in hepatic tumorigenesis are conserved between zebrafish and human [67]. Unexpectedly, zebrafish embryos appear more sensitive to N-methyl-N'-nitro-N-nitrosoguanidine and 7,12-dimethyl-benz-[alpha]-anthracene than juveniles in developing neoplasia [68,69].

Zebrafish mutants of tumor suppressor genes develop tumors at a higher rate than wild type. *Tp53* is the most important tumor suppressor gene, which is mutated in more than 50% human cancers [70]. Berghmans et al. identified zebrafish mutants carrying missense mutations in the DNA binding domain of *tp53* by using a target-selected mutagenesis strategy [71]. Homozygous *tp53* mutants failed to undergo apoptosis upon γ-irradiation, and displayed malignant peripheral nerve sheath tumors after 8.5 months postfertilization. Adenomatous polyposis coli (APC) is another tumor suppressor gene that is a pivotal component in canonical Wnt pathway [72]. Mutated APC constitutively activates the Wnt pathway that is frequently implicated in human colorectal cancers. A nonsense zebrafish APC mutant was isolated by Hurlstone et al.

by screening an ENU-mutagenized zebrafish library [73]. Homozygous APC mutants died between by 96 hours postfertilization, exhibiting multiple defects as in the mouse APC mutants. Heterozygous APC mutant embryos developed normally but had highly proliferative intestinal, hepatic, and pancreatic neoplasias at ages older than 15 months [74]. This zebrafish phenotype is associated with the accumulation of β-catenin and expression of Wnt target genes, resembling the features of human colorectal cancers. The chemical carcinogen 7,12-dimethylbenz[a]anthracene promoted the occurrence of these lesions. Further investigation in the zebrafish APC mutant disclosed a new role of APC in regulating retinoic acid level [75,76].

For mimicking the cancers that are closely related to upregulation of certain oncogenes, transgenic zebrafish is a suitable tool. T-cell acute lymphoblastic leukemia (T-ALL) was modeled by expressing a chimeric mouse *c-myc* fused to GFP or mouse *c-myc* alone under the control of the zebrafish *rag2* promoter in transgenic zebrafish [77]. After average latencies of 52 days (*zRag2-EGFP-mMyc*) or 44 days (*zRag2-mMyc*) (range, from 30 to 131 days), leukemias arose in the thymus, then spread into gill arches, retro-orbital soft tissue, skeletal muscle, and abdominal organs. The GFP expressing leukemic cells could cause new T-ALL in irradiated recipient fish after transplantation. This T-ALL model was improved by the same research group, in which the Cre-lox system was introduced to control the mouse *c-myc* expression [78]. At least two more transgenic zebrafish blood cancer models have been created. They are myeloid leukemias [79] and pre-B-cell acute lymphoblastic leukemia [80].

Melanoma is the most dangerous type of skin cancer and often carries the activating mutations in the serine/threonine kinase BRAF. To study the role of BRAF in melanoma formation, Patton et al. made a transgenic line expressing the most common mutant form of BRAF (V600E) driven by the melanocyte specific *mitfa* promoter [81]. Highly visible patches of ectopic melanocytes were observed in the adult *mitfa-BRAF*^{V600E} line. On a *tp53* deficient background, activated BRAF-induced formation of melanoma was similar to human melanomas and transplantable between zebrafish, indicating BRAF and tp53 interact genetically to develop melanoma.

5.4   ZEBRAFISH AS A NOVEL PLATFORM FOR DRUG DISCOVERY

5.4.1   Introduction of Drug Discovery

In the early history of drug discovery, a large portion of medicine was discovered through serendipitous exposure of animals or humans to naturally occurring molecules. For example, in 1785, William Withering recorded that leaves of the common foxglove plant (*Digitalis purpurea*) were able to treat heart failure. From these leaves digitalis was isolated to strengthen the contraction of the heart muscle [82]. Today, cardiac glycosides (the effective ingredient of digitalis) are still used in the treatment of congestive heart failure and cardiac arrhythmia. Another example is dicumarol, which was found in the 1930s when the internal bleeding of cattle caused by spoiled sweet clover hay was investigated [83]. Dicumarol and its derivatives are still frequently prescribed in modern medicine. Although the benefits of whole organism drug discovery are obvious, the application of this strategy has been limited by ethical and practical considerations. Designed exposure of animals to large numbers of chemical compounds is expensive, laborious, time-consuming, and could provoke potential ethical problems.

In the 1970s the pharmaceutical industry turned to target-based drug discovery, in which cell, cell extracts, or purified proteins were used to systematically screen compounds for modifiers of biological events. The major advantages of this approach are that target-based discovery can be well planned and performed in high-throughput fashion with automated instruments. By using this approach, a number of "blockbuster" medicines have been invented, including HIV protease inhibitors and the c-Abl kinase inhibitor Gleevec. However, target-based discovery also has its disadvantages. First, it requires sufficient understanding of the target biological process. Before Gleevec was discovered, the function of c-Abl in CML (chronic myelogenous leukemia) was already very well known. Second, it is difficult to target the biological processes in an integrated physiological context. For instance, angiogenesis involves complicated cell to cell and cell to extracellular matrix interactions [50], and therefore it's very difficult to screen for inhibitors in the target-based approach. Third, specificity and toxicity of initial hits in a target-based approach are not scrutinized thoroughly enough. This requires further testing in whole animal models. It is highly desirable to have toxicity data as early as possible in the drug discovery process since toxicity testing could take a long time and many of the initial promising hits have failed due to toxicities [84,85].

5.4.2 Zebrafish as an Emerging Model for Drug Discovery

If an animal model is small and accessible, one can combine the advantages of whole organism drug discovery and high-throughput screening together. Established model systems such as *C. elegans, Drosophila*, and zebrafish (embryo) are suitable for this purpose as they are small enough to grow in microformat plates. Among them, zebrafish is the most appropriate one for drug discovery because it is the only vertebrate animal capable of producing large numbers of transparent embryos available for easy access.

One concern is that whether compounds identified by zebrafish screening will have the same activity in mammals. Because of the short history of using zebrafish as a platform for drug discovery, clinically applicable new drugs have yet to be identified. However, some compounds with known effects in humans have been tested in zebrafish and most of them produced similar effects. Milan et al. reported that 22 out of 23 drugs known to prolong the QT interval (a part of the cardiac cycle) in human prolonged the QT interval in zebrafish as well [86]. Chan et al. reported that a well-characterized anti-angiogenic small molecule PTK787/ZK222584 blocked blood vessel formation in zebrafish [87]. Langheinrich reviews other compounds regulating cholesterol synthesis, coagulation, and vasodilation with analogous effects in both human and zebrafish [88]. It is therefore quite reasonable to conclude that compounds with an activity in conserved biological processes would behave very similarly in human and zebrafish.

The workflow of zebrafish based drug discovery is simple and straightforward. Embryos (3–6) are first arrayed in each well of microtiter plates (96 well or 384 well format) and individual compounds are then added. At selected developmental stages, treated embryos are visually examined for interesting phenotypes (Figure 5.2) under a microscope or an automated instrument.

The zebrafish platform has several advantages. First, as a whole organism system, zebrafish offer the possibility of identifying in vivo modifiers of all biological processes available during embryogenesis. In contrast, target-based approaches are only able to identify modifiers of pre-selected targets in vitro. Second, a single embryo can provide a great amount of morphological information during development. Multiple organs including the skin (pigmentation), heart, eye, ear, and brain can be easily examined at the same time. By using tissue-specific GFP transgenic lines, many internal organs can be

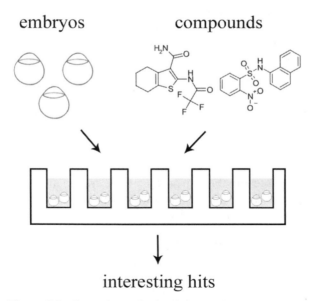

Figure 5.2   Procedure of zebrafish based drug discovery.

conveniently examined as well. Third, zebrafish offers a physiological context, which eliminates compounds with undesirable toxic effects at the very beginning of the screening process [84].

Once a new effective compound is found and characterized, the next step is to identify its biological targets. Although no systematic method is currently available, several approaches have been successfully explored to isolate targets of chemical compounds, including candidate gene methods, expression cloning, and affinity chromatography [89].

We screened a library of 1120 compounds consisting of 85% FDA-approved drugs (Prestwick Chemical, Inc.) for inhibition of angiogenesis, using *flk1:GFP* transgenic zebrafish expressing GFP specifically in blood vessels. One anti-angiogenic compound, mycophenolic acid (MPA), was found to effectively inhibit new blood vessel formation in the trunk [90]. MPA is a known immunosuppressive drug by targeting inosine monophosphate dehydrogenase (IMPDH) (Figure 5.3*F*). In MPA-treated embryos, sprouting of ISVs was severely blocked (Figure 5.3*B*), and blood circulation was limited in the dorsal aorta and caudal vein (Figure 5.3*E*). Consistent with our findings, Huang et al. and Chong et al. also reported that MPA inhibited angiogenesis of cultured endothelial cells [91,92]. Homologous alignment revealed that zebrafish have 3 IMPDH genes. Expression patterns detected by whole mount in situ hybridization showed that IMPDH1a and IMPDH1b were mainly expressed in superficial epithelial cells (Figure 5.3*G* and *H*), while IMPDH2 was expressed in the head and ventral trunk region through where ISVs develop (Figure 5.3*I*). Antisense morpholino oligos were designed against the translation start codons of IMPDH1b and IMPDH2. As expected, knockdown of IMPDH1b didn't produce any anti-angiogenic defects, while IMPDH2 knockdown induced the phenotypes of defective angiogenesis that are indistinguishable from those caused by MPA treatment (Figure 5.3*C*). In addition a synergistic action between IMPDH2 knockdown and MPA treatment was observed.

Recently Yu et al. reported the first small molecule inhibitor of bone morphogenetic proteins (BMP) signaling: dorsomorphin, which was identified from screening compounds that disrupted dorsalventral axis of zebrafish embryo. Dorsomorphin selectively inhibits the type I BMP receptors ALK2, ALK3, and ALK6. Further investigation with dorsomorphin revealed that BMP signaling was important in iron-hepcidin homeostasis [93].

In conclusion, the zebrafish is an emerging platform for drug discovery. Reasonably high-throughput screens of small molecules conducted in zebrafish yielded both drugs and developmental modifiers. Hence zebrafish-based screening has the ability to discover novel drug candidates for treating human diseases.

ACKNOWLEDGMENT

We thank Sharina Palencia Desai for reading the manuscript.

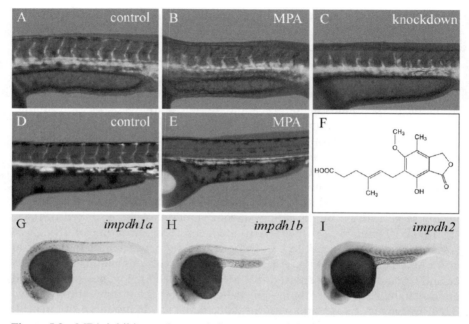

Figure 5.3   MPA inhibits angiogenesis in zebrafish. (*A*) 32 hpf control embryo. Blood vessels appear as green fluorescence. (*B*) 32 hpf embryo treated with 0.9 μmol/L MPA. Shorter fluorescent ISVs were observed. (*C*) Transgenic embryo (32 hpf) injected with 5 ng of IMPDH2-MO. Shorter fluorescent ISVs similar to the panel B were observed. (*D*) 48 hpf control wild-type embryo analyzed by microangiography with injection of fluorescein dextran ($MW = 2,000,000$ Da; Sigma, catalogue #FD-2000S) into the common cardinal vein as previously described. Green fluorescent dye is seen in the circulation, revealing all connected blood vessels. (*E*) 48 hpf embryo treated with 0.9 μmol/L MPA followed by microangiography analysis. No circulation in ISVs was observed, although circulation in the aorta and the posterior cardinal vein is seen. (*F*) Structure of mycophenolic acid [chemical name: 6-(4-Hydroxy-6-methoxy-7-methyl-3-oxo-5-phthalanyl)-4-methyl-4-hexenoic acid]. (*G* to *I*). Embryos at 26 hpf showing expression patterns of IMPDH1a (*G*), and IMPDH1b (*H*), and IMPDH2 (*I*), as detected by RNA whole mount in situ hybridization. Only IMPDH2 has major expression in the somites where the ISVs are present. (See color insert.)

REFERENCES

1. Hamilton F. *An account of the fishes found in the river ganges and its branches*. Edinburgh, 1822.

2. Shrestha J. *Fishes of Nepal*. Tribhuvan University, Kathmandu, 1981.

3. Westerfield M. *The zebrafish book*. University of Oregon Press, Eugene, Oregon, 2000.

4. Daga RR, Thode G, Amores A. Chromosome complement, C-banding, Ag-NOR and replication banding in the zebrafish *Danio rerio*. *Chromosome Res* 1996;4:29–32.

5. Hinegardner R, Rosen D. Cellular DNA content and the evolution of teleostean fishes. *Am Nat* 1972;106:621–44.

6. Laale HW. The biology and use of zebrafish, *Brachydanio rerio* in fisheries research—literature review. *J Fish Biol* 1977;10:121–173.

7. Streisinger G, Walker C, Dower N, Knauber D, Singer F. Production of clones of homozygous diploid zebra fish (*Brachydanio rerio*). *Nature* 1981;291: 293–6.

8. Eisen JS. Zebrafish make a big splash. *Cell* 1996;87:969–77.

9. Driever W, Solnica-Krezel L, Schier AF, Neuhauss SC, Malicki J, Stemple DL, et al. A genetic screen for mutations affecting embryogenesis in zebrafish. *Development* 1996;123:37–46.

10. Haffter P, Granato M, Brand M, Mullins MC, Hammerschmidt M, Kane DA, et al. The identification of genes with unique and essential functions in the development of the zebrafish, *Danio rerio*. *Development* 1996;123:1–36.

11. Patton EE, Zon LI. The art and design of genetic screens: zebrafish. *Nat Rev* 2001;2:956–66.

12. Amsterdam A, Hopkins N. Mutagenesis strategies in zebrafish for identifying genes involved in development and disease. *Trends Genet* 2006;22:473–8.

13. Sivasubbu S, Balciunas D, Amsterdam A, Ekker SC. Insertional mutagenesis strategies in zebrafish. *Genome Biol* 2007;8(suppl1):S9.

14. Grunwald DJ, Streisinger G. Induction of recessive lethal and specific locus mutations in the zebrafish with ethyl nitrosourea. *Genet Res* 1992;59:103–16.

15. Mullins MC, Hammerschmidt M, Haffter P, Nusslein-Volhard C. Large-scale mutagenesis in the zebrafish: in search of genes controlling development in a vertebrate. *Curr Biol* 1994;4:189–202.

16. Solnica-Krezel L, Schier AF, Driever W. Efficient recovery of ENU-induced mutations from the zebrafish germline. *Genetics* 1994;136:1401–20.

17. Jin SW, Herzog W, Santoro MM, Mitchell TS, Frantsve J, Jungblut B, et al. A transgene-assisted genetic screen identifies essential regulators of vascular development in vertebrate embryos. *Dev Biol* 2007;307:29–42.

18. McCallum CM, Comai L, Greene EA, Henikoff S. Targeting induced local lesions IN genomes (TILLING) for plant functional genomics. *Plant Physiol* 2000;123: 439–42.

19. Stemple DL. TILLING—a high-throughput harvest for functional genomics. *Nat Rev* 2004;5:145–50.

20. Zhang J, Talbot WS, Schier AF. Positional cloning identifies zebrafish one-eyed pinhead as a permissive EGF-related ligand required during gastrulation. *Cell* 1998;92:241–51.

21. Geisler R, Rauch GJ, Geiger-Rudolph S, Albrecht A, van Bebber F, Berger A, et al. Large-scale mapping of mutations affecting zebrafish development. *BMC Genom* 2007;8:11.

22. Wienholds E, Schulte-Merker S, Walderich B, Plasterk RH. Target-selected inactivation of the zebrafish rag1 gene. *Science* 2002;297:99–102.

23. Wienholds E, Plasterk RH. Target-selected gene inactivation in zebrafish. *Meth Cell Biol* 2004;77:69–90.

24. Draper BW, McCallum CM, Stout JL, Slade AJ, Moens CB. A high-throughput method for identifying *N*-ethyl-*N*-nitrosourea (ENU)-induced point mutations in zebrafish. *Meth Cell Biol* 2004;77:91–112.

25. Lin S, Gaiano N, Culp P, Burns JC, Friedmann T, Yee JK, et al. Integration and germ-line transmission of a pseudotyped retroviral vector in zebrafish. *Science* 1994;265:666–9.

26. Gaiano N, Amsterdam A, Kawakami K, Allende M, Becker T, Hopkins N. Insertional mutagenesis and rapid cloning of essential genes in zebrafish. *Nature* 1996;383:829–32.

27. Amsterdam A, Burgess S, Golling G, Chen W, Sun Z, Townsend K, et al. A large-scale insertional mutagenesis screen in zebrafish. *Genes Dev* 1999;13: 2713–24.

28. Amsterdam A, Nissen RM, Sun Z, Swindell EC, Farrington S, Hopkins N. Identification of 315 genes essential for early zebrafish development. *Proc Nat Acad Sci USA* 2004;101:12792–7.

29. Wang D, Jao LE, Zheng N, Dolan K, Ivey J, Zonies S, et al. Efficient genome-wide mutagenesis of zebrafish genes by retroviral insertions. *Proc Nat Acad Sci USA* 2007;104:12428–33.

30. Gall JG, Pardue ML. Formation and detection of RNA-DNA hybrid molecules in cytological preparations. *Proc Nat Acad Sci USA* 1969;63:378–83.

31. Jin L, Lloyd RV. In situ hybridization: methods and applications. *J Clini Lab Anal* 1997;11:2–9.

32. Krauss S, Johansen T, Korzh V, Moens U, Ericson JU, Fjose A. Zebrafish pax [zf-a]: a paired box-containing gene expressed in the neural tube. *EMBO J* 1991;10:3609–19.

33. Thisse C, Thisse B. High-resolution in situ hybridization to whole-mount zebrafish embryos. *Nat Protocols* 2008;3:59–69.

34. Summerton J, Weller D. Morpholino antisense oligomers: design, preparation, and properties. *Antisense Nucleic Acid Drug Dev* 1997;7:187–95.

35. Nasevicius A, Ekker SC. Effective targeted gene "knockdown" in zebrafish. *Nat Genet* 2000;26:216–20.

36. Huang HG, Vogel SS, Liu NG, Melton DA, Lin S. Analysis of pancreatic development in living transgenic zebrafish embryos. *Mol Cell Endocrinol* 2001; 177:117–24.

37. Liu NA, Liu Q, Wawrowsky K, Yang Z, Lin S, Melmed S. Prolactin receptor signaling mediates the osmotic response of embryonic zebrafish lactotrophs. *Mol Endocrinol* 2006;20:871–80.

38. Gong Z, Korzh V. *Fish development and genetics the zebrafish and medaka models*. Hackensack, NJ: World Scientific, 2004.

39. Meng A, Tang H, Ong BA, Farrell MJ, Lin S. Promoter analysis in living zebrafish embryos identifies a cis-acting motif required for neuronal expression of GATA-2. *Proc Nat Acad Sci USA* 1997;94:6267–72.

40. Higashijima S, Hotta Y, Okamoto H. Visualization of cranial motor neurons in live transgenic zebrafish expressing green fluorescent protein under the control of the islet-1 promoter/enhancer. *J Neurosci* 2000;20:206–18.

41. Yang Z, Jiang H, Chachainasakul T, Gong S, Yang XW, Heintz N, et al. Modified bacterial artificial chromosomes for zebrafish transgenesis. *Methods* 2006;39: 183–8.

42. Penberthy WT, Shafizadeh E, Lin S. The zebrafish as a model for human disease. *Front Biosci* 2002;7:D1439–53.

43. Shin JT, Fishman MC. From Zebrafish to human: modular medical models. *Ann Rev Genomics Human Genet* 2002;3:311–40.

44. Kari G, Rodeck U, Dicker AP. Zebrafish: an emerging model system for human disease and drug discovery. *Clin Pharmacol Therapeut* 2007;82:70–80.

45. Orkin SH, Zon LI. Genetics of erythropoiesis: Induced mutations in mice and zebrafish. *Ann Rev Genet* 1997;31:33–60.

46. Amatruda JF, Zon LI. Dissecting hematopoiesis and disease using the zebrafish. *Dev Biol* 1999;216:1–15.

47. Weinstein BM, Schier AF, Abdelilah S, Malicki J, Solnica-Krezel L, Stemple DL, et al. Hematopoietic mutations in the zebrafish. *Development* 1996;123:303–9.

48. Ransom DG, Haffter P, Odenthal J, Brownlie A, Vogelsang E, Kelsh RN, et al. Characterization of zebrafish mutants with defects in embryonic hematopoiesis. *Development* 1996;123:311–9.

49. Risau W. Mechanisms of angiogenesis. *Nature* 1997;386:671–4.

50. Carmeliet P. Angiogenesis in life, disease and medicine. *Nature* 2005;438:932–6.

51. Isogai S, Horiguchi M, Weinstein BM. The vascular anatomy of the developing zebrafish: an atlas of embryonic and early larval development. *Dev Biol* 2001;230:278–301.

52. Childs S, Chen JN, Garrity DM, Fishman MC. Patterning of angiogenesis in the zebrafish embryo. *Development* 2002;129:973–82.

53. Stainier DY, Weinstein BM, Detrich HW, 3rd, Zon LI, Fishman MC. Cloche, an early acting zebrafish gene, is required by both the endothelial and hematopoietic lineages. *Development* 1995;121:3141–50.

54. Cross LM, Cook MA, Lin S, Chen JN, Rubinstein AL. Rapid analysis of angiogenesis drugs in a live fluorescent zebrafish assay. *Arterioscler Thromb Vasc Biol* 2003;23:911–2.

55. Zhong TP, Rosenberg M, Mohideen MA, Weinstein B, Fishman MC. gridlock, An HLH gene required for assembly of the aorta in zebrafish. *Science* 2000;287:1820–4.

56. Spagnoli FM. From endoderm to pancreas: a multistep journey. *Cell Mol Life Sci* 2007;64:2378–90.

57. Zorn AM, Wells JM. Molecular basis of vertebrate endoderm development. In: *International review of cytology*. Academic Press, 2007, p. 49–111.

58. Song J, Kim HJ, Gong Z, Liu N-A, Lin S. Vhnf1 acts downstream of Bmp, Fgf, and RA signals to regulate endocrine beta cell development in zebrafish. *Dev Biol* 2007;303:561–75.

59. Sun ZX, Hopkins N. Vhnf1, the MODY5 and familial GCKD-associated gene, regulates regional specification of the zebrafish gut, pronephros, and hindbrain. *Genes Dev* 2001;15:3217–29.

60. Sellick GS, Barker KT, Stolte-Dijkstra I, Fleischmann C, Coleman RJ, Garrett C, et al. Mutations in PTF1A cause pancreatic and cerebellar agenesis. *Nat Genet* 2004;36:1301–5.

61. Krapp A, Knofler M, Ledermann B, Burki K, Berney C, Zoerkler N, et al. The bHLH protein PTF1-p48 is essential for the formation of the exocrine and the correct spatial organization of the endocrine pancreas. *Genes Dev* 1998;12: 3752–63.

62. Lin JW, Biankin AV, Horb ME, Ghosh B, Prasad NB, Yee NS, et al. Differential requirement for ptf1a in endocrine and exocrine lineages of developing zebrafish pancreas. *Dev Biol* 2004;270:474–86.

63. Lieschke GJ, Currie PD. Animal models of human disease: zebrafish swim into view. *Nat Rev* 2007;8:353–67.

64. Goessling W, North TE, Zon LI. New waves of discovery: modeling cancer in zebrafish. *J Clin Oncol* 2007;25:2473–9.

65. Stanton MF. Diethylnitrosamine-Induced hepatic degeneration and neoplasia in the aquarium fish, *Brachydanio Rerio*. *J Nat Cancer Inst* 1965;34:117–30.

66. Beckwith LG, Moore JL, Tsao-Wu GS, Harshbarger JC, Cheng KC. Ethylnitrosourea induces neoplasia in zebrafish (*Danio rerio*). *Lab Invest J Tech Meth Pathol* 2000;80:379–85.

67. Lam SH, Wu YL, Vega VB, Miller LD, Spitsbergen J, Tong Y, et al. Conservation of gene expression signatures between zebrafish and human liver tumors and tumor progression. *Nat Biotechnol* 2006;24:73–5.

68. Spitsbergen JM, Tsai HW, Reddy A, Miller T, Arbogast D, Hendricks JD, et al. Neoplasia in zebrafish (*Danio rerio*) treated with *N*-methyl-*N*'-nitro-*N*-nitrosoguanidine by three exposure routes at different developmental stages. *Toxicol Pathol* 2000;28:716–25.

69. Spitsbergen JM, Tsai HW, Reddy A, Miller T, Arbogast D, Hendricks JD, et al. Neoplasia in zebrafish (*Danio rerio*) treated with 7,12-dimethylbenz[a]anthracene by two exposure routes at different developmental stages. *Toxicol Pathol* 2000;28:705–15.

70. Beroud C, Soussi T. The UMD-p53 database: new mutations and analysis tools. *Human Mutat* 2003;21:176–81.

71. Berghmans S, Murphey RD, Wienholds E, Neuberg D, Kutok JL, Fletcher CD, et al. tp53 mutant zebrafish develop malignant peripheral nerve sheath tumors. *Proc Nat Acad Sci USA* 2005;102:407–12.

72. Logan CY, Nusse R. The Wnt signaling pathway in development and disease. *Ann Rev Cell Dev Biol* 2004;20:781–810.

73. Hurlstone AF, Haramis AP, Wienholds E, Begthel H, Korving J, Van Eeden F, et al. The Wnt/beta-catenin pathway regulates cardiac valve formation. *Nature* 2003;425:633–7.

74. Haramis AP, Hurlstone A, van der Velden Y, Begthel H, Van den Born M, Offerhaus GJ, et al. Adenomatous polyposis coli-deficient zebrafish are susceptible to digestive tract neoplasia. *EMBO Rep* 2006;7:444–9.

75. Eisinger AL, Nadauld LD, Shelton DN, Peterson PW, Phelps RA, Chidester S, et al. The adenomatous polyposis coli tumor suppressor gene regulates expression of cyclooxygenase-2 by a mechanism that involves retinoic acid. *J Biol Chem* 2006;281:20474–82.

76. Shelton DN, Sandoval IT, Eisinger A, Chidester S, Ratnayake A, Ireland CM, et al. Up-regulation of CYP26A1 in adenomatous polyposis coli-deficient vertebrates via a WNT-dependent mechanism: implications for intestinal cell differentiation and colon tumor development. *Cancer Res* 2006;66:7571–7.

77. Langenau DM, Traver D, Ferrando AA, Kutok JL, Aster JC, Kanki JP, et al. Myc-induced T cell leukemia in transgenic zebrafish. *Science* 2003;299:887–90.

78. Langenau DM, Feng H, Berghmans S, Kanki JP, Kutok JL, Look AT. Cre/lox-regulated transgenic zebrafish model with conditional myc-induced T cell acute lymphoblastic leukemia. *Proc Nat Acad Sci USA* 2005;102:6068–73.

79. Onnebo SM, Condron MM, McPhee DO, Lieschke GJ, Ward AC. Hematopoietic perturbation in zebrafish expressing a tel-jak2a fusion. *Exp Hematol* 2005;33:182–8.

80. Sabaawy HE, Azuma M, Embree LJ, Tsai HJ, Starost MF, Hickstein DD. TEL-AML1 transgenic zebrafish model of precursor B cell acute lymphoblastic leukemia. *Proc Nat Acad Sci USA* 2006;103:15166–71.

81. Patton EE, Widlund HR, Kutok JL, Kopani KR, Amatruda JF, Murphey RD, et al. BRAF mutations are sufficient to promote nevi formation and cooperate with p53 in the genesis of melanoma. *Curr Biol* 2005;15:249–54.

82. Luderitz B. Cardiac glycosides: William Withering (1741–1799). *J Interv Card Electrophysiol* 2005;14:61–2.

83. Mueller RL, Scheidt S. History of drugs for thrombotic disease: discovery, development, and directions for the future. *Circulation* 1994;89:432–49.

84. MacRae CA, Peterson RT. Zebrafish-based small molecule discovery. *Chem Biol* 2003;10:901–8.

85. Sams-Dodd F. Target-based drug discovery: is something wrong? *Drug Discov Today* 2005;10:139–47.

86. Milan DJ, Peterson TA, Ruskin JN, Peterson RT, MacRae CA. Drugs that induce repolarization abnormalities cause bradycardia in zebrafish. *Circulation* 2003;107:1355–8.

87. Chan J, Bayliss PE, Wood JM, Roberts TM. Dissection of angiogenic signaling in zebrafish using a chemical genetic approach. *Cancer Cell* 2002;1:257–67.

88. Langheinrich U. Zebrafish: a new model on the pharmaceutical catwalk. *Bioessays* 2003;25:904–12.

89. King RW. Chemistry or biology: which comes first after the genome is sequenced? *Chem Biol* 1999;6:R327–33.

90. Wu X, Zhong H, Song J, Damoiseaux R, Yang Z, Lin S. Mycophenolic acid is a potent inhibitor of angiogenesis. *Arterioscler Thromb Vasc Biol* 2006;26:2414–6.

91. Huang Y, Liu Z, Huang H, Liu H, Li L. Effects of mycophenolic acid on endothelial cells. *Int Immunopharmacol* 2005;5:1029–39.

92. Chong CR, Qian DZ, Pan F, Wei Y, Pili R, Sullivan DJ, Jr, et al. Identification of type 1 inosine monophosphate dehydrogenase as an antiangiogenic drug target. *J Med Chem* 2006;49:2677–80.

93. Yu PB, Hong CC, Sachidanandan C, Babitt JL, Deng DY, Hoyng SA, et al. Dorsomorphin inhibits BMP signals required for embryogenesis and iron metabolism. *Nat Chem Biol* 2008;4:33–41.

6

TOXICITY PATHWAYS AND MODELS: MINING FOR POTENTIAL SIDE EFFECTS

Sean Ekins and Josef Scheiber

Contents

6.1   INTRODUCTION

In recent years there has been considerable research into developing better in silico, in vitro, and in vivo methods and models for toxicology [1]. This is desirable, as the pharmaceutical industry needs to prospectively identify molecules as early as possible that might fail in the clinic due to toxicity. Of particular concern are molecules that reach the market but may require recall due to idiosyncratic toxicities (e.g., hepatotoxicity) that were not observed in

Drug Efficacy, Safety, and Biologics Discovery: Emerging Technologies and Tools,
Edited by Sean Ekins and Jinghai J. Xu

clinical trials. It is therefore imperative to avoid such compounds. Subsequently our biology knowledge has greatly expanded, to the regulation of drug-metabolizing enzymes and transporters via nuclear hormone receptors (NHRs), for example. Nevertheless, our understanding of which molecules bind to these receptors or the impact of their gene interaction networks has lagged behind. Toxicogenomics, proteomics, metabonomics, pharmacogenomics, and chemogenomics represent the experimental approaches that can be combined with high-throughput molecular screening to provide a global view of the complete biological system being modulated by a compound. For example, the utilization of human tissues or cells in vitro, and in particular, hepatocytes, which are the gold standard for understanding likely hepatotoxicity of a compound, has been important for ascertaining the effect of compounds on multiple NHRs [2–4]. Functional interpretation and relevance of the complex multidimensional in vitro data that result from such analysis to the observed phenotype in humans is the focus of current research in toxicology. However, the generation of such data, including microarray gene expression studies, is still relatively expensive and there are important issues with experimental protocols, throughput, and variability, all affecting reproducibility. This pattern could be repeated for other toxicities. The present chapter describes how the integration of different experimental, molecular and computational technologies could enable the mining of toxicology pathways. One may, for example, define the likely toxicity of a compound using a network or biological fingerprint interaction signature developed from high-throughput data. Focused nuclear hormone receptor gene expression data from assay of human hepatocytes treated with a compound in vitro could yield important networks from which to infer likely hepatotoxicity. Such an approach may enable us to understand not only whether a new molecule or its predicted metabolites bind to a particular gene, such as a NHR, which could impact its own metabolism and disposition, but also whether it binds to other downstream proteins that result in hepatotoxicity (or other toxicities).

6.2 TOXICITY PATHWAYS

A better understanding of small molecule–protein interactions should improve our ability to predict the possible toxic consequences [5,6] that have been responsible for the withdrawal of numerous marketed drugs and late stage failures [7]. The focus is now on preclinical toxicity. Because of the complexities of different model systems, better predictive approaches [8] are needed [9,10]. A first step toward identifying toxicity pathways can be to identify and annotate targets that are known to cause undesired effects if they are hit by small molecules [11]. In vitro testing then ensures a certain predictivity for toxic measures. Accurate predictions for toxicity mechanisms in vivo are certainly complicated as the whole organism is highly integrated, with thousands of endobiotic and xenobiotic molecules interacting in different cellular organelles of tissues. Species differences in protein expression and ligand specificity should also be considered. Methods are therefore needed to account for the complexity of biological data and to enable prediction of the complete system incorporating metabolic, regulatory, signaling, and transport processes [12,13]. Interpreting toxicity in this systems context may improve our understanding and ultimate predictions but may require collection and integration of "high-throughput" data, including global gene expression, protein content, and metabolic profiles for the same samples, along with genetic, clinical, and phenotypic data.

The generation of both biological and chemical data using high-throughput methods in drug discovery necessitates the use of computational technologies, including databases and data-mining algorithms, in order to store, analyze, interpret, and learn from this information [14]. Within drug disposition and toxicology in vitro approaches for generating data with drug-metabolizing enzymes, transporters, ion channels, and receptors can be used for predictive computer model generation [15]. Many of these proteins are known to be regulated by NHRs or other transcription factors [3,4,16–23] affecting endogenous metabolism, cell growth, proliferation and oxidative stress [24,25]. The effect of these NHRs and other transcriptional factors on the toxic response and drug metabolism is itself complex and overlapping in a species-specific manner [26], with the same compounds working as agonists and antagonists on different receptors [24]. Understanding the interactions of diverse ligands with these receptors [27–31] and their impact on regulation of proteins has resulted in a schematic of the cross-talk [32]. The NHRs induce gene expression of drug-metabolizing enzymes and transporters to control steroid, heme, carcinogen, and xenobiotic metabolism [33–35]. There have been some preliminary approaches to mining these data [36–39] that are likely to continue in the future.

6.3 ALGORITHMS FOR DATA ANALYSIS

Traditionally functional organization of a biological system was described in terms of pathways. Pathways were thought of as relatively small linear chains of biochemical reactions or signaling interactions that lead from a defined starting point (e.g., cell surface receptor) to a target effector (e.g., transcriptional factor). Such a description is in part due to the nature of biological research that until recently was inherently low throughput, with data scattered in many tens of thousands of individual publications. In recent years, however, several key developments have taken place in this area in terms of pathway databases, natural language processing algorithms for automatic extraction of pathway information, online abstracts and high-throughput techniques for determining potential protein–protein interactions. Based on the data available from these technologies, it has become clear that organization of intra- and intercellular molecular processes is much more complex. Contrary to the previous model of fairly independent small pathways, it is now evident that known molecular processes can be linked into rather large, highly interconnected networks. A recent review has described in considerable detail the theory behind network models and their architecture and how they can be used to provide insight into the functional organization of the cell [40].

Several approaches have been developed for a more advanced, functional analysis of high-throughput data. In particular, there have been considerable advances in the availability of software for visualizing complex gene networks. To date several algorithms have been described in the literature for combining protein interaction information and expression data to find condition-specific modules in protein networks (e.g., clustering algorithms, simulated annealing, probabilistic graphical models, Monte Carlo optimization). These algorithms can be used for combining protein interaction information and expression data to find condition-specific modules in protein networks. More recently "signature networks" have been proposed that combine comprehensive databases [40]. These powerful analytical and network building tools have enabled the development of the commercially available integrated high-throughput data-mining suites described previously such as Ingenuity Pathway Analysis™ (Ingenuity Inc), PathArt™ (Jubilant Biosys), Pathways Studio™ (Ariadne Inc), MetaCore™, MetaDrug™ (GeneGo Inc), ToxShield (Gene Logic), and ToxWiz (Cambridge Cell Networks). As a result it is possible to visualize the global cellular mechanisms behind differences in expression as most of these tools use manually curated content on human physical protein–protein interactions at different levels of cellular functionality, which are captured as maps of current biological knowledge or custom-built interaction networks. In recent years several of these tools have added curated content relevant to toxicology [41–44]. For example, Ingenuity Pathway Analysis (IPA) and MetaCore contains toxicity-related pathways (Table 6.1, Figure 6.1), and for each there are associated gene lists as shown in the literature (Figure 6.2). If a user generates a network with the data that is enriched in these genes, it should be possible to infer the probability of the presence of a particular toxicity. For example, a recent study used IPA, MetaCore, and ToxShield to analyze microarray data from liver slices after treatment with acetaminophen and carbon tetrachloride [45]. Both IPA and MetaCore were able to correctly identify pathologies associated with these compounds and IPA was able to identify a fibrotic response from 3 h in vitro slice culture data, indicating that combination of computational and in vitro experimental approaches may aid in predicting hepatotoxicity responses seen in vivo [45].

6.4 DATABASES, MODELING, AND PREDICTIVE TOOLS

Since the 1970s industry and academia have organized databases on proteins, enzyme-encoding genes, metabolic, and cell signaling pathways [43]. Similarly there has been the creation of molecule structure databases such as

TABLE 6.1 Hepatotoxicity Related Endpoints and the Respective Gene Content in Ingenuity Pathway Analysis and MetaCore Version 4.5

Effect	IPA	MetaCore
Steatosis	+	+
Fibrosis	+	+
Hyperbilirubinemia	+	+
Steatohepatitis	+	−
Fibrogenesis	+	−
Oxidative stress	+	−
Necrosis	+	+
Calcium deposition	+	−
Mitochondrial damage	+	−
Bile acid transport	+	−
Lipid peroxidation	−	−
CYP induction, metabolism, interaction	+	−
Proliferation	+	−
Hyperglycemia	−	+
Hypertriglyceridemia	−	+

Note: For genes associated with cholestasis, see Figure 6.3.

ChemSpider and PubChem, drug databases such as DrugBank [46], as well as databases of biology data (PDSP Ki database [47–49], BioPrint [50], etc., see e.g., http://depth-first.com/articles/2007/01/24/thirty-two-free-chemistry-databases). There have also been limited efforts to organize toxicity data in commercial databases, Vitic (Lhasa), MDL Toxicity Database, TOXNET, ToxLine, and DSSTox. However, with the initiation of the REACH initiative in Europe and TOXCAST in the United States, we envisage that a substantial quantity of toxicology data will be available in the public domain in the near future. Already developed are separate databases of absorption, distribution, metabolism, and excretion (ADME) associated proteins or pathways such as PharmGKB [51], the nuclear receptor database [52], human membrane transporter database [53], and the ADME-AP database [54]. Several companies are marketing content databases of expression profiles, as well as histopathology, multiparameter clinical chemistry tests, and morphology in organs after treatment with several hundred marketed drugs and toxicants using different array platforms [55,56], and there are also some freely available databases with gene expression profiles following treatment with different toxic molecules [57,58]. We are aware of at least one gene expression database, the Connectivity Map (http://www.broad.mit.edu/cmap/), that is publicly available and relates to the treatment of human cells with compounds that can be used to aid in the prediction of toxicity [59–61], though we are not aware of a similar database focused on hepatotoxicity mediated via NHRs in particular. To date the Connectivity Map has been used for finding drug-like molecules with

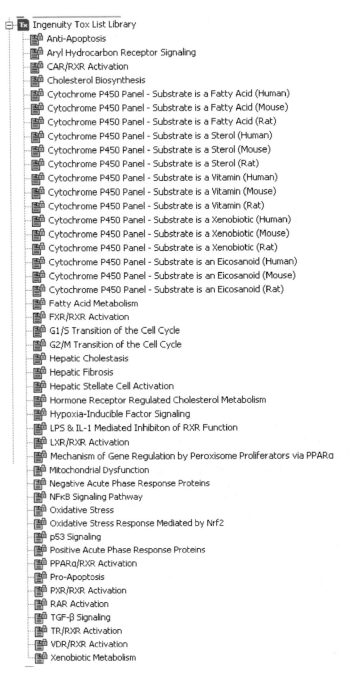

Figure 6.1   Toxicity pathways in Ingenuity Pathway Analysis.

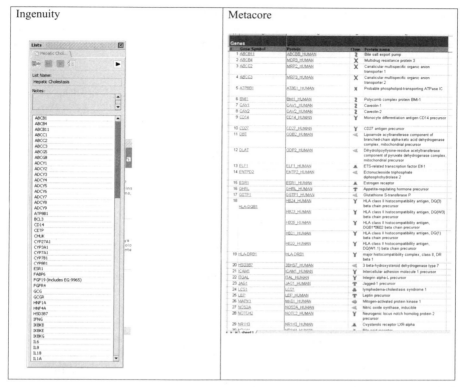

Figure 6.2 Gene list associated with hepatic cholestasis in Ingenuity Pathway Analysis and MetaCore version 4.5. (See color insert.)

similar gene-expression fingerprints, identifying new molecules for diseases as well as rapid identification of novel uses for existing approved drugs. The Connectivity Map could be supplemented with expression profiles from compounds that are known to have liver toxicity, and perhaps other compounds could be annotated with different toxicities or additional off-target effects. If a gene signature for a new compound retrieved multiple molecules that were ranked similarly and that were known hepatotoxins, then there would be a high probability that the test compound shared similar off-target effects. The broad use of microarray approaches and database development [56] provides valuable methods and data for understanding toxicity, which is increasingly seen as important for future submissions to regulatory authorities, so development of such databases integrating knowledge from very different areas is urgently needed [62].

Computational models have become widely available for predicting human ADME/Tox properties [10,43]. These systems are generally based on quantitative structure activity relationships (QSAR) that generate descriptors based on the input molecular structure, and then use computational algorithms to relate the key descriptors to the biological activity [15]. To date we are aware of a QSAR developed for predicting hepatotoxicity that uses 382 molecules with binary descriptions of toxicity and an ensemble decision tree method [63]. Following both internal and external testing, the authors suggest that the molecular descriptor-based approach has an 80% accuracy level [63]. Similarly a second group has used SIMCA with CoMFA generated fields for 654 drugs along with data after treating HepG2 cells in vitro. However, the prediction accuracy was poor, and a local model for NSAID and LDH leakage performed better [64]. Other commercially available, knowledge-based tools or mechanistic tools are available. Computational approaches for toxicity prediction have been infrequently studied [9,65] but would be complementary to research on ADME parameters [15]. These methods for individual toxicology properties have tended to be rule-based systems like DEREK™, Hazard Expert™, LeadScope™ or the mechanistic methods COMPACT [66] and MultiCASE™. There is a need for predictive toxicity tools that incorporate the high-content data from modern experimental methods performed on human and animal cells. This would enable us to understand whether a molecule interferes with endogenous metabolic, regulatory, or transport proteins. As xenobiotics and their metabolites influence multiple genes and pathways simultaneously, the prediction of a response in a heterogeneous population dependent on drug dose, genes, physiological state, and other factors is complex. Therefore the combination of different experimental and predictive approaches will aid in explaining metabolism and toxicity for compounds.

Each of the technologies described above still face some considerable challenges. These include controlling the experimental variability followed by effective verification, storage, utilization, and dissemination of the massive amount of data that can be generated. The data derived in animals or even human in vitro models must be extrapolated to humans in vivo, and this is another complex process. The development of new technologies would certainly benefit from the incorporation of relevant high-throughput type content to provide identification of the specific interaction networks for groups of new chemical entities and toxins. A further challenge is in effectively comparing multiple networks (with a database of signatures for a toxicity, response, etc.) that could be generated with network software like that described above. It has been recently suggested that methods and concepts applied to one area, such as sequence analysis, may be key for network analysis as it progresses [67]. The idea is to find faithful reductions of complex 3D data by 2D or 1D representations such that efficient data mining and analysis are possible. Recent studies have compared 1D and 3D representations of molecules and found the 1D representations and similarity calculations to have some advantages for mining different data sets [68] and likely some utility for ADME/Tox datasets [69]. An additional simple fast alignment of metabolic pathways has suggested the exploitation of local diversity with an algorithm called

FIT-MATCH using networks where the edge is labeled with the EC number of the catalyzing enzyme. This algorithm has been made freely available in METAPAT [70]. Areas still to be addressed by the research community include reliable methods for scoring statistically such alignments of networks and storage of networks in a freely accessible data repository. First steps have been taken in this direction by the Human Metabolome database [71] (www. hmdb.ca), Reactome (http://www.reactome.org/), MetaCyc, and others (e.g., see http://www.bmrb.wisc.edu/metabolomics/external_metab_links.html). The availability of such network comparison, searching, scoring, and rebuilding tools will become a necessity as the biological data deluge continues. The next step would be how a user could then retrieve the answer to a query in a format that would not require a network visualization. For example, it would need to answer the question, What is the closest network to compound X that contains genes that are associated with hepatotoxicity endpoints (Table 6.1)? Or, What networks are known to interfere with compounds that are similar to mine?

QSAR algorithms could be used for generating quantitative structure–gene interaction relationship (QS-GIR) predictive models using microarray data and machine learning algorithms to complement gene signature network databases. These combined approaches would then allow interpretation of possible interactions with these or other genes related to hepatotoxicity for a large series of molecules. A signature could be created simply by the presence or absence of genes (binary) or levels of expression of the genes (continuous), for example, for each molecule used, a string of genes in the gene signature that could be used as an input for a multivariate recursive partitioning model. For the same molecules molecular descriptors could also be calculated [72–74] and used with the gene signatures to derive the QS-GIR to, in turn, predict hepatotoxicity (Figure 6.3). This model would then be used to predict the likely gene interaction profile for a new molecule from the input of a molecular structure.

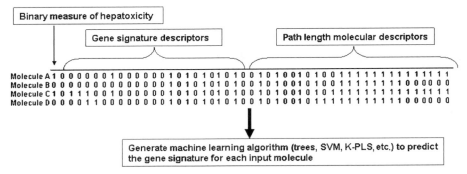

Figure 6.3 Schematic for generation of a quantitative structure–gene interaction relationship.

6.5 EXAMPLES

Several studies have combined large databases of molecules with machine learning algorithms, and these give proof of what could be achieved to enrich our knowledge of potential toxicities. A network approach may assist in designing drugs with affinity for multiple targets [75] or avoid off- or anti-targets. For example, recently an interaction network between 25 nuclear receptors was constructed from an annotated chemical library containing 2033 molecules [37], and revealed potential cross-pharmacologies for the side-effect prediction of small molecules. There have also been several attempts to establish relationships between molecular structure and broad biological activity and off-target effects (toxicity) [76–78]. For example, Fliri et al. presented the biological spectra for a cross section of the proteome [79]. Using hierachical clustering of the spectra similarity they could create a relationship between structure and bioactivity. This work was further extended to identify agonist and antagonist profiles at various receptors, correctly classifying similar functional activity in the absence of drug target information [80]. A similar probabilistic approach has been applied to link adverse effects for drugs (obtained from the drug labeling information) with biological spectra. In one case, clustering molecules by side-effect profile showed that similar molecules had overlapping profiles, in the same way that they had similar biological spectra, ultimately linking preclinical with clinical effects [81]. This work could lead to the prediction of a biospectra profile, functional activity, and a side-effect profile for a new molecule based on similarity alone. A global mapping of pharmacological space has been presented focusing on a polypharmacology network of 200,000 molecules with activity against 698 proteins [82] from which Bayesian binary models were created (for molecules active at $<10\,\mu M$ or inactive), suggesting that they would be useful for predicting primary pharmacology. The further assessment of 617 approved oral drugs in 2D molecular property space (molecular weight vs. cLogP) showed that many of them had cLogP > 5 and MW > 500. Despite this, their associated targets were potentially druggable but had yet to realize their potential [82]. This group did not appear to address the potential of their approach to understand or predict toxicity.

A more recent study created a drug-target network using approved drug data for 890 molecules from DrugBank and OMIM, and over half of these molecules formed the largest connected network with multiple target proteins (polypharmacology or promiscuity) while drugs acting on single targets were in the minority [83]. Such networks might help us understand likely nodes involved in toxicity and add to the similarity maps for enzymes and receptors [84] and human polypharmacology networks [82] that have been developed.

For example, it is possible to simultaneously interpret high-throughput data and predictions on interaction networks, providing a better approach to predicting and understanding potential undesirable off target effects. An example data set uses percentage of inhibition data for clotrimazole and ticonazole, which are screened against many different assays at a single concentration [79]. The data for 10 assays has been arbitrarily encoded as inhibitors (>50% inhibition) or noninhibitors (<50% inhibition) analyzed with MetaCore [41]. The analyzed network algorithm was then used to produce a statistically significant network for the different proteins ($p = 2.838e^{-31}$, Figure 6.4). This network also mapped to many Gene Ontology processes indicating how molecules of the same or different therapeutic classes could be evaluated for effects that would be useful to identify structurally dissimilar molecules with similar network patterns. This type of visualization of high-throughput screening data illustrated how the target proteins could be connected as a network to infer the possible downstream effects of inhibition [41].

Several studies have used different databases, different molecular descriptors, and QSAR algorithms to build predictive models for pharmacology data.

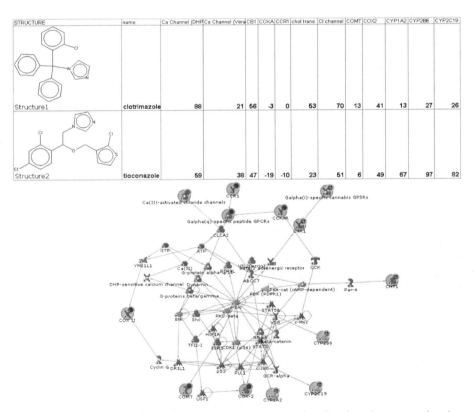

Figure 6.4 High-throughput data analysis on a net work using data for two molecules from Fliri et al. [79]. (See color insert.)

One study has used probabilistic neural networks with 24 atom-type descriptors to classify 799 molecules from the MDL Drug Data Reports (MDDR) database with activity against one of 7 targets (GPCRs, kinases, enzymes, nuclear hormone receptors, and zinc peptidases) [85]. Similarly 21 targets related to depression were selected, and molecules from the MDDR database were used to create support vector machine (SVM) classification models from atom-type descriptors [86]. SVM filters could be useful for virtual screening due to their speed. Others have used similarity searching of the MDDR database with reference inhibitors for several different targets and showed variable enrichment factors greater than random [87].

Another recently published approach identified chemical substructures that are relevant for toxicology-related adverse effects [88] using naïve Bayesian statistics with Scitegic's ECFP_4-descriptors. Using approximately 4000 molecules with side-effect information from the World Drug Index, it was shown that large-scale modeling of adverse effects delivers encouraging results. Along with these models the WOMBAT database was used to establish models that can predict whether a compound interacts with a certain target. Consequently this approach can also be used to annotate targets with unknown side effects by computing model correlations in chemical space. The information can then be used for predictive in vitro modeling of whether a compound will show a certain effect. A similar approach has been taken by Azzaoui et al. to relate the promiscuity of compounds to their safety [89], and this makes use of the fact that compounds hitting several targets cause more undesired effects, ultimately enabling the computation of a promiscuity score for a molecule that varies with the number of targets hit.

Structure-based approaches to small molecule–protein interactions include flexible docking of molecules into multiple proteins, often called inverse docking (e.g., INVDOCK). This approach was recently applied for identifying potential adverse reactions using a database of 147 proteins related to toxicities (DART). This method has been recently demonstrated with 11 marketed anti-HIV drugs, resulting in reasonable accuracy against the DNA polymerase beta and DNA topoisomerase I [90]. A fully structure-based approached has been presented by Xie et al. [91]. They have developed a method to compare the binding sites of different proteins using new shape descriptors that are fast to calculate and therefore are able to use the approach to predict additional compounds for the targets under scrutiny. Thereby side effects could be annotated to targets based on the binding pocket similarities.

These computational chemogenomic approaches [92] may supplement the in vitro methods that are used to detect off-target effects, especially high-throughput screening, which is being quite widely used to detect new uses for drugs [49] that are utilized for other indications [93,94]. Computational approaches may simultaneously speed up this process and ensure that potential toxicity is minimized.

6.6 FUTURE

The public availability of data on drugs and drug-like molecules may make the types of analyses described above possible for scientists outside the private sector. For example chemical repositories such as DrugBank (http://redpoll. pharmacy.ualberta.ca/drugbank/) [46], PubChem (http://pubchem.ncbi.nlm. nih.gov/), PDSP (http://pdsp.med.unc.edu/pdsp.php), ChemSpider (www. chemspider.com) [47,48], and others consist of target and small-molecule data that could be used for computational toxicology approaches. These may also be linked to pathway analysis tools or gene expression databases like the Connectivity Map. In the future we envisage that the pathway analysis tools will need to be integrated with other informatics tools in order to fully leverage their content and present the results to the user in a simple manner. Access to toxicology data within a pharmaceutical company is particularly difficult due to software validation, legal requirements, and the like, so efforts to leverage all available literature data from sources such as publications, databases, and patents would be particularly valuable. As described in some of the examples of this chapter, there have been some early efforts in this direction. But as yet the curation of such data is not straightforward and is highly context dependent.

A key issue will be, beside an integration of tools, the integration and federation of various data sources. One can imagine a data environment where all data from toxicogenomics to every biochemical assay around a compound is streamlined and easily accessible to the researcher. Having this kind of global molecule profile should make it possible to see all the differences among compounds in full detail and perhaps highlight ways to improve the compounds to ultimately get better drugs.

ACKNOWLEDGMENT

Peter Olinga is gratefully acknowledged for collaboration on network software comparison.

REFERENCES

1. Ekins S. *Computational toxicology: risk assessment for pharmaceutical and environmental chemicals*. Hoboken, NJ: Wiley, 2007.
2. LeCluyse E, Rowlands JC, eds. *Cross-species differences in receptor-mediated gene regulation*. Hoboken, NJ: Wiley, 2007.
3. LeCluyse EL. Pregnane X receptor: molecular basis for species differences in CYP3A induction by xenobiotics. *Chem Biol Interact* 2001;134:283–9.

4. LeCluyse EL. Human hepatocyte culture systems for the in vitro evaluation of cytochrome P450 expression and regulation. *Eur J Pharm Sci* 2001;13:343–68.

5. Ekins S, Kirillov E, Rakhmatulin E, Nikolskaya T. A novel method for visualizing nuclear hormone receptor networks relevant to drug metabolism. *Drug Metab Dispos* 2005;33:474–81.

6. Nikolsky Y, Ekins S, Nikolskaya T, Bugrim A. A novel method for generation of signature networks as biomarkers from complex high throughput data. *Tox Lett* 2005;158:20–9.

7. Rawlins MD. Cutting the cost of drug development? *Nat Rev* 2004;3:360–4.

8. FDA. *Innovation stagnation: challenge and opportunity on the critical path to new medicinal products*. Washington, DC: GPO. 2004.

9. Ekins S. In silico approaches to predicting metabolism, toxicology and beyond. *Biochem Soc Trans* 2003;31:611–14.

10. van de Waterbeemd H, Gifford E. ADMET in silico modelling: towards prediction paradise? *Nat Rev Drug Discov* 2003;2:192–204.

11. Whitebread S, Hamon J, Bojanic D, Urban L. Keynote review: in vitro safety pharmacology profiling: an essential tool for successful drug development. *Drug Discov Today* 2005;10:1421–33.

12. Ekins S, Boulanger B, Swaan PW, Hupcey MAZ. Towards a new age of virtual ADME/TOX and multidimensional drug discovery. *J Comput Aided Mol Des* 2002;16:381–401.

13. Bugrim A, Nikolskaya T, Nikolsky Y. Early prediction of drug metabolism and toxicity: systems biology approach and modeling. *Drug Discov Today* 2004;9: 127–35.

14. Navarro JD, Niranjan V, Peri S, Jonnalagadda CK, Pandey A. From biological databases to platforms for biomedical discovery. *Trends Biotechnol* 2003;21: 263–8.

15. Ekins S, Swaan PW. Computational models for enzymes, transporters, channels and receptors relevant to ADME/TOX. *Rev Comp Chem* 2004;20:333–415.

16. Akiyama TE, Gonzalez FJ. Regulation of P450 genes by liver-enriched transcription factors and nuclear receptors. *Biochim biophy acta* 2003;1619:223–34.

17. Goodwin B, Moore LB, Stoltz CM, McKee DD, Kliewer SA. Regulation of the human CYP2B6 gene by the nuclear pregnane X receptor. *Mol Pharmacol* 2001;60:427–31.

18. Staudinger J, Liu Y, Madan A, Habeebu S, Klaassen CD. Coordinate regulation of xenobiotic and bile acid homeostasis by pregnane X receptor. *Drug Metab Dispos Biol Fate Chem* 2001;29:1467–72.

19. Staudinger JL, Goodwin B, Jones SA, Hawkins-Brown D, MacKenzie KI, LaTour A, et al. The nuclear receptor PXR is a lithocholic acid sensor that protects against liver toxicity. *Proc Natl Acad Sci USA* 2001;98:3369–74.

20. Xie W, Barwick JL, Downes M, Blumberg B, Simon CM, Nelson MC, et al. Humanized xenobiotic response in mice expressing nuclear receptor SXR. *Nature* 2000;406:435–9.

21. Moore JT, Kliewer SA. Use of the nuclear receptor PXR to predict drug interactions. *Toxicology* 2000;153:1–10.

22. Waxman DJ. P450 gene induction by structurally diverse xenochemicals: central role of nuclear receptors CAR, PXR, and PPAR. *Arch Biochem Biophys* 1999;369:11–23.

23. Mankowski DC, Ekins S. Prediction of human drug metabolizing enzyme induction. *Curr Drug Metab* 2003;4:381–91.

24. Ulrich RG. The toxicogenomics of nuclear receptor agonists. *Curr Opin Chem Biol* 2003;7:505–10.

25. Ulrich RG, Rockett JC, Gibson GG, Pettit SD. Overview of an interlaboratory collaboration on evaluating the effects of model hepatotoxicants on hepatic gene expression. *Environ Health Perspect* 2004;112:423–7.

26. Sonoda J, Rosenfeld JM, Xu L, Evans RM, Xie W. A nuclear receptor-mediated xenobiotic response and its implication in drug metabolism and host protection. *Curr Drug Metab* 2003;4:59–72.

27. Tabb MM, Kholodovych V, Grun F, Zhou C, Welsh WJ, Blumberg B. Highly chlorinated PCBs inhibit the human xenobiotic response mediated by the steroid and xenobiotic receptor (SXR). *Environ Health Perspect* 2004;112: 163–9.

28. Sueyoshi T, Kawamato T, Zelko I, Honkakoski P, Negishi M. The repressed nuclear receptor CAR responds to phenobarbital in activating the human CYP2B6 gene. *J Biol Chem* 1999;274:6043–6.

29. Spink BC, Pang S, Pentecost BT, Spink DC. Induction of cytochrome P450 1B1 in MDA-MB-231 human breast cancer cells by non-ortho-substituted polychlorinated biphenyls. *Toxicol In vitro* 2002;16:695–704.

30. Mimura J, Fujii-Kuriyama Y. Functional role of the AhR in the expression of toxic effects by TCDD. *Biochim Biophys Acta* 2003;1619:263–8.

31. Hartley DP, Dai X, He YD, Carlini EJ, Wang B, Huskey SE, et al. Activators of the rat pregnane X receptor differentially modulate hepatic and intestinal gene expression. *Mol Pharmacol* 2004;65:1159–71.

32. Ekins S, Mirny L, Schuetz EG. A ligand-based approach to understanding selectivity of nuclear hormone receptors PXR, CAR, FXR, LXRa and LXRb. *Pharm Res* 2002;19:1788–800.

33. Xie W, Yeuh MF, Radominska-Pandya A, Saini SP, Negishi Y, Bottroff BS, et al. Control of steroid, heme, and carcinogen metabolism by nuclear pregnane X receptor and constitutive androstane receptor. *Proc Natl Acad Sci USA* 2003;100:4150–5.

34. Sahi J, Stern RH, Milad MA, Rose KA, Gibson G, Zheng X, et al. Effects of avasimibe on cytochrome P450 2C9 expression in vitro and in vivo. *Drug Metab Dispos Boil Fate Chem* 2004;32:1370–6.

35. Sahi J, Milad MA, Zheng X, Rose KA, Wang H, Stilgenbauer L, et al. Avasimibe induces CYP3A4 and multiple drug resistance protein 1 gene expression through activation of the pregnane X receptor. *J Pharmacol Exp Therapeut* 2003;306: 1027–34.

36. Cases M, Garcia-Serna R, Hettne K, Weeber M, van der Lei J, Boyer S, et al. Chemical and biological profiling of an annotated compound library directed to the nuclear receptor family. *Curr Topics Med Chem* 2005;5:763–72.

37. Mestres J, Couce-Martin L, Gregori-Puigjane E, Cases M, Boyer S. Ligand-based approach to in silico pharmacology: nuclear receptor profiling. *J Chem Info Model* 2006;46:2725–36.

38. Ekins S, Kirillov E, Rakhmatulin EA, Nikolskaya T. A novel method for visualizing nuclear hormone receptor networks relevant to drug metabolism. *Drug Metab Dispos Boil Fate Chem* 2005;33:474–81.

39. Apic G, Ignjatovic T, Boyer S, Russell RB. Illuminating drug discovery with biological pathways. *FEBS Lett* 2005;579:1872–7.

40. Barabasi A-L, Oltvai ZN. Network biology: understanding the cell's functional organization. *Nat Rev Genet* 2004;5:101–13.

41. Ekins S. Systems-ADME/Tox: resources and network approaches. *J Pharmacol Toxicol Meth* 2006;53:38–66.

42. Ekins S, Andreyev S, Ryabov A, Kirillov E, Rakhmatulin EA, Sorokina S, et al. A combined approach to drug metabolism and toxicity assessment. *Drug Metab Dispos Biol Fate Chem* 2006;34:495–503.

43. Ekins S, Bugrim A, Nikolsky Y, Nikolskaya T. Systems biology: applications in drug discovery. In: Gad SC, ed. *Drug discovery handbook*. New York: Wiley, 2005. p. 123–83.

44. Ekins S, Nikolsky Y, Bugrim A, Kirillov E, Nikolskaya T. Pathway mapping tools for analysis of high content data. *Meth Mol Biol* 2007;356:319–50.

45. Olinga P, Ekins S, Elferink MGL, Bauerschmidt S, Polman J, Schoonen WGEJ, et al. Gene network analysis of acetaminophen and carbon tetrachloride treated rat liver slices identifies hepatotoxicity mechanisms observed in vivo. *Drug Metab Rev* 2007;39: S1. pages 1–388.

46. Wishart DS, Knox C, Guo AC, Shrivastava S, Hassanali M, Stothard P, et al. DrugBank: a comprehensive resource for in silico drug discovery and exploration. *Nucleic Acids Res* 2006;34:D668–72.

47. Roth BL, Lopez E, Beischel S, Westkaemper RB, Evans JM. Screening the receptorome to discover the molecular targets for plant-derived psychoactive compounds: a novel approach for CNS drug discovery. *Pharmacol Ther* 2004;102:99–110.

48. Strachan RT, Ferrara G, Roth BL. Screening the receptorome: an efficient approach for drug discovery and target validation. *Drug Discov Today* 2006;11: 708–16.

49. O'Connor KA, Roth BL. Finding new tricks for old drugs: an efficient route for public-sector drug discovery. *Nat Rev* 2005;4:1005–14.

50. Mao B, Gozalbes R, Barbosa F, Migeon J, Merrick S, Kamm K, et al. QSAR modeling of in vitro inhibition of cytochrome P450 3A4. *J Chem Info Model* 2006;46:2125–34.

51. Oliver DE, Rubin DL, Stuart JM, Hewett M, Klein TE, Altman RB. Ontology development for a pharmacogenetics knowledge base. *Pac Symp Biocomp* 2002:88–99.

52. Nakata K, Yukawa M, Komiyama N, Nakano T, Kaminuma T. A nuclear receptor database that maps pathways to diseases. *Genome Infomat* 2002;13: 515–16.

53. Yan Q, Sadee W. Human membrane transporter database: a Web-accessible relational database for drug transport studies and pharmacogenomics. *AAPS Pharmsci* 2000;2:E20.

54. Sun LZ, Ji ZL, Chen X, Wang JF, Chen YZ. ADME-AP: a datbase of ADME associated proteins. *Bioinformatics* 2002;18:1699–700.

55. Ganter B, Tugendreich S, Pearson CI, Ayanoglu E, Baumhueter S, Bostian KA, et al. Development of a large-scale chemogenomics database to improve drug candidate selection and to understand mechanisms of chemical toxicity and action. *J Biotechnol* 2005;119:219–44.

56. Castle AL, Carver MP, Mendrick DL. Toxicogenomics: a new revolution in drug safety. *Drug Discov Today* 2002;7:728–36.

57. Tong W, Cao X, Harris S, Sun H, Fang H, Fuscoe J, et al. Arraytrack—supporting toxicogenomic research at the U.S. Food and Drug Administration National Center for Toxicological Research. *Environ Health Perspect* 2003;111:1819–26.

58. Thomas RS, Rank DR, Penn SG, Zastrow GM, Hayes KR, Pande K, et al. Identification of toxicologically predictive gene sets using cDNA microarrays. *Mol Pharmacol* 2001;60:1189–94.

59. Hieronymus H, Lamb J, Ross KN, Peng XP, Clement C, Rodina A, et al. Gene expression signature-based chemical genomic prediction identifies a novel class of HSP90 pathway modulators. *Cancer Cell* 2006;10:321–30.

60. Lamb J, Crawford ED, Peck D, Modell JW, Blat IC, Wrobel MJ, et al. The connectivity map: using gene-expression signatures to connect small molecules, genes, and disease. *Science* 2006;313:1929–35.

61. Wei G, Twomey D, Lamb J, Schlis K, Agarwal J, Stam RW, et al. Gene expression-based chemical genomics identifies rapamycin as a modulator of MCL1 and glucocorticoid resistance. *Cancer Cell* 2006;10:331–42.

62. Hackett JL, Lesko LJ. Microarray data- the US FDA, industry and academia. *Nat Biotechnol* 2003;21:742–3.

63. Cheng A, Dixon SL. In silico models for the prediction of dose-dependent human hepatotoxicity. *J Comput Aid Mol Des* 2003;17:811–23.

64. Clark RD, Wolohan PR, Hodgkin EE, Kelly JH, Sussman NL. Modelling in vitro hepatotoxicity using molecular interaction fields and SIMCA. *J Mol Graph Model* 2004;22:487–97.

65. Greene N. Computer systems for the prediction of toxicity: an update. *Adv Drug Del Rev* 2002;54:417–31.

66. Lewis DFV. *Cytochromes P450*. Bristol: Taylor and Francis, 1996.

67. Sharan R, Ideker T. Modeling cellular machinery through biological network comparison. *Nat Biotechnol* 2006;24:427–33.

68. Cheng A, Diller DJ, Dixon SL, Egan WJ, Lauri G, Merz KM Jr. Computation of the physico-chemical properties and data mining of large molecular collections. *J Comput Chem* 2002;23:172–83.

69. Wang N, DeLisle RK, Diller DJ. Fast small molecule similarity searching with multiple alignment profiles of molecules represented in one-dimension. *J Med Chem* 2005;48:6980–90.

70. Wernicke S, Rasche F. Simple and fast alignment of metabolic pathways by exploiting local diversity. *Bioinformatics* 2007;23:1978–85.

71. Wishart DS, Tzur D, Knox C, Eisner R, Guo AC, Young N, et al. HMDB: the Human Metabolome Database. *Nucleic Acids Res* 2007;35:D521–6.

72. Ekins S, Berbaum J, Harrison RK. Generation and validation of rapid computational filters for CYP2D6 and CYP3A4. *Drug Metab Dispos Biol Fate Chem* 2003;31:1077–80.

73. Young SS, Gombar VK, Emptage MR, Cariello NF, Lambert C. Mixture deconvolution and analysis of Ames mutagenicity data. *Chemo Intell Lab Sys* 2002;60: 5–11.

74. Young SS, Ekins S, Lambert C. So many targets, so many compounds, but so few resources. *Curr Drug Discov* 2002;December:17–22.

75. Csermely P, Agoston V, Pongor S. The efficiency of multi-target drugs: the network approach might help drug design. *Trends Pharmacol Sci* 2005;26:178–82.

76. Kauvar LM, Higgins DL, Villar HO, Sportsman JR, Engqvist-Goldstein A, Bukar R, et al. Predicting ligand binding to proteins by affinity fingerprinting. *Chem Biol* 1995;2:107–18.

77. Kauvar LM, Laborde E. The diversity challenge in combinatorial chemistry. *Curr Opin Drug Discov Dev* 1998;1:66–70.

78. Kauvar LM, Villar HO, Sportsman JR, Higgins DL, Schmidt DEJ. Protein affinity map of chemical space. *J Chromatog B* 1998;715:93–102.

79. Fliri AF, Loging WT, Thadeio PF, Volkmann RA. Biological spectra analysis: Linking biological activity profiles to molecular structure. *Proc Natl Acad Sci USA* 2005;102:261–6.

80. Fliri AF, Loging WT, Thadeio PF, Volkmann RA. Biospectra analysis: model proteome characterizations for linking molecular structure and biological response. *J Med Chem* 2005;48:6918–25.

81. Fliri AF, Loging WT, Thadeio PF, Volkmann RA. Analysis of drug-induced effect patterns to link structure and side effects of medicines. *Nat Chem Biol* 2005;1:389–97.

82. Paolini GV, Shapland RH, van Hoorn WP, Mason JS, Hopkins AL. Global mapping of pharmacological space. *Nat Biotechnol* 2006;24:805–15.

83. Yildirim MA, Goh KI, Cusick ME, Barabasi AL, Vidal M. Drug-target network. *Nat Biotechnol* 2007;25:1119–26.

84. Keiser MJ, Roth BL, Armbruster BN, Ernsberger P, Irwin JJ, Shoichet BK. Relating protein pharmacology by ligand chemistry. *Nat Biotechnol* 2007;25: 197–206.

85. Niwa T. Prediction of biological targets using probabilistic neural networks and atom-type descriptors. *J Med Chem* 2004;47:2645–50.

86. Lepp Z, Kinoshita T, Chuman H. Screening for new antidepressant leads of multiple activities by support vector machines. *J Chem Info Model* 2006;46: 158–67.

87. Hert J, Willett P, Wilton DJ, Acklin P, Azzaoui K, Jacoby E, et al. Comparison of fingerprint-based methods for virtual screening using multiple bioactive reference structures. *J Chem Info Comput Sci* 2004;44:1177–85.

88. Bender A, Scheiber J, Glick M, Davies JW, Azzaoui K, Hamon J, et al. Analysis of pharmacology data and the prediction of adverse drug reactions and off-target effects from chemical structure. *ChemMedChem* 2007;2:861–73.

89. Azzaoui K, Hamon J, Faller B, Whitebread S, Jacoby E, Bender A, et al. Modeling promiscuity based on in vitro safety pharmacology profiling data. *ChemMed-Chem* 2007;2:874–80.

90. Ji ZL, Wang Y, Yu L, Han LY, Zheng CJ, Chen YZ. In silico search of putative adverse drug reaction related proteins as a potential tool for facilitating drug adverse effect prediction. *Toxicol Lett* 2006;164:104–12.

91. Xie L, Bourne PE. A robust and efficient algorithm for the shape description of protein structures and its application in predicting ligand binding sites. *BMC Bioinform* 2007;8(suppl 4):S9.

92. Bredel M, Jacoby E. Chemogenomics: an emerging strategy for rapid target and drug discovery. *Nat Rev* 2004;5:262–75.

93. Chong CR, Chen X, Shi L, Liu JO, Sullivan DJ, Jr. A clinical drug library screen identifies astemizole as an antimalarial agent. *Nat Chem Biol* 2006;2:415–16.

94. Chong CR, Xu J, Lu J, Bhat S, Sullivan DJ, Jr., Liu JO. Inhibition of angiogenesis by the antifungal drug itraconazole. *ACS Chem Biol* 2007;2:263–70.

7

COMPUTATIONAL SYSTEMS BIOLOGY MODELING OF DOSIMETRY AND CELLULAR RESPONSE PATHWAYS

QIANG ZHANG, YU-MEI TAN, SUDIN BHATTACHARYA, AND MELVIN E. ANDERSEN

Contents

7.1 INTRODUCTION

A major goal of toxicological and human health risk research is to obtain accurate dose–response relationships between the exposure levels of environmental chemicals or pharmaceutical drugs and the magnitude of

Drug Efficacy, Safety, and Biologics Discovery: Emerging Technologies and Tools,
Edited by Sean Ekins and Jinghai J. Xu
Copyright © 2009 by John Wiley & Sons, Inc.

disruptions associated with various biological endpoints. Such quantitative descriptions of the cause–effect relationships will not only assist regulatory agencies in establishing safety guidelines for drug adverse effects and chemical exposures but also in predicting and evaluating confidently the potential health risk imposed on human populations under varied exposure scenarios.

Dose–response curves delineating various adverse effects at multiple levels of biological organization can be obtained experimentally or from well-documented clinical experiments and occupational or accidental exposures. These dose–response curves alone, however, are often insufficient for regulatory and risk assessment purposes. Frequently they do not cover the full range of exposure, especially in the low-dose area, which is the more environmentally and occupationally relevant region for human exposure. In most circumstances risks in the low-dose area have to be estimated by extrapolating from high-dose data using linear assumptions with or without threshold consideration. Despite its simplicity and widespread usage, this default extrapolation scheme receives increasing challenges from other empirical or hypothetical alternatives including hormesis, in which nonlinearity and nonmonotonicity dominates the low-dose region [1]. Regardless of the type of extrapolation performed, reliable and accurate predictions made for low-dose risk require sufficient understanding of the mechanistic underpinnings that mediate the adverse responses throughout the full dose range. To this end a mathematical modeling approach is often required. A computational model implementing the correct biological mechanism, and adequately validated with high-dose experimental data, can reliably predict the low-dose effect, which a priori is unknown or uncertain. A second reason arguing for a modeling approach in risk assessment is that the dose–response curves obtained experimentally only represent a small set of simple exposure scenarios. In contrast, realistic exposure can be complex as exposure levels vary in time and space, and many chemicals and drugs co-exist as a mixture. Since it is unlikely for experiments to be able to reproduce these exposure situations exactly, and impractical to design experiments to test all the possibilities exhaustively, assessing the adverse effects and hazards brought about by these complex situations ultimately depends on mechanistically based modeling approaches.

Evaluating dose–response relationship using a modeling approach consists of two basic components: pharmacokinetic (PK) and pharmacodynamic (PD) modeling. Environmental chemicals and therapeutic drugs entering the human body via various routes are first metabolized and converted into inactive or active metabolites. Tissue or cellular exposure to the chemicals and their major metabolites are functions of time determined by the pharmacokinetics and dosing paradigm. This dosimetric relationship between exposure dose and tissue dose, containing time and space variables, can be captured by physiologically based pharmacokinetic (PBPK) models [2]. Once the tissue dose is known, the biological impacts of the chemicals on the target cells, tissues, and organs can be assessed by physiologically based pharmacodynamic (PBPD) models. Integration of PBPK and PBPD modeling provides a powerful tool to quantitatively evaluate human health risk for various exposure paradigms.

A major obstacle hindering a wide adoption of this modeling approach has been the absence of adequate knowledge of the intracellular signaling networks that mediate the disrupting effects of a chemical. In the past decade, a new wave of technology in the areas of genome-wide functional screening, bioinformatics tools, and network mapping, has motivated reverse-engineering of biological networks at molecular and cellular levels with increased resolution, and identified the molecular targets for many environmental chemicals. However, the behavior of these networks, spanning multiple cellular compartments and executing various biological functions, can only be understood fully with the aid of computational models. Computational systems biology is an emerging interdisciplinary science that obtains and organizes large-scale experimental data to develop mechanistically based systems-level models of biological networks, and studies the network behaviors and their implications for biological functions.

7.2 PHYSIOLOGICALLY BASED PHARMACOKINETIC MODELING

PBPK modeling was developed by chemical engineers, primarily by Kenneth Bischoff [3] and Robert Dedrick [4], and was first applied to environmental health and pharmaceutical research. As part of a systems approach, PBPK modeling has been used broadly over the past 25 years to assess tissue dose in relation to administered dose for a wide variety of human health risk-related chemicals and therapeutic drugs. The process of developing a PBPK model for dose–response assessment starts with identifying adverse or toxic effects of the chemical of interest in animals and humans. Available experimental and clinical data are then evaluated for the metabolism, pharmacokinetics, and mode of action of the parent compound and its metabolites. Mode of action is the sequence of events by which the active form of the chemical interacts with the tissue and leads to adverse responses. Next a PBPK model is developed by describing the body as compartments that correspond to separate tissues or groups of similar tissues with appropriate volumes and blood flows. The process of model development is iterative—the model structure and parameters are refined and tested repeatedly until the model is capable of fitting the entire suite of experimental observations (Figure 7.1). The refined model is used to estimate tissue dose and human health risk based on the assumption that similar tissue response arises from equivalent target tissue dose across species.

When performing dose–response assessment using the equivalent-dose approach, one key element that determines the relevance of a particular toxic endpoint in animal to human health is mode of action. Information on mode

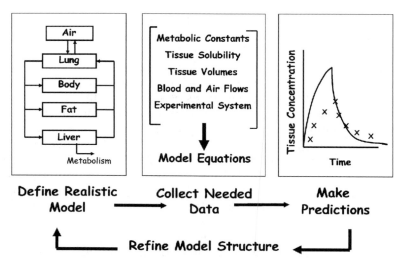

Figure 7.1 Iterative process of PBPK model development.

of action is also critical for describing tissue dosimetry with a PBPK model. For example, the carcinogenicity of vinyl chloride is mediated by its reactive metabolites that enhance mutagenicity by reacting with DNA. Thus the PBPK model for vinyl chloride describes metabolism of the compound in liver by two saturable pathways to predict both total metabolism and glutathione depletion [5]. Chloroform, on the other hand, promotes tumorigenesis through a nongenotoxic mode of action. Reactive metabolites of chloroform induce cytotoxic and regenerative cell proliferation that leads to tumor formation. The PBPK model for chloroform incorporates this mode of action to predict cell killing resulting from the covalent binding of chloroform metabolites to macromolecules [6]. The use of PBPK modeling makes it possible to evaluate a nonlinear mode of action in a quantitative manner.

PBPK modeling integrates diverse information from chemistry, biochemistry, and physiology to simulate tissue dose over a wide variety of exposure conditions. It is capable of supporting extrapolations in the following aspects: high doses to low doses; route-to-route (e.g., inhalation, oral, dermal); across classes of chemicals; in vitro to in vivo; and between species. Scaling up animal data to estimate human health risk or to develop rational clinical protocols is the ultimate goal of PBPK modeling. Applying PBPK modeling to dose–response assessment reduces uncertainty, since model uncertainty and sensitivity can be assessed, identified, and quantified in the process of organizing model parameters [7]. In a sense, PBPK modeling can be viewed as an example of a systems approach at the level of cells, tissues, organs, and organisms to determine the systemic disposition of chemicals. It will remain as an important front-end for modeling cellular responses in dose–response assessment.

7.3 PHYSIOLOGICALLY BASED PHARMACODYNAMIC MODELING

PBPK modeling in conjunction with experimental measurement establishes tissue-level concentrations of xenobiotics and their major metabolites, which are a prerequisite for further quantifying the hazardous effects occurring in the cell. Chemicals and their active metabolites exert adverse effects either by cellular reactivity to cause structural damage to critical cellular constituents and signaling molecules, as with many oxidative chemical stressors, or by interacting with specific molecular targets to enhance or suppress their functions, as with most pharmaceutical compounds. In many circumstances a chemical will act on multiple yet distinct intracellular sites to simultaneously affect more than one biological process. Furthermore the cellular impact brought about by chemical stressors rarely remains at the original sites of interaction, since the perturbed molecular components are invariably embedded in large signaling networks that are interweaved with others to form even larger networks. The initial local disruption can propagate through the networks to affect multiple biological functions. Thus the biological consequences of a chemical cannot be fully assessed by merely examining the initial impingement. Rather, the impact must be evaluated in the context of biological networks, whose systems-level behavior can be different from those of the individual components comprising the networks. For example, if a component embedded in a molecular feedback loop is affected by a chemical, both upstream and downstream components will be affected. As a result the property of the feedback circuit as a whole becomes altered. In such situations or those that are more complicated, a qualitative description of tissue response to chemical disruption is usually inadequate to address the risk issue. Nonlinearities and complex dynamics arising from these networks, which are often beyond intuitive comprehension based on simple logical reasoning, can only be fully captured by exploiting mathematical models.

The early need for PD modeling has been addressed by biologically based dose–response (BBDR) models that capture the dose–response relationship in an empirical way, and have been capable of reproducing and even predicting adverse biological effects for a variety of chemical exposures [8–10]. However, a significant drawback of these models is the lack of sufficient biological details about the operating mechanisms underlying pathway disruption by chemicals. Due to the large degree of empiricism, BBDR models lack the flexibility to readily scale to different exposure scenarios, including varied dosing paradigms and mixed exposures targeting the same biological process but at different sites. The integration of multiple BBDR models is difficult, if not impossible, since the lack of biological details makes it challenging to locate cross-talking nodal points that will couple the different models.

The focus on BBDR models was due largely to the void of knowledge in the molecular pathways and networks initiating the adverse effects of chemicals. In the past decades, however, the emerging high-throughput, high-content technologies spanning areas of genomics, proteomics, and metabonomics have accelerated the process of identifying the molecular components and interconnections comprising the intracellular signaling networks. Although we are still far from completely mapping these networks and understanding their specific regulatory functions, the increased resolution has enabled significant advances in computational modeling approaches for cellular response pathways. Mechanistically based biological models have proven to be insightful both qualitatively and quantitatively for understanding systems-level behaviors [11,12].

7.4 COMPONENTS OF COMPUTATIONAL SYSTEMS BIOLOGY

The systems approach for predicting dose–response relationships at the cell, tissue, and organism levels is an iterative process involving cycled interactions between laboratory experiments and in silico simulations. It typically consists of the following interactive steps, although in practice these steps may not always be as well delineated as described here (Figure 7.2).

1. *Conceptualization.* The objective of this initial step is to identify intracellular or extracellular chemical target sites and biological networks/processes that are perturbed by the chemicals. It starts with an initial thorough literature search, followed by targeted laboratory experiments, if necessary, to complement the existing knowledge about the target sites and cellular networks affected. As mentioned above, high-content "omics" experiments with gain of function and loss of function manipulation of the biological system [13,14], are efficient ways of identifying the intracellular pathways and their constituents perturbed by the chemicals. This system-oriented approach can also suggest pathway components and gene regulatory networks not known previously. This step, primarily involving experimental biologists, generates a directed graph-like connection or network map—a conceptual model that lays out the backbone structure of the intracellular pathways and networks most significantly affected by the studied chemical (Figure 7.3*a*).

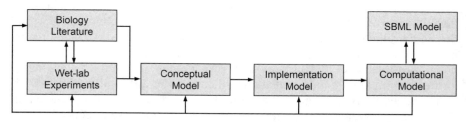

Figure 7.2 Iterative process of PBPD model development.

a.

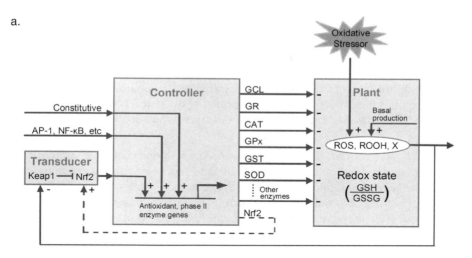

b.

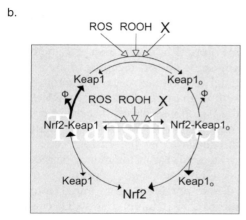

Figure 7.3 (*a*) A conceptual model for the Nrf2-mediated adaptive response to oxidative stress. It consists of three distinct functional modules—a stress-sensing transducer module consisting of Keap1 and Nrf2, a controller module consisting of basal and Nrf2-driven gene expression of anti-oxidant and phase II enzymes, and a biochemical plant module consisting of relevant metabolic reactions catalyzed by antioxidant and phase II enzymes, which remove reactive oxygen species (ROS), peroxides (ROOH), and electrophiles (X). (*b*) An implementation model for the Keap1-Nrf2 transducer module.

2. *Implementation.* With the conceptual model, experimental biologists and computational biologists then need to work together to determine the details of molecular interactions and biochemical reactions to be explicitly modeled (Figure 7.3*b*). The resulting implementation model will include all the molecular processes implied in the conceptual model and deemed

necessary to be modeled, the parameter values obtained experimentally or assumed, and the flow rates governing each reaction.

3. *Computation.* The implementation model is then coded in a programming language to generate the computational model, which is essentially an executable computer program residing in a simulation environment. Modern modeling tools are able to automatically generate the computational model from an implementation model developed with the same tools [15].

4. *Model calibration and validation.* Newly constructed computational models need to be tuned both structurally and parametrically to accommodate available experimental data. These data include time-course studies and dose responses obtained under control and various manipulated conditions. Provided that the experimental data are reliable, there are two possible outcomes after model tuning. One is that there is no single parameter set in the biologically reasonable range that can reproduce the experimental results properly. Should this occur, a minor structural adjustment within the scope of existing knowledge, at either the conceptual or implementation level, may be necessary to arrive at an initial parameter suite. For example, if the first version of a model simulating steroid hormone receptor mediated gene expression is constructed with omission of receptor dimerization for simplicity, the inability of the model to fit a sharp experimental dose–response curve may justify the inclusion of the dimerization step, which can in theory increase the steepness of dose–response curve. In certain circumstances similar minor modifications may be inadequate to recapitulate the experimental result. This failure would suggest that the current conceptual model is incomplete or incorrect. Major structural adjustment may be required to incorporate pathways initially neglected or ones that are yet to be discovered by additional experiments. The second possibility from initial tuning of the model is that there may exist one or more parameter sets that can give rise to reasonable fits to experimental data. This consequence suggests that the structure of the model in its current form may be correct, and the number of parameter sets will be further pruned as new experimental data become available.

5. *Prediction.* The model developed through the first four steps can now be used to generate theoretical predictions for new exposure conditions. To the extent possible, these predictions need to be verified by experiments to further test the validity of the model. If the new experimental data agree with model prediction, the value and reliability of the model for risk assessment is further solidified, and confidence is gained in the predictive power of the model for exposure situations that are not experimentally accessible. If the experimental data do not agree with the model prediction, procedures similar to those described in step 4 would again be followed, using the data as a new training set to further refine the model. Such model refinement is often based

on in vitro or animal experiments. For these models to be useful for human health risk assessment, model translation has to be done to incorporate relevant known differences between in vivo and in vitro conditions, and between human and the modeled animal.

Modern modeling tools are able to export and import biological models through the systems biology markup language (SBML) [16]. This universal markup language greatly expedites model exchange between biological researchers who often use different simulation programs. In addition SBML facilitates model integration, a process that required laborious manual work in the past.

7.5   MODELING THE DOSE–RESPONSE RELATIONSHIP— SIGNIFICANCE OF THE INDIVIDUAL CELL

A common assumption in most experiments is that the averaged mRNA or protein level changes in a population of cells, obtained with bulk assays, are representative of the behavior of each individual cell in that population. This logic has been fundamental to the current degree of success in biological research. However, the behavior of individual cells in an isogenic cell population is often very heterogeneous [17,18]. Gene expression in many cells, in response to physiological or xenobiotic stimuli, can occur in a binary, all-or-none fashion, contrasting with the continuous changes observed with bulk assays such as Northern and Western blots [19,20]. This quantal nature is more prominent with higher level biological responses, including cell division, differentiation, and apoptosis. It is likely that combinations of binary expression of suites of genes may dictate these discrete cellular fates.

With respect to gene expression, smooth dose–response curves at the population level can be achieved in two different ways (Figure 7.4). In a graded fashion, gene expression in individual cells is continuous and increases with higher inducer doses. For this response mode the behavior of individual cells is comparable to that assayed at the population level. In a binary fashion, gene expression in individual cells is all-or-none: only the percentage of cells fully expressing the gene increases in response to higher doses. For this binary mode the behavior of individual cells could be completely different from that assayed at the population level. Since a large part of mechanistic modeling is to simulate the biochemical networks in single cells, models need to be constructed to reproduce single cell behavior rather than the population average. If a computational model representing the behavior of a cell reproduces the experimental dose response obtained at the population level, while gene expression in individual cells actually proceeds in an all-or-none manner, then the model is mechanistically incorrect, and may lead to erroneous predictions.

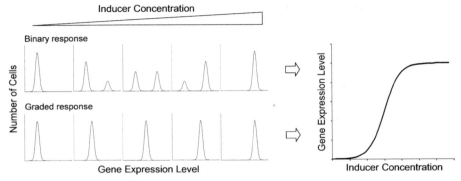

Figure 7.4 Binary and graded mode of gene expression in individual cells. In a binary response, gene expression in an individual cell is either fully induced or uninduced. Two cell populations exist accordingly, and the relative numbers of cells in each population vary as inducer concentration increases. In a graded response, only one cell population exists, gene expression in individual cells is induced at continuously higher levels as inducer concentration increases. Regardless of the response mode, dose responses at the entire population level can be similarly graded.

It is becoming increasingly apparent that studies of pathways and pathway perturbation by chemicals need to focus on responses of individual cells. To this end, the current technologies include microscopy, flow cytometry, and recently, optical fiber well arrays, which allows uninterrupted simultaneous monitoring of gene expression in multiple individual cells [21,22].

With respect to all-or-none type of gene expression in individual cells, at least two mechanisms may explain the binary phenomenon: stochastic gene activation [18,23,24] and switch-like molecular circuit [25,26]. The stochastic view holds that the promoter of a gene template can assume only one of two discrete transcriptional states, active or inactive. Transitions between the two states are random events, and transcription factors (TF) regulate the probability with which the transitions occur. In this operating mode, gene expression in individual cells is likely to be all-or-none for conditions when the downstream mRNA and protein are degraded at a faster rate than promoter transitions. At the cell population level, however, the dose–response curve can still be graded, since proportionally more cells are recruited to express the gene as the inducer concentration increases.

For the switch-like mechanism often an all-or-none type of molecular circuit with a threshold exists between the inducer and TF, while the gene template itself can transcribe at continuously varying levels. Graded inducer concentrations are converted to an all-or-none type of response at the TF level, rendering a binary mode of gene expression in the cell. The shape of the dose–response curve at the population level can vary, however, depending on the degree of cell-to-cell variation in the threshold and/or inducer concentrations [27,28].

Notably, in a homogeneous cell population, where concentrations of the inducer or threshold values do not differ much, the dose–response curve at the population level is also switch-like because most cells switch gene expression on or off at about the same threshold inducer concentrations. In contrast, if the inducer concentrations and/or threshold values have a broad distribution among cells, a more graded dose–response relationship will be observed as incrementally more cells are activated in response to increasing inducer concentrations. Cell-to-cell variation in threshold values can result from variations in the abundance of the molecular components comprising the switch circuit. Concentrations of proteins can also fluctuate considerably over time and vary significantly between cells, due to intrinsic and extrinsic noise in gene expression [29].

It is important to differentiate the two mechanisms of binary gene regulation, not only for the purpose of implementing the correct biology in the model. From a technical perspective, random binary gene activation requires a stochastic simulation algorithm, whereas for a switch-like circuit a deterministic method is often adequate.

7.6 NONLINEAR DOSE–RESPONSE RELATIONSHIPS

Although regulatory agencies, including the US EPA, have largely adopted a low-dose linear assumption for carcinogens and presumed thresholds with multiple uncertainty factors for most noncancer responses, in the real world, the dose–response relationship between a chemical and its adverse biological consequences often follows a nonlinear fashion, and in many cases it is even nonmonotonic [30]. At cell and tissue levels, where chemicals and their major metabolites interact with endogenous molecular targets, nonlinear signaling is commonplace. One major form of nonlinearity is ultrasensitivity, which is operationally defined as dose responses that are more sensitive than a hyperbolic, Michaelis–Menten form. Within a defined range of an ultrasensitive dose–response curve, the change in the input dose causes a greater percentage change in the output response. Ultrasensitivity is ubiquitous in signaling pathways in the cell, serving a basic amplifier function during the course of signal propagation. Extreme ultrasensitivity, arising from a switch-like circuit, may mediate binary decision making such as proliferation, differentiation, survival, and apoptosis [28]. In many cases ultrasensitive circuits are part of a larger network capable of multi-stability and oscillation, and so on.

Several arrangements of signaling modules can give rise to ultrasensitivity. One form is multiple inputs by the same signal affecting a common response. In the case of MAP kinase activation an upper level kinase dual-phosphorylates the immediate downstream kinase in two separate collisions rather than one. In this distributive process the appropriate choice of the reaction kinetics such as K_m values can give rise to mild ultrasensitivity in the absence of conditions for zero-order ultrasensitivity [31]. Positive cooperative binding is another form of multiple inputs, in which a receptor can bind with several ligand molecules with increasing affinities for sequential binding. Homo-dimerization, as occuring with steroid hormone receptors, can also be categorized as a special form of multiple inputs, which effectively increases the Hill coefficient of the dose–response curve.

A second source of ultrasensitivity is zero-order reactions discovered by Goldbeter [32]. In its classical form zero-order ultrasensitivity occurs with a pair of coupled enzymatic reactions that interconvert a protein between two different forms (e.g., phosphorylated vs. dephosphorylated), and at least one of the two converting enzymes operates close to saturation by its substrate. Zero-order ultrasensitivity may occur in different variations embedded in a larger molecular circuit, which may not be immediately recognized.

Positive feedback, a common arrangement of biochemical networks, can also produce ultrasensitivity and may exhibit bistability under certain conditions. Kinetically, biological positive feedback loops can be either fast or slow, depending on the type of biochemical reactions involved. A fast loop that turns on activation promptly but is subject to fluctuation due to signaling noise, is less robust; a slow loop that turns on activation in a more delayed manner, but can better resist fluctuation, is more robust [33].

It appears that cells often exploit different forms of ultrasensitive circuits in various combinations to achieve the desired signaling properties that cannot be realized otherwise, and simultaneously these impose less biophysical and biochemical strain on individual ultrasensitive variants. For example, the MAP kinase signaling in 3T3 fibroblasts utilizes multistep phosphorylation, zero-order sensitivity, stacked cascade, as well as positive feedback to achieve both switch-like signal transduction and bistability [11].

Another important consideration in dose–response modeling is the idea of nonmonotonicity. Largely two mechanisms have been proposed to explain nonmonotonicity. In one mechanism, a chemical regulates a biological response through two separate pathways. The two pathways have opposite influences and differ in their sensitivity to the chemical. The adenosine analog phenyl-isopropyladenosine (PIA) regulates the activity of adenylyl cyclase (AC) with a U-shaped dose–response relationship in the striatum [34]. This is because PIA inhibits AC activity through the A1 adenosine receptor and activates it through the A2 receptor, while the former has a higher affinity for PIA than the latter does. A second mechanism behind nonmonotonicity is related to overcompensation for cellular perturbation in an adaptive response mediated via negative feedback. To maintain a homeostatic intracellular environment, cells are often equipped with complex negative feedback networks to cope with perturbations caused by physical or chemical stressors. The feedback action is usually carried out by activation of a suite of genes that are responsible for counteracting the perturbation to regain homeostasis [35]. Transcription-mediated adaptive response is a common defensive scheme for a variety of cellular stresses, including radiation-induced DNA damage, oxidative stress, and heat shock [36–38]. Depending on the strength of the negative feedback, a low-level stress may cause the system to overreact by activating gene expression in excess, leading to overcorrection of the perturbed state. In oxidative stress response, exposure to oxidative stressors initially causes a decrease in reduced glutathione (GSH), a crucial intracellular antioxidant non-protein thiol. However, the oxidative stressor also up-regulates gene expression of glutamylcysteine ligase (GCL), the rate-limiting enzyme for de novo GSH synthesis. Increased expression of GCL accelerates GSH production and replenishes the diminished GSH pool over time. This replenishment can lead to GSH concentrations greater than present in the basal condition (Figure 7.5a). Nevertheless, further increases in the strength of the stress consume more GSH than can be compensated for through overexpression of GCL, resulting in GSH depletion, and pushing the cell from an adaptive state to stressed state. As shown in Figure 7.5b, a bell-shaped dose–response curve between the intensity of oxidative stress and GSH concentration can appear, once the gene induction of GCL is fully engaged.

The organization of the molecular components in any biological network can take on very complex pathway structures. Even with a small set of components, different combinations of possible interactions and kinetics can generate network behaviors surpassing immediate recognition and comprehension. The complex behavior of cellular dynamics such as multistability, oscillation, and frequency selection have all been observed in various cellular systems [39–41]. These diverse properties undoubtedly play significant roles

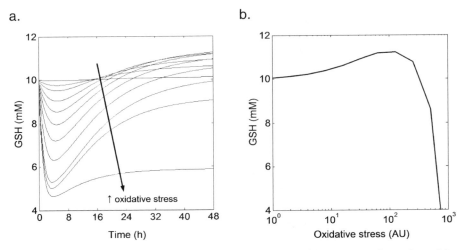

Figure 7.5 Computer-simulated results for intracellular GSH content from the oxidative stress–response model shown in Figure 3.3. (a) The temporal changes in GSH content in response to varied levels of oxidative stress. (b) The dose response of GSH compared with the level of oxidative stress. AU: arbitrary unit.

in accounting for the adverse effects of many xenobiotics. To capture and understand these basic biological properties and to assist in analyzing results from the laboratory bench, we have to rely increasingly on mathematically modeling approaches.

7.7 MODULARIZATION IN COMPUTATIONAL MODELS

Mechanistic modeling of signaling pathways and gene regulatory networks for the purpose of human health risk evaluation inevitably implies that as we gain more knowledge about the molecular details of the biological processes mediating the adverse effects of xenobiotics, the corresponding models developed will become increasingly large and complex. Additionally, with increasing use of PBPK, BBDR, and computational systems biology models of cellular signaling pathways, model management and computational standardization will become important. Prior to requiring specific rules for model simplification and parsimonious design, a systematic strategy should be in place at the very beginning of model development. This strategy should ease the processes of model construction, modification, and expansion in the life cycle of model development. We foresee that rather than constructing models as a single inseparable entity, large-scale models need to be partitioned and modularized at the early stage of design, and built up using a bottom-up approach.

In the field of computer science, programming practice has evolved from procedural languages to the current object-oriented (OO) languages. The key characteristic of OO design is the existence of class libraries that host sets of predefined objects and functions. Programmers only need to know what an object/function can do and the input/output (I/O) interface, and are less concerned with implementation details encapsulated beneath the interface. With class libraries, programming practice largely involves building new classes using predefined objects and functions.

The hierarchical building scheme and avoidance of repeated coding in computer programming can be equally applied to modeling large-scale biological networks. Sets of molecular components and interactions can be organized to form pre-built functional modules with distinct signal transduction and control properties. These modules can then be linked through interfaces to constitute large biological networks displaying desired systems-level behavior. These modules are likely to be recurring signaling or regulatory motifs that are frequently used by cells for signal transduction and gene regulation [41]. For example, NF-κB activation by IKK, the MAP kinase cascade, and the NMDA receptor-mediated Ca^{2+} influx are all within the scope of biochemical interactions or reactions that can be pre-built as signaling modules. A module may exist in several variants, each equipped with a set of parameter values that affords the variant a characteristic I/O or dose–response relationship. Certain important regulatory elements in the module can be also interfaced as controls, which can modify the I/O behavior of the module.

Figure 7.6 gives two examples of functional modules. In the module of the MAP kinase cascade there is an ultrasensitive relationship under certain parameter conditions between the input small G protein Ras and the output dual-phosphorylated ERK. The module also has two control points at the interface including phosphatase PP2A and MKP. Manipulating the amount of the phosphatase can transform the module from an ultrasensitive switch to a graded relay station [11,42]. Another module example is a generic gene induction module. The steady state relationship between the input inducer and output protein is determined by the specific mechanism of gene induction implemented within the module. This I/O relationship can be modulated by the control elements including co-activator and co-repressor.

Although it is unnecessary for module users to delve into the implementation details inside a module, the encapsulated molecular components and specific interactions should be available to users, along with time-course responses and I/O relationships under characteristic sets of parameter conditions. Construction of functional modules is generally facilitated by a number of graphic interface-based, user-friendly modeling tools that have emerged in recent years such as the Systems Biology Workbench [15]. In addition these tools ease the work of assembling these modules into larger network models, as the required adjustments for mass action of the interfacing molecular species from different modules are taken care of automatically.

When constructing a biological model, we are faced with two opposite challenges. On one hand, we are challenged with the scarcity of specific biological knowledge; on the other hand, there is a plethora of detailed knowledge available for a variety of signaling pathways, that is not organized quantitatively. To a large degree, the amount of biological detail needed in a module or

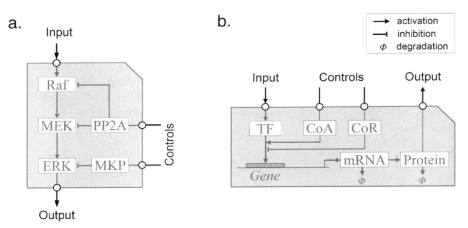

Figure 7.6 Illustrations of prebuilt functional modules for ERK activation (*a*) and generic gene induction (*b*).

model depends on the specific research questions being addressed. For example, if the process from G-protein coupled receptor (GPCR) activation to cAMP production is the main focus of the study, the intermediate steps in between should be explicitly modeled in order to reveal the subtlety of the signaling process. On the other hand, if cAMP is only an upstream element in a much larger network, implementation of GPCR-induced cAMP elevation may be subject to rule of simplification, as long as the I/O relationship and timing is in line with the actual biology.

In dealing with lack of or insufficient knowledge of a pathway, a black box modular approach may be followed. Usually experimental data can provide enough quantitative descriptions of the I/O relationship, even though what mediates this relationship may be unclear. As long as the module can re-establish this relationship, despite use of mechanisms still debatable or purely hypothetical, it should serve well as a functional unit in the context of a larger network model. As more structural details are known, they can be gradually incorporated into the module, without affecting the behavior of the network model, since the I/O relationship remains largely the same. For instance, in the oxidative stress response, how exactly the Kelch-like ECH-associated protein-1 (Keap1) senses reactive oxygen species and transduces this signal to NF-E2-related factor 2 (Nrf2) is not completely clear, and several mechanisms have been proposed [43]. This situation should not hinder us from modeling the adaptive response as a whole in which Keap1-Nrf2 is the sensor module (Figure 7.3). Experimental data are available for the relationship between the stressor level and Nrf2 activation, and construction of a module that will reproduce this relationship using either of the proposed mechanisms or in combination, will suffice for the current modeling purpose. As the mechanism of the Keap1 sensor becomes better established, it will replace the existing implementation of the module.

A convenient benefit from mechanistically modeling the biological networks responsible for dose response to chemical exposure and drug administration is the ease with which models for different chemicals can potentially be integrated into single models for mixed exposure studies. Models developed separately for each chemical can be joined at locations where the two models share the same signaling and regulatory components. Behaviors such as synergism and antagonism may emerge from the joined models, and could help explain the mixed exposure and drug–drug interaction data.

7.8 CONCLUSION

We are in an era in which knowledge about the underlying details of the molecular machinery controlling cellular functions has increased exponentially owing to a vast array of experimental technology breakthroughs. However, understanding how these molecular components work together to give rise to systems-level behaviors, and how perturbation of cellular pathways by xenobiotics alter their behaviors, is presently beyond the means of traditional biological research. Overcoming this challenge requires increased interactions between mathematicians, interdisciplinary biological modelers, and experimentalists. Complementing laboratory experiments with mechanistically based modeling is becoming increasingly relevant to toxicology and risk/safety assessment, since most chemicals disrupt biological functions through interacting with the existing biochemical networks within the cell. Systems-level computational modeling is providing an opportunity to understand dose–response relationships in a way that was previously impossible.

REFERENCES

1. Calabrese EJ. Toxicological awakenings: the rebirth of hormesis as a central pillar of toxicology. *Toxicol Appl Pharmacol* 2005;204:1–8.
2. Leung HW. Development and utilization of physiologically based pharmacokinetic models for toxicological applications. *J Toxicol Environ Health* 1991;32:247–67.
3. Bischoff KB, Dedrick RL, Zaharko DS, Longstreth JA. Methotrexate pharmacokinetics. *J Pharm Sci* 1971;60:1128–33.
4. Dedrick RL. Animal scale-up. *J Pharmacokinet Biopharm* 1973;1:435–61.
5. Clewell HJ, Gentry PR, Gearhart JM, Allen BC, Andersen ME. Comparison of cancer risk estimates for vinyl chloride using animal and human data with a PBPK model. *Sci Total Environ* 2001;274:37–66.
6. Reitz RH, Mendrala AL, Corley RA, Quast JF, Gargas ML, Andersen ME, et al. Estimating the risk of liver cancer associated with human exposures to chloroform using physiologically based pharmacokinetic modeling. *Toxicol Appl Pharmacol* 1990;105:443–59.
7. Clewell HJ, Clewell RA, 3rd. Development and specification of physiologically based pharmacokinetic models for use in risk assessment. *Regul Toxicol Pharmacol* 2008;50:129–43.
8. Leroux BG, Leisenring WM, Moolgavkar SH, Faustman EM. A biologically-based dose-response model for developmental toxicology. *Risk Anal* 1996;16:449–58.
9. Moolgavkar SH, Luebeck G. Two-event model for carcinogenesis: biological, mathematical, and statistical considerations. *Risk Anal* 1990;10:323–41.
10. Whitaker SY, Tran HT, Portier CJ. Development of a biologically-based controlled growth and differentiation model for developmental toxicology. *J Math Biol* 2003;46:1–16.
11. Bhalla US, Ram PT, Iyengar R. MAP kinase phosphatase as a locus of flexibility in a mitogen-activated protein kinase signaling network. *Science* 2002;297: 1018–23.
12. Nelson DE, Ihekwaba AE, Elliott M, Johnson JR, Gibney CA, Foreman BE, et al. Oscillations in NF-kappaB signaling control the dynamics of gene expression. *Science* 2004;306:704–8.
13. Lum L, Yao S, Mozer B, Rovescalli A, Von Kessler D, Nirenberg M, et al. Identification of Hedgehog pathway components by RNAi in *Drosophila* cultured cells. *Science* 2003;299:2039–45.

14. Chanda SK, White S, Orth AP, Reisdorph R, Miraglia L, Thomas RS, et al. Genome-scale functional profiling of the mammalian AP-1 signaling pathway. *Proc Natl Acad Sci USA* 2003;100:12153–8.

15. Sauro HM, Hucka M, Finney A, Wellock C, Bolouri H, Doyle J, et al. Next generation simulation tools: the Systems Biology Workbench and BioSPICE integration. *Omics* 2003;7:355–72.

16. Hucka M, Finney A, Sauro HM, Bolouri H, Doyle JC, Kitano H, et al. The systems biology markup language (SBML): a medium for representation and exchange of biochemical network models. *Bioinformatics* 2003;19:524–31.

17. Elowitz MB, Levine AJ, Siggia ED, Swain PS. Stochastic gene expression in a single cell. *Science* 2002;297:1183–6.

18. Blake WJ, M KA, Cantor CR, Collins JJ. Noise in eukaryotic gene expression. *Nature* 2003;422:633–7.

19. Broccardo CJ, Billings RE, Chubb LS, Andersen ME, Hanneman WH. Single cell analysis of switch-like induction of CYP1A1 in liver cell lines. *Toxicol Sci* 2004;78:287–94.

20. Ferrell JE, Jr. Building a cellular switch: more lessons from a good egg. *Bioessays* 1999;21:866–70.

21. Kuang Y, Biran I, Walt DR. Simultaneously monitoring gene expression kinetics and genetic noise in single cells by optical well arrays. *Anal Chem* 2004;76:6282–6.

22. Biran I, Walt DR. Optical imaging fiber-based single live cell arrays: a high-density cell assay platform. *Anal Chem* 2002;74:3046–54.

23. Raser JM, O'Shea EK. Control of stochasticity in eukaryotic gene expression. *Science* 2004;304:1811–4.

24. Zhang Q, Andersen ME, Conolly RB. Binary gene induction and protein expression in individual cells. *Theor Biol Med Model* 2006;3:18.

25. Rossi FM, Kringstein AM, Spicher A, Guicherit OM, Blau HM. Transcriptional control: rheostat converted to on/off switch. *Mol Cell* 2000;6:723–8.

26. Fiering S, Northrop JP, Nolan GP, Mattila PS, Crabtree GR, Herzenberg LA. Single cell assay of a transcription factor reveals a threshold in transcription activated by signals emanating from the T-cell antigen receptor. *Genes Dev* 1990;4:1823–34.

27. Bagowski CP, Besser J, Frey CR, Ferrell JE, Jr. The JNK cascade as a biochemical switch in mammalian cells: ultrasensitive and all-or-none responses. *Curr Biol* 2003;13:315–20.

28. Ferrell JE, Jr., Machleder EM. The biochemical basis of an all-or-none cell fate switch in Xenopus oocytes. *Science* 1998;280:895–8.

29. Kaern M, Elston TC, Blake WJ, Collins JJ. Stochasticity in gene expression: from theories to phenotypes. *Nat Rev Genet* 2005;6:451–64.

30. Calabrese EJ, Baldwin LA. The hormetic dose-response model is more common than the threshold model in toxicology. *Toxicol Sci* 2003;71:246–50.

31. Huang CY, Ferrell JE, Jr. Ultrasensitivity in the mitogen-activated protein kinase cascade. *Proc Natl Acad Sci USA* 1996;93:10078–83.

32. Goldbeter A, Koshland DE, Jr. Ultrasensitivity in biochemical systems controlled by covalent modification: interplay between zero-order and multistep effects. *J Biol Chem* 1984;259:14441–7.

33. Brandman O, Ferrell JE, Jr., Li R, Meyer T. Interlinked fast and slow positive feedback loops drive reliable cell decisions. *Science* 2005;310:496–8.

34. Ebersolt C, Premont J, Prochiantz A, Perez M, Bockaert J. Inhibition of brain adenylate cyclase by A1 adenosine receptors: pharmacological characteristics and locations. *Brain Res* 1983;267:123–9.

35. Zhang Q, Andersen ME. Dose response relationship in anti-stress gene regulatory networks. *PLoS Comput Biol* 2007;3:e24.

36. El-Samad H, Kurata H, Doyle JC, Gross CA, Khammash M. Surviving heat shock: control strategies for robustness and performance. *Proc Natl Acad Sci USA* 2005;102:2736–41.

37. Motohashi H, Yamamoto M. Nrf2-Keap1 defines a physiologically important stress response mechanism. *Trends Mol Med* 2004;10:549–57.

38. Pollycove M, Feinendegen LE. Radiation-induced versus endogenous DNA damage: possible effect of inducible protective responses in mitigating endogenous damage. *Hum Exp Toxicol* 2003;22:290–306; discussion 7, 15–7, 19–23.

39. Smolen P, Baxter DA, Byrne JH. Frequency selectivity, multistability, and oscillations emerge from models of genetic regulatory systems. *Am J Physiol* 1998;274:C531–42.

40. Bhalla US, Iyengar R. Emergent properties of networks of biological signaling pathways. *Science* 1999;283:381–7.

41. Tyson JJ, Chen KC, Novak B. Sniffers, buzzers, toggles and blinkers: dynamics of regulatory and signaling pathways in the cell. *Curr Opin Cell Biol* 2003;15:221–31.

42. Mackeigan JP, Murphy LO, Dimitri CA, Blenis J. Graded mitogen-activated protein kinase activity precedes switch-like c-Fos induction in mammalian cells. *Mol Cell Biol* 2005;25:4676–82.

43. Itoh K, Tong KI, Yamamoto M. Molecular mechanism activating Nrf2-Keap1 pathway in regulation of adaptive response to electrophiles. *Free Radic Biol Med* 2004;36:1208–13.

STEM CELL TECHNOLOGY FOR EMBRYOTOXICITY, CARDIOTOXICITY, AND HEPATOTOXICITY EVALUATION

Julio C. Davila, Donald B. Stedman, Sandra J. Engle, Howard I. Pryor II, and Joseph P. Vacanti

Contents

Drug Efficacy, Safety, and Biologics Discovery: Emerging Technologies and Tools,
Edited by Sean Ekins and Jinghai J. Xu
Copyright © 2009 by John Wiley & Sons, Inc.

8.1   INTRODUCTION

Drug safety issues are still the main cause of attrition during drug discovery and development. Traditionally drug safety is assessed firstly in terms of animal and in vitro toxicology testing [1–3]. A critical concern regarding the use of these models for toxicological studies is whether the response to exposure of animals or cells isolated from animal tissues to new chemical entities truly reflects the response in the human population. Preclinical species and humans have in fact inherent physiological and pharmacological differences. Cellular models based on human tissues, such as immortalized and primary cells represent the desired systems for predicting or anticipating target-organ toxicity of new drugs in humans during the early stages of drug development [4–6]. However, these cell-based models have limitations. For example, most of the human cell lines available today are tumor-derived and have been genetically transformed in order to maintain their "abnormal" proliferative capacity in culture; their representative cell functions that reflect the tissue of origin have, in many cases, been lost in culture and therefore conclusions based on gene function could be limiting and its clinical relevancy questionable. On the other hand, while primary human cell cultures represent the relevant model system for drug metabolism and toxicological studies, their limited supply, variable quality, and inter-individual differences hinder routine use. Therefore new strategies and better predictive assays to assess drug safety earlier during pharmaceutical development continue to be in high demand. Recent and continuous technological advances in the development of stem cell systems suggest results that may be beneficial in this respect.

Stem cell technology provides unprecedented opportunities not only for investigating new ways to prevent and treat a vast array of diseases but also for changing the way we identify new molecular targets, discover and develop new drugs, and test drugs for safety [7–10]. Stem cells can be classified into two major categories, according to their developmental status: embryonic and adult stem cells. Embryonic stem cells are obtained from the inner cell mass of 5- to 6-day-old blastocyst, and are considered to have characteristics of pluripotent stem cells. Pluripotent cells are capable of giving rise to most tissues of the organism, including the germ line during development. Adult stem cells, also known as mesenchymal stem cells, are present in somatic tissues and have characteristics of multipotent adult progenitor cells (MAPCs). Multipotent cells are capable of giving rise to several different cell types but not all cell types in the organism (see Figure 8.1).

Stem cells either from an embryonic or adult source have unique properties that make them very valuable and advantageous in the area of investigational toxicology [6–13]: (1) Stem cells are capable of dividing and self-renewing for long periods of time in culture. In contrast to primary hepatocytes derived from human donors, stem cells can generate an unlimited reliable supply of quality human cells without losing their functions and characteristics

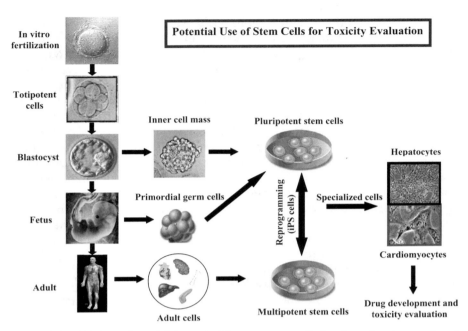

Figure 8.1 Origin and establishment of human stem cells for drug development and toxicity evaluation. When a sperm fertilizes an egg, a single cell is created; in few hours this fertilized egg divides into identical cells, capable of forming an entire organism (totipotent cells). Approximately four days after fertilization, these totipotent cells begin to form a hollow sphere of cells called blastocyst. This blastocyst has an outer layer containing a cluster of cells called inner cell mass. This inner cell mass can be isolated and cultured, and it has the potential to form colonies of cells with embryonic and pluripotent characteristics. Pluripotent stem cells can also be obtained from fetal tissues commonly known as primordial germ cells. Pluripotent stem cells may undergo further specialization to give rise to more specialized cells known as multipotent stem cells such as hepatocytes and cardiomyocytes. Multipotent stem cells can also be isolated from adult tissues and be reprogrammed in vitro to cells that have cell surface markers and genes characteristic of pluripotent stem cells (induced pluripotent stem [iPS] cells). Although the predictive value of the technology is still in the developmental and validation stage, the stem cell approach hold great promise for developing unique in vitro model systems to test drugs and chemicals and potentially anticipate and predict toxicity in humans. (See color insert.)

of the tissue of origin in culture. In addition there is no longer the need for either continuous isolation of cells from human tissue donors or the use of transformed cell lines that can have significant disadvantages for screening. (2) Stem cells are unspecialized cells and can give rise to more specialized tissue-specific cell types. For example, stem cells obtained from heart tissues have the potential to differentiate into pacemaker, atrium, and ventricular-like cells. Under appropriate culture conditions these specialized cells will resemble primary cells and therefore are able to mimic complex biological and biochemical functions characteristic of a mature and fully functional differentiated cell type; moreover they are capable of synthesizing clinically relevant tissue biomarkers. (3) Stem cells have plasticity properties; that is, stem cells from one tissue or organ can be induced to differentiate into cells of other organs, either in vitro or after transplantation in vivo. For example, stem cells from bone marrow, blood, or placenta can differentiate into hepatic-like cells; this striking property of the stem cells provides new opportunities for overcoming the limitation of procuring human tissues such as liver for evaluating toxic potentials of novel therapeutics. (4) Stem cells with a specific ethnic genome could be used to develop specific ethnic cell lines, reducing some of the concerns about genetic diversity of the human population, rather than relying solely on inbred strains of animals for preclinical screening. (5) The use of stem cells may allow the development of very sensitive functional cell-based toxicity assays for high-throughput screening (HTS) applications, therefore reducing the required amounts of test compounds, increasing the efficiency, and reducing time and cost of developing safe and effective drugs. (6) Stem cells can be scaled up and banked for a readily available and constant source of cells of both nondifferentiated and differentiated cell types. (7) The use of stem cells will facilitate the standardization of manufacturing protocols and methods for consistent differentiation of stem cells into a more stable homogeneous population of specialized cell types suitable for toxicological testing. (8) Stem cell technology has the potential to reduce the use of animals for toxicological testing, therefore gaining both scientific and, most important, public acceptance.

For many years stem cells had been just a concept in mammalian biology until murine embryonic stem cell culture was established in 1981 [14]. Major improvements on the isolation and purification of mouse embryonic stem (ES) cells, genetic engineering techniques, and the application of molecular markers make these cell systems an alternative source of a wide number of tissue-specific cell types and therefore an ideal in vitro tool for drug discovery and toxicity [9,14–19]. For example, murine embryonic stem cells have been a valuable tool for drug and chemical embryotoxicity screening [20–23]. Although the mouse stem cells have been a valuable screening tool in drug discovery and development, the challenge now is to improve our ability to manipulate human stem cells in vitro for biomedical applications. In 1998 a breakthrough was reported in this area when Thompson and coworkers [24] demonstrated that human embryonic stem cells (hESC) could be isolated and continuously maintained in culture for long periods of time. This group, and subsequently other scientists in the field, demonstrated that hESC were able to retain the same unique properties as mouse ES cells; for example, the ability to differentiate into several somatic or somatic-like functional cells such as cardiomyocytes, hepatocytes, and neuronal, [24–27]. This important and significant finding has been the subject of increasing scientific interest because of the unprecedented opportunities and impact that this technology may provide to biomedical research and toxicology.

Ideally human stem cells and derived materials must balance several criteria in order to be useful for toxicity studies: (1) The procurement of the human tissue as well as the initial isolation of the stem cells should be without complication by technical and ethical issues. (2) The material should be routinely available and come from pathology-free donors. (3) The proliferative capacity of a stem cell or committed progenitor should be high. (4) Spontaneous differentiation should be minimal, and controlled differentiation should be robust and reproducible. (5) Induced, terminal differentiation should lead to a homogeneous population of fully functional mature cells of the desired phenotype. (6) The mature phenotype should be stable and yield reproducible responses over a given period of time and comparable to those of in vivo. (7) Cells should be easily cryopreserved and restored to culture. (8) Culture of the cells should be amenable to automation.

The use of human stem cells for toxicity testing and mechanistic approaches is still in the developmental and validation stages. Currently the most successful development of human stem cells as an in vitro model for toxicity testing is probably in human cardiac tissue. In contrast, developing stem cell models of fully functional hepatocytes have been more difficult, but they have remained a main focus of many researchers and companies working in this area today. In this chapter we briefly overview some of the potential applications, advantages, and disadvantages that the stem cell technology may offer to the field of toxicology today. The focus will be on the use of mammalian stem cell models for embryotoxicity, cardiotoxicity, and hepatotoxicity.

8.2   STEM CELL TECHNOLOGY FOR EMBRYOTOXICITY EVALUATION

One of the many challenges facing the pharmaceutical industry is the high rate of drug candidate failure prior to reaching market. As the industry starts to explore more novel drug targets, these rates are only likely to rise. One common underlying cause of preclinical candidate attrition is toxicity, of which developmental toxicity is a subset and accounts for about 7%. Because developmental toxicity-related attrition normally occurs later in the drug development timeline, its effects are more catastrophic. To provide developmental toxicity risk assessments earlier in the drug development process will require predictive in vitro assays. One such proposed assay is the Embryonic Stem Cell Test (EST).

8.2.1   Embryotoxic Potential of Teratogenic Compounds

Embryonic stem cells (ESC) isolated from the inner cell mass of a blastocyst have a number of important characteristics [18]. They have the capacity of self-renewal, can be induced to differentiate into cell types of all three germ lineages, and, following their injection into blastocyst, can colonize the germ line. This ability to differentiate can be facilitated in vitro by allowing ESC to form aggregates, called "embryoid bodies" (EBs). These EBs have been shown to recapitulate gene expression patterns of embryos during early development [28,29]. Marker genes for cell lineages representing ectoderm, endoderm, and mesoderm are all present. Additionally many studies have focused on ESC differentiation as a model for studying developmental biology, while others are investigating ways to take advantage of these remarkable cells as potential tools for drug or chemical embryotoxicity screening.

It was Laschinski et al. [30] who first published data that demonstrated a differential response of embryotoxic compounds on undifferentiated murine ESC versus differentiated mouse fibroblasts. Following a workshop on screening chemicals for reproductive toxicity, the Center for Documentation and Evaluation of Alternative Methods to Animal Experiments (ZEBET) within the European Center for the Validation of Alternative Methods (ECVAM) began the development of the Embryonic Stem Cell Test (EST). Their objective was the validation of three in vitro assays, one of which was the murine embryonic stem cell test (EST). The aim of the EST assay is to discriminate among non, weak and strong embryotoxic compounds [20–23]. The EST assay utilizes two permanent mouse cell lines, 3T3 fibroblasts and D3 murine ES cells, to predict the embryotoxic potential of a given compound. The strategy is to find the drug concentrations that cause a 50% inhibition of differentiation into contracting cardiomyocytes and growth of ESC (ID_{50} and IC_{50}, respectively). A similar value for inhibition of growth (IC_{50}) is determined for 3T3 cells. These three concentrations are inserted into three linear discriminant functions that define the embryotoxicity class: non, weak, and strong. The equation that yields the largest number defines the embryotoxicity. For example, if the first equation (non) is largest it is predicted as a non.

A blinded validation study of the EST assay was conducted at four independent laboratories using 20 coded compounds, and a detailed report was issued [20]. Comparing the predicted in vitro classifications to the "true" in vivo classifications assigned by Brown [31] showed an overall accuracy of 78%. With the predictivity of strongly embryotoxic compounds at 100%, it was the weak compounds (69%) that proved to be the most difficult to classify correctly. Recent attempts to replicate some of the results obtained from ECVAM using a subset of their validation compounds resulted in very similar overall accuracy, of 73% [32]. Additionally a number of pharmaceutical compounds were tested in this in vitro system; these compounds fell into three general classes: FDA pregnancy category B (nonembryotoxic and nondevelopmentally toxic), category C compounds (embryotoxic), and category C compounds (developmentally toxic) [32]. Based on the review of available data, each compound was assigned a "true class" of non, moderate, or strong. However, none of these pharmaceutical compounds were classified as strong. Results from the linear discriminant model are shown in Table 8.1. The EST assay

TABLE 8.1 The 3 × 3 Contingency Table for Pharmaceutical Compounds: Precision, Predictability, and Overall Accuracy of the EST for Low-, Moderate-, and High-risk Developmentally Toxic Compounds

EST	EST Predicted Low	EST Predicted Moderate	EST Predicted High	Precision
True class non	Acebutolol hydrochloride Camphorsulfonic acid Chlorthalidone Cefotaxime Cyclobenzaprine hydrochloride Glyburide Disopyramide phosphate salt Sulfasalazine Hydrochlorothiazide Loratadine Norepinephrine (11)	Metoclopramide monohydrochloride (1)	0	92%
True class moderate	Dimethadione Warfarin (2)	1-3-Chlorophenyl piperazine Propafenone hydrochloride Trazadone hydrochloride Ropinirole Carbamazepine Mirtazapine propranolol Hydrochloride Metoprolol tartrate salt Nitrofen (9) 0	Fluoxetine Duloxetine (2)	69%
True class strong (multiple species teratogen)	0	0	0	N/A
Predictability	85%	90%	0%	Accuracy 80%

181

had an overall accuracy 80%. The predictability of low and moderate was 85% and 90%, while the precision was 92% and 69%, respectively. This was a slight improvement over the subset of validation compounds from ECVAM (accuracy 73%, predictability low and moderate 50% and 63%, precision 50% and 79%). These data further validate the utility of the EST assay for estimating the developmental risk of chemicals used as pharmaceutical drugs. The EST assay has proved to be reproducible, both within and among laboratories. Its predictivity for strongly embryotoxic compounds was excellent and should lead to a low rate of erroneous calls for "true" strong.

The need for low-bulk (mg) amounts of compound will enable use of the EST assay early in the drug development process and will help reduce the total number of laboratory animals needed in research. The weakness of the assay, however, is that it is labor intensive, with a relatively low throughput of 3 to 6 compounds a month. Additionally it fails to discriminate non from weak embryotoxins as well as would be desired; this might be aided by measuring more sensitive markers of cardiac function and/or cells of noncardiac lineages.

Indeed the evolution of the EST began even before the final report was issued by ECVAM. Attempts are being made to build in vitro models based on appropriate tissue and developmental stage-specific molecular endpoint markers. Bremer et al. [33] constructed a genetically modified ESC that contained a green fluorescent protein (GFP) reporter under the control of the cardiac-specific gene α-actin promoter and used quantitative fluorescence-activated cell sorting to build a model to predict the effects of chemicals on ESC differentiation into cardiomyocytes. In Bigot et al. [34] and zur Nieden et al. [35], a real-time reverse transcription polymerase chain reaction (RT-PCR) method was utilized to examine the cardiomyocyte-specific marker α- and β-myosin heavy chain gene expression following exposure to test compounds. Both papers demonstrated that a molecular marker method held promise for faster, more quantitative and higher throughput assays. Zur Nieden followed up with a new study evaluating multiple molecular endpoints designed to assess potential effects of teratogenic compounds on osteogenic, chondrogenic, neural, and cardiomyocyte differentiation [36]. These pilot studies concluded that additional molecular endpoints may improve the overall predictive value of the EST assay. A further study monitored selected genes, including cardiac markers (NK×2.5 and α-MHC), a "Stemness" marker (OCT-4) and an early mesoderm marker (Brachyury) over a time course of EB differentiation after exposure to retinoic acid and lithium chloride [37]. The resulting data suggested that changes in the pattern of gene expression could be helpful in determining the potential embryotoxicity of a compound.

Recently Festag and coworkers established a protocol for differentiating ES cells into endothelial cells using a multifaceted process that involved culturing EBs in the presence of VEGF alone or a with a cocktail consisting of VEGF, bFGF, IL-6, and Epo [38]. Both treatments resulted in an increase in the expression of endothelial cell-specific genes (PECAM-1, VE-Cadherin, Flk-1, Tie-2, and sFit) as compared to untreated EBs. This group subsequently tested the disturbance of endothelial differentiation in their EB model by measuring the reduction in expression of PECAM-1 and VE-Cadherin as a basis for predicting the embryotoxic potential of known teratogenic compounds [39]. In this study disruption of endothelial differentiation proved to be sufficient to correctly classify all six compounds tested.

Our laboratory's approach [32] was to measure the expression of a panel of genes (Table 8.2) that are characteristic of undifferentiated cells and differentiated cells from all three germ layers in EBs at the end of the EST assay (day 10). Then, by following changes of multiple molecular endpoints, we created a predictive statistical model for developmental toxicity that allowed us to both classify and rank the relative risk of a compound. Changes in gene expression following treatments were measured by RT-PCR, and the resulting data were incorporated into a multivariate "normal reference distribution" from known nonteratogenic compounds. Using the normal reference distribution, we computed the dimension-scaled Mahalanobis distance (MHD) across a range of concentrations and cytotoxicity [32]. By computing the rate of increase with concentration, we obtain a slope. Our hypothesis is that we would expect the slope for teratogenic compounds to increase rapidly with increasing concentrations. Ideally the rate will correspond to the relative teratogenic potential. The results from this modeling approach are provided in Table 8.3. Although this model gave results similar to the EST model, two compounds cycobenzaprine and loratadine moved classes from predicted low to moderate, and one compound move from predicted moderate to low. Clearly, the MHD model still had difficulty separating weak embryotoxic from nonembryotoxic compounds and was not an improvement over other methods.

8.2.2 Future Directions

The development of an in vitro model to accurately predict the response of mammalian embryos in vivo to chemical exposure has been the dream of many for more than 20 years. However, because of the complexity of mammalian development, it has proved to be an elusive goal. Difficulties persist even when these efforts have been confined to cover only a limited period of development, namely organogenesis. No single assay will be sufficient to cover all manifestations of development, and a testing battery will be necessary. As our understanding of the developmental process for both the embryo and ESC is enhanced by the availability of masses of genomic, proteomic, and metabolomic data, we anticipate that we will step closer to improving in vitro developmental toxicity testing.

Although all current testing assays use murine embryonic stem cells, the establishment of human embryonic stem cells (hESC) by Thomson in 1998 [24] and the subsequent formation of stem cell banks throughout the world

TABLE 8.2 Genes Currently Used to Support the Mahalanobis Distance Model

Category	Group	Gene Symbol	Gene Name	Marker For:
Extracellular matrix	Carbohydrate kinase	Gpc3	Glypican 3	Extracellular matrix
Cell adhesion molecule	Other cell adhesion molecule	Postn	Periostin, osteoblast specific factor	Osteoblast
Cytoskeletal protein	Actin family cytoskeletal protein	Myh6	Myosin, heavy polypeptide 6, cardiac muscle, alpha	Cardiac
Protease	Cam family adhesion molecule	Cpe	Carboxypeptidase E	Neural
Signaling molecule	Cytokine	Nodal	Nodal	Stemness
Molecular function unclassified	Miscellaneous function	Prnp	Prion protein	Neural
Transfer/carrier protein	Other cytoskeletal proteins	Afp	Alpha fetoprotein	Yolk sac endoderm
Cytoskeletal protein	Actin family cytoskeletal protein	Actc1	Actin, alpha, cardiac	Cardiac

TABLE 8.3 The 3 × 3 Contingency Table for Pharmaceutical Compounds: Precision, Predictability, and Overall Accuracy for Changes in Gene Expression Using the MHD Model for Low-, Moderate-, and High-risk Developmentally Toxic Compounds

EST	MHD Predicted Low	MHD Predicted Moderate	EST Predicted High	Precision
True class non	Acebutolol hydrochloride Camphorsulfonic acid Chlorthalidone Cefotaxime Glyburide Disopyramide phosphate salt Sulfasalazine Hydrochlorothiazide (8)	Metoclopramide monohydrochloride Cyclobenzaprine hydrochloride Loratadine (3)	0	73%
True class moderate	Dimethadione Warfarin Metoprolol tartrate salt (3)	1-3-Chlorophenyl piperazine Propafenone hydrochloride Trazadone hydrochloride Carbamazepine Mirtazapine Propranolol hydrochloride nitrofen Fluoxetine (8) 0	Duloxetine (1)	67%
True class strong (multiple species teratogen)	0	0	0	N/A
Predictability	73%	73%	0%	Accuracy 70%

185

has provided both basic and applied researchers a powerful tool to study both normal and abnormal development. As with mouse there is mounting evidence that hESC differentiation can recapitulate early embryonic development [38].

The value in utilizing hESC in vitro to help identify possible developmental toxicants lies in several areas: (1) it provides a second species against which to judge possible toxicity; (2) there are many teratogens for which animals overestimate the developmental hazard, and using hESC will allow a direct comparison of mouse and human in vitro models; (3) it allows one to take advantage of the enormous amount of human genomic data available; and (4) hESC may provide a more relevant risk assessment of developmental toxicity and give us an earlier more accurate identification of safer drugs and chemicals.

A new player in the world of development and stem cells is microRNAs (miRNA). MicroRNAs are endogenous single-stranded RNA molecules of approximately 22 nucleotides, thought to negatively and positively regulate the expression of other genes. MicroRNA has been shown to play an essential role in multiple biological processes, particularly embryonic development. Their expression profile in stem cells is different from that in other tissues [40]. The current understanding is that one miRNA could regulate a number of target genes, thereby affecting a number of biological processes simultaneous. One could imagine that a small set of miRNA's might be used as biomarkers for developmental toxicity, just as protein-coding messenger RNAs are used today.

8.3 STEM CELL TECHNOLOGY FOR CARDIOTOXICITY EVALUATION

Cardiotoxicity is estimated to account for roughly 20% of postmarketing adverse reactions resulting in changes to the physician's guidance for use, black box warnings, or withdrawal of the new chemical entities from the market [1–3,41]. Noncardiac drugs shown to induce cardiotoxicity encompass a wide variety of drugs such as immunomodulating drugs, antidiabetic drugs, antimigraine drugs, appetite suppressants, antipsychotic drugs, antidepressant drugs, glucocorticoids, antifungal drugs, and anticancer agents [42]. Few, if any, of the cardiotoxic effects of these drugs were predicted by preclinical or early clinical trials. Today the mechanism of toxicity associated with these drugs still is poorly understood in humans. Given the potential risks to large numbers of patients from such a broad category of drugs, new, more predictive models for cardiotoxicity are essential.

Models of cardiotoxicity currently in use depend heavily on engineered, artificial systems or nonhuman species. For example, to comply with the International Conference on Harmonization (ICH) guidelines for preclinical evaluation of compounds that may cause drug-induced changes in action potential duration (APD) such as QT prolongation syndrome and the potentially life-threatening arrhythmias termed *torsades de pointes* (TdP), the pharmaceutical industry has adopted a cascade of assays [43]. Initial, high-throughput in vitro assays rely on the use of a transformed, noncardiac cell system overexpressing human ether-a-go-go (hERG or KCNE2), the ion channel most closely associated with drug-induced QT prolongation, at nonphysiological levels and in the absence of other ion channels known to contribute to APD in the heart [44–46]. The standard ex vivo assay uses directly isolated Purkinje fibres or papillary muscle from guinea pig, rabbit, or dog to functionally assess changes in APD. While this assay uses species with ion channel profiles similar to humans and evaluates the hERG channel in its native environment, it is labor intensive and has very low throughput. Additionally one cannot be certain that the lack of APD changes in these species is predictive of human arrhythmia potential since small changes in physiology and biology often produce significant differences in APD. In vivo APD assessment relies on assays using conscious or anaesthetized guinea pigs, dogs, or monkeys, which are expensive and labor intensive models. The collection of assays used for evaluating QT prolongation is emblematic of the difficulties associated with cardiotoxicity testing in general. None of the assays in the cascade are performed with normal human material, nor do the assays reproduce human physiology or the clinical setting in which cardiotoxicity occurs.

Primary isolated cardiomyocytes from a variety of species, including humans, are also used for in vitro cardiotoxicity studies [47–49]. The primary advantage of these cells is that they can be obtained in pure populations of specific cardiomyocyte subtypes (e.g., atrial or ventricular). However, these cells retain their normal morphology and function for only a short period (generally <72 hours) before they lose their characteristic rod-shaped, striated morphology and show changes in contraction and relaxation. Isolation of the cells can be time-consuming, and their terminally differentiated nature means they have a limited capacity to divide. Furthermore it is often hard to obtain human tissue in sufficient amounts for large-scale studies, and the clinical background of the samples may contribute significant variability to experiments.

The goal of preclinical cardiac safety pharmacology studies is to predict the risk of toxicity of potential new drug candidates prior to entering the clinic. Given the potential for large numbers of compounds that must be screened, there is a need for inexpensive, validated in vitro assays that overcome the species differences and more closely mimic the complex cellular situation in the human heart. Similarly in vivo screens that place human cardiomyocytes in their normal organ and physiological context are essential to understanding the impact of different body systems on the functioning cardiomyocyte. Cardiomyocytes derived from stem cells offer a promising opportunity to address gaps in the systems currently used for cardiotoxicology testing.

8.3.1   Stem Cell Sources of Cardiomyocytes

A variety of functional cardiomyocytes have been generated from human adult, gestational, and embryonic stem cell sources. Adult human heart tissue offers the most obvious stem cell source for generating cardiomyocytes. Beltrami and colleagues demonstrated in 2001 the existence of a slowly dividing population of cells, termed cardiac stem cells (CSC), in the normal, hypertrophied, and postinfarcted human heart [50–52]. These cells most likely represent a population of cells responsible for normal homeostasis in the heart that are mobilized upon tissue damage. Later work isolated a rare, c-kit+, Sca-1+, MDR1+, Lin-, telomerase positive population of small cells from adult heart in a variety of species including human [50,53–56]. These cells maintained a stable phenotype over months of passage (self-renewing), generated the three main cell types found in the heart (cardiomyocytes, smooth muscle cells, and endothelial cells), and recapitulated both the self-renewal and multipotency from single cells at low frequency (clonogenic). Human CSC induced to differentiate in vitro with dexamethasone expressed cardiac associated transcription factors (GATA-4, Nk×2.5, MEF2c) and structural proteins (α-sarcomeric actin, myosin heavy chain [MHC]). Unlike in vitro differentiated rat CSC in which sarcomeres were not observed and myocytes failed to contract spontaneously or in response to a variety of chemicals or electrical stimulation, human CSC developed sarcomeric striations and, after stimulation at 1 Hz, showed contractile activity [53]. Co-culture of human CSC with rat neonatal myocytes further increased the percentage of cells responding to electrical stimulation and exhibiting calcium transients [53]. When injected into infarcted immunodeficient mouse or immunosuppressed rat hearts, human CSC integrated into the rodent hearts, developed structural proteins (MHC, trononin I) consistent with mature myocytes, and formed connexin 43 positive gap junctions with rodent myocytes [53]. Ex vivo analysis of chimeric rodent–human hearts identified synchronic calcium transients indicating functional integration of the human cells [53].

Messina and colleagues reported the shedding of endogenous CSC from enzymatically digested explants of human atrial ventricular biopsy specimens [57]. These c-kit+, Sca-1+, CD34+, Flk-1+ cells formed nonadherent or loosely adherent clusters of cells termed cardiospheres. Based on expression of a variety of markers associated with stem cells, endothelial cells, smooth muscle cells, and committed cardiomyocytes, cardiospheres appear to consist of a mixture of CSC, differentiating progenitors, and spontaneously differentiated cardiomyocytes. Disassociated cardiospheres were capable of forming new cardiospheres (self-renewing) and were clonogenic. When human cardiospheres were co-cultured with rat cardiomyocytes, they formed connexin 43-positive gap junctions with the rat cardiomyocytes and spontaneously contracted. Undifferentiated human cardiospheres engrafted into immunodeficient mouse hearts after ischemic damage, developed MHC and connexin 43 expression, and appeared to contribute to the regenerating myocardium.

Isl1, a LIM homeodomain transcription factor, has also been used to identify a resident cardiac progenitor population in early postnatal rat, mouse, and human [58]. These cells likely represent the remnants of multipotent embryonic cells that contribute to the formation of the right ventricle, both atria, the outflow tract, and parts of the left ventricle of the developing heart [59]. Isl1+ cells do not express markers normally associated with stem cells such as c-kit or Sca-1. However, Isl1+ cells can be clonally expanded in co-culture with a cardiac mesenchymal feeder layer while maintaining their ability to subsequently differentiate into smooth muscle, endothelial cells, and cardiomyocytes. Subsequent co-culture of isl1+ cells with neonatal cardiomyocytes leads to expression of transcription factors and structural proteins consistent with fully mature cardiomyocyte. Additionally a small fraction of the differentiated cells respond to β-adrenergic agonists [58].

Despite the obvious relevancy the use of endogenous cardiac stem/progenitor cells directly isolated from adult human heart is hindered by several limitations. Healthy adult heart tissue is not readily available. Biopsy samples are generally small and associated with clinical pathologies that may compromise yield or quality of the isolated stem cells or the experimental results derived from these cells. Stem cells isolated from cadaver specimens have not been fully explored and may be suboptimal. The need for co-culture with rodent neonatal cardiomyocytes either in vitro or in vivo to induce full differentiation further complicates the use of these cells. It is also unclear what is the long-term proliferative capacity of these cells.

Bone marrow-derived stromal stem cells or mesenchymal stem cells (MSC), extracted from the iliac crest of healthy volunteers, are a more readily available source of human adult stem cells and are less likely to have a clinical pathology [60]. Human MSC express CD44, CD105, CD73, Stro-1, and CD106 (VCAM-1) and are negative for hematopoietic and endothelial cell lineages. Although MSC represent only a small percentage of cells in the bone marrow, they are highly proliferative at low density in early passages, thus allowing for a significant expansion of the cell population prior to in vitro induction of differentiation. The cells have a propensity for forming adipocytes, chondroblasts, and osteoblasts. However, cardiomyocyte formation has been induced in vitro with 5-azacytidine, dexamethasone/insulin/ascorbic acid, or co-culture with cardiomyocytes or in vivo following engraftment [61–63]. Two to three weeks following in vitro induction of differentiation, MSC gradually increase in size and develop a ball or stick morphology prior to connecting with adjoining cells to form spontaneously beating myotubule-like structures. A small proportion of differentiated cells express cardiac-specific transcription factors and structural proteins as well as late-stage cardiac differentiation markers (MLC2a and MLC2v). In vitro MSC-derived cardiomyocytes display action potentials similar to pacemaker cells and ventricular cells and respond to β-adrenergic and muscarinic receptors [64]. MSC- or MSC-derived cardiomyocytes injected into areas of myocardial infarct integrate into the damaged tissue, develop characteristics of cardiomyocytes, and appear to improve functional recovery of the heart [65,66]. This has spurred much interest in these cells as a therapy for myocardial infarct with less attention directed toward generating large in vitro populations for assay develop [67].

More recently white adipose stromal cells have been shown to exhibit spontaneous cardiogenic potential [68–70]. At low frequency these cells spontaneously beat and express cardiac-specific transcription factors, structural proteins, and late-stage differentiation makers. Additionally the contracting cells respond to β-adrenergic and cholinergic stimulation with increased and decreased beating, respectively [69]. The relative ease with which subcutaneous white adipose tissue can be obtained via liposuction makes this an attractive source of stem cells, although human adipose-derived cardiomyocytes have yet to be described. Brown adipose tissue from mouse has also been found to contain higher numbers of cells capable of differentiating into cardiomyocytes; however, the small amount of brown adipose in humans limits it usefulness [68–70].

Additional reports have suggested that cardiomyocytes may be derived from other adult tissues. Human skeletal muscle has been shown to possess a population of cells capable of differentiating in vitro in the presence of a low dose (10^{-9}M) of 9-cis-retinoic acid (RA) into cardiomyocytes as determined by expression of cardiac-specific genes and proteins [71]. Spontaneously beating cells exhibited calcium transients and RA-treated skeletal muscle cells formed connexin 43-expressing gap junctions when co-cultured with mouse cardiac cells. Similarly endothelial progenitor cells derived from human peripheral blood have been reported to form cardiomyocytes in co-culture with rat neonatal cardiomyocytes [72]. These cardiomyocyte-like cells arise at low frequency but express structural proteins of cardiomyocytes, form active gap junctions, and demonstrate calcium transients. The emphasis for use of these cells has again focused on applications for cell therapy with less effort on developing efficient in vitro differentiation protocols [67].

Several human gestational or fetal sources of stem cells for cardiomyocyte differentiation have been investigated. Both CD133+ hematopoietic stem cells and mesenchymal stem cells derived from human umbilical vein have been shown to differentiate into cardiomyocyte-like cells as determined by expression of cardiac-specific transcription factors and structural proteins, although no functional studies were done [73–75]. Similarly placental-derived stem cells have been shown to differentiate into cardiomyocytes following co-culture with fetal cardiomyocytes or ascorbic acid treatment. These cells, when differentiated, express cardiac-specific genes and have action potentials similar to working cardiomyocytes [76,77]. Stem cells with broad differentiation capacity have also been isolated from amniotic fluid [78]. Although the cells were not specifically differentiated into cardiomyocytes, the cells could be induced to form multiple mesoderm lineages including osteocytes, adipocytes, and myocytes. Fetal-derived stem cells are an attractive choice for generating differentiated cardiomyocytes. The source for these cells is plentiful and routinely discarded as medical waste. Additionally there are few ethical and legislative considerations surrounding the use of these cells.

hESC have been shown by multiple laboratories to generate cardiomyocytes. Beating clusters of cells appear spontaneously when hESC-derived embryoid bodies are allowed to adhere to gelatin-coated plates or endoderm-like feeder cells [27,47,79–81]. When isolated from the mixed population of cells by microdissection, the contracting areas were shown to express numerous cardiac-specific transcription factors and structural proteins, display the organized sarcomeres, and develop spontaneous, rhythmic contractions. Patch-clamp electrophysiology on dissociated hESC-derived cardiomyocytes shows action potentials consistent with pacemaker, atrial, and ventricular cardiomyocytes, although ventricular myocytes seemed to predominant in some models [80]. hESC-derived cardiomyocytes responded with increased beating with β-adrenoreceptor agonists and with decreased beating following treatment with an L-type calcium channel blocker and a muscarinic agonist. When injected into immunocompromised rat and mouse models of ischemic injury, hESC-derived cardiomyocytes engrafted into the heart tissue at the site of injection, expressed markers of mature cardiomyocytes and mitigated the progressive decreases in cardiac function normally seen at 4 weeks after infarction [82,83]. In the mouse model the beneficial effects of the hESC cardiomyocytes was lost after 12 weeks, and electron microscopy studies demonstrated that while the hESC cardiomyocytes were coupled to each other by desmosomes, a thin layer of extracellular matrix separated them from mouse cardiomyocytes.

Technical hurdles as well as the current social and legislative environment have slowed the application of all hESC to large-scale cardiotoxicity testing. Theoretically hESC can be propagated in unlimited numbers before being induced to differentiate; however, culture techniques often require time-consuming and laborious manual dissection to both propagate the undifferentiated hESC and to generate EBs. In vitro differentiation techniques are costly, require many steps, and are neither robust nor reliable. Stem cell derived cardiomyocytes rarely represent more than roughly 30% of the cells present in any given culture and often less than 1%. The cardiomyocyte subtype (pacemaker, atrial, ventricular) is usually mixed as well. The phenotype of the differentiated cells more closely resembles fetal or neonatal cardiomyocytes than the desired adult cardiomyocyte. Additionally the differentiated cells have not been well characterized in terms of stability of basal parameters, reproducibility of responses, or functional integrity in response to known cardiotoxic agents.

8.3.2 Future Directions

Human stem cell derived cardiomyocytes appear to present channels and proteins of interest at physiological levels in their normal context, thus making it possible to envision high-throughput in vitro cardiotoxicity assays in a physiologically relevant human system. In vitro cardiotoxicology assays such as those used to detect responses to oxidative stress, resistance to apoptosis, and protection from ischemia, which are currently performed in heterologous or transformed cell systems and already formatted for high-throughput analysis, could be adapted to stem cell derived cardiomyocytes with minimal modifications. hESC-derived cardiomyocytes have been shown to express functional hERG/KCNE2 channels, opening up the possibility of high-throughput testing for inhibition in human cardiomyocytes [81]. Manually isolated, beating hESC-derived cardiomyocytes have been applied to micro-electrode arrays (MEA) [84,85]. MEA consist of 60 evenly spaced electrodes that allow assessment of electrical activity in networks of cells with high spatial and temporal resolution. By this technique hESC-derived cardiomyocytes were shown to form a functional syncytium with stable conductive properties and D-sotalol-induced delayed repolarization could be detected. MEA can be used to detect multiple facets of cardiomyocyte function, including rhythmicity, the origin and route of excitation, repolarization, and conduction in a semiautomated fashion. Spontaneously contracting stem cell derived cardiomyocytes can be maintained in culture for extended periods of time (up to three months), potentially allowing repeated, noninvasive analysis or multiple analyses progressing from noninvasive to invasive. Furthermore stem cell derived cardiomyocytes appear to recapitulate cardiomyocyte development, which opens a window for studying cardiotoxicity at each stage of cell development [86].

Genetic manipulation of the stem cell population may address many of the concerns associated with heterogeneity of the differentiated population. Huber and colleagues generated a stable transgenic hESC line expressing a hygromycin resistance-enhanced green fluorescent (eGFP) fusion protein under the control of the myosin light chain 2v promoter [87]. Following differentiation, fluorescence-activated cell sorting (FACS) of dispersed cells yielded relatively pure populations (>93%) of eGFP positive cells that were also positive for cardiac-specific markers. MEA studies showed that areas initiating electrical activity and propagating the action potential were associated with eGFP, and whole cell patch-clamp studies of the eGFP-expressing cells demonstrated the presence of cardiac-specific action potentials. The eGFP-expressing cells could engraft into the hearts of immunosuppressed rats and remain detectable for at least four weeks [87]. Similarly Anderson and colleagues used a transgene containing a neomycin cassette and a MHC promoter driven GFP-IRES-puramycin resistance cassette to select for relatively pure populations (>91%) of hESC-derived cardiomyocytes [88]. Zwaka and Thomson showed that homologous recombination, in which endogenous DNA is specifically replaced with an exogenous DNA construct, occurs in hES cells, and stably modified stem cells retaining multipotency can be obtained [89]. Taken together, these data make it likely that relatively pure populations of specific cardiomyocyte subtypes can be isolated through genetic manipulation.

The application of human stem cells to the generation of two and/or three-dimensional (2D/3D) cell configuration, engineered heart tissue, may make it possible to replace nonhuman ex vivo studies with studies directly in a reconstituted human system. Earlier work with neonatal rat cardiomyocytes has shown that cardiomyocytes seeded into various natural or synthetic scaffolds, released from temperature sensitive surfaces or delaminated, and allowed to self-assemble formed 3D, contracting structures with the properties of endogenous heart tissue [90]. More recently Feinberg and colleagues engineered 2D anisotropic polydimethylsiloxane elastomer thin films that, when seeded with rat neonatal cardiomyocytes, formed 3D conformations during the synchronous shortening of contraction and returned to their original shape during relaxation [91]. These "muscular thin films" could be electrically paced and force measurements could be obtained. Although not yet reported, it is likely that stem cell derived human cardiomyocytes would function similarly in the "muscular thin films." In fact hESC derived cardiomyocytes seeded into 50% poly-L-lactic acid/50% polylactic-glycolic acid scaffolds with human endothelial cells and embryonic fibroblasts formed spontaneously contracting, highly vascularized engineered cardiac muscle [92]. The engineered 3D tissue exhibited typical structural properties of early cardiac tissue and responded appropriately to β-adrenergic and muscarinic agonists. The presence of all three major cells types normally found in the heart (cardiomyocytes, endothelial cells, and smooth muscle cells differentiated from the embryonic fibroblasts) allows for the investigation of interactions between the cells that was not previously accessible in vitro.

Human-animal chimeric studies may make possible, the in vivo investigation of complex biological processes leading to cardiotoxicity. As described previously, the direct injection of stem cells or stem cell-derived cardiomyocytes into the hearts of immunocompromised or immunosuppressed rodents is routinely carried out to evaluate the functional potential of the cells and their capacity to improve damaged heart tissue. While current technology has so far yielded only small patches of engrafted cells that generally function autonomously from the surrounding heart, improved engraftment through better engineered rodent models [93] and better understanding of how to generate cells for engraftment may make it possible to generate sizable patches of human tissue in an intact heart. Assuming that the human cardiac tissue can adjust to the rapid beating of the rodent heart, this makes it possible to study new chemical entities delivered through their likely route of administration and subject to metabolism, albeit rodent metabolism [93]. Large animal models, which better mimic human heart function and metabolism, are possible as suggested by work showing that hESC-derived cardiomyocytes can engraft and function as pacemakers when injected into hearts of immunosuppressed swine with complete atrioventricular block [94].

8.4   STEM CELL TECHNOLOGY FOR
HEPATOTOXICITY EVALUATION

Over the past decade there has been a great deal of interest in the use of stem cells for the evaluation of hepatotoxicity. Early determination of hepatotoxicity during drug discovery could save millions of dollars in drug development costs [1–3]. Early toxicity screening studies therefore focus on the liver during screening and nonclinical safety assessment, and during this phase of testing approximately 40% of new drug development failures are due to toxicity [95]. Only one out of five drugs that advances to a clinical phase of testing will reach the market place, and most of the remainder fail due to hepatotoxicity [95]. Obviously, having a candidate drug fail due to hepatotoxicity at a late stage of development could be financially disastrous, so any screening method that would eliminate hepatotoxic compounds earlier in development would be very advantageous [5,6,96].

As early as the 1970s it was recognized that animal studies were an expensive and cumbersome method for testing compounds for toxicity [97]. In addition, while animal studies correlate well for cardiovascular, hematologic, and gastrointestinal toxicity, they correlate very poorly for hepatotoxicity in humans [41]. Over the past three decades, a host of sophisticated cellular assays have been developed to evaluate prelethal mechanistic hepatotoxicity that obviates the need for animal studies as a first step in the identification of several forms of basic hepatotoxicity. An in-depth review of these methods is beyond the scope of this discussion and can be found in several classic toxicology textbooks, including Zimmerman's *Hepatotoxicity* [4–6,96,98,99].

Currently primary human hepatocytes and genetically engineered human cell lines are the in vitro model systems of choice for understanding further the potential mechanisms of drug-induced liver injury (DILI) [6]; some of these DILI mechanisms include altered lipid metabolism, causing fatty liver, increased oxidative stress leading to cellular injury, decreased mitochondrial function leading to apoptosis or necrosis, cytotoxic T cell-mediated cell killing, decreased bile salt clearance causing cholestasis, and incomplete or dysregulated tissue repair [5,6,98,100]. Unfortunately, human hepatic tissue is available in extremely limited quantities, and immortalized human cells such as HepG2 have relatively poor predictive value due to their abnormal metabolic profile [6]. Hepatocytes derived from stem cell sources show promise for providing a human-derived population of cells that can bridge the gap between these cellular models [6,8].

Stem cells have been discovered and characterized in a wide range of species; however, the cell types that will be applicable for use in hepatotoxicity screening are derived exclusively from mammalian species. Mammalian stem cell populations from embryonic, gestational, and adult tissues will be briefly examined below, and the important developments leading toward their application in hepatotoxicity will be specifically emphasized.

8.4.1 Mouse Embryonic Stem Cells

Through early studies of embryological development, mouse embryonic stem cells (mESC) were identified in the early 1980s, and methods were described for isolating these cells and evaluating their characteristics in vitro and in vivo [101,102]. Over the ensuing decade these cells were evaluated for many basic properties, and it was discovered that mESC can divide in vitro for long periods of time. This division is asymmetric, yielding a genetically identical stem cell and a daughter cell with the potential to differentiate into many embryonic cell types [103,104]. As the understanding of these cells advanced, investigators began to examine them for their ability to develop into a highly specific cell type.

Some of the early reports evaluating the ability of mESC to develop into hepatocytes centered on the expression of known hepatocytes genetic products such as α-fetoprotein (AFP), albumin (ALB), and the family of hepatocyte nucleofactors (HNF) [105,106]. From these investigations it became clear that mESC had the capacity to progress down the hepatocyte lineage, but only a fraction of the cells in culture would naturally progress toward a hepatocyte genotype [107–109]. In addition mESC would stop developing at an immature phenotype in vitro without the addition of growth factors such as hepatocyte growth factor (HGF) and activin [107,110–112]. Several protocols have been evaluated for the systematic application of sequential growth factors such as fibroblast growth factor-1 (FGF-1), fibroblast growth factor-4 (FGF-4), and HGF followed by oncostatin M (OSM) in order to drive mESC towards a mature hepatocyte genotype [113–115]. Further, attempts to improve conversion efficiency included the addition of cues common in embryonic development such as the presence of cardiac mesoderm, transfection with lineage specific genes, or co-culturing with cells that promote hepatocyte differentiation [116–121]. Work on these in vitro differentiation techniques has demonstrated that hepatocyte-like cells can be generated from mESC and these findings have been further validated in vivo.

One of the earliest in vivo studies of differentiated mESC was presented by Choi et al. in 2002. In this study, they injected mESC into the spleen of immunosuppresed nude mice and observed phenotypic hepatic differentiation. The phenotypic hepatocytes were then isolated and found to be expressing several liver-specific antibodies [122]. Using the carbon tetrachloride intoxication model, Yamamoto et al. demonstrated that mESC differentiated in vitro to hepatocyte-like cells and would engraft to an injured liver to perform several liver-specific functions including measurable improvements to prothrombin time, serum ALB, and serum ammonia levels [113]. The ability of these cells to perform their expected postdifferentiation function in vivo validates their use as a cell source for evaluating the hepatotoxic effect of drugs. In pursuit of that specific aim, Tsutsui et al. have demonstrated that mESC in vitro have the capability to metabolize drugs through the identification of expressed CYP450 genes, measurement of testosterone hydroxylation activity, and determination of phenobarbital inducibility of selective CYP450 enzymes [123]. Soto-Gutierrez et al. have demonstrated that mESC cultured with growth factors, followed by co-culture with liver nonparenchymal cells will develop into hepatocyte-like cells that secrete ALB and metabolize ammonia, lidocaine, and diazepam. Further, when implanted into mice with induced liver failure, the hepatocyte-like cells improved liver function [121].

Clearly, the accumulation of such a large volume of quality studies using mESC is the direct result of the ubiquitous nature of the mouse animal model in scientific research. The availability of murine cells in large quantities caused mESC to be one of the earliest mammalian embryonic stem cells types identified. An enormous amount of work has been done to develop sophisticated culturing techniques and differentiation strategies for these cells over the past two decades. The result is that mESC are the stem cell type with the most advanced knowledgebase, which could lead to potential promising short-term applications. While animal-derived cells can serve as a ready supply of cells for testing, subtle differences in animal and human responses are known to exist and these differences can prove costly if discovered late in the drug development process [124]. Therefore, the ideal in vitro method to test human hepatotoxicity would clearly be based on the use of human tissue derived hepatocytes.

8.4.2   Human Embryonic Stem Cells

The identification and characterization of mESC have led to the discovery of primate and eventually hESC [24,125]. However, three separate articles have addressed the ethical, moral, and political implications of such a discovery [126–128]. To date, the investigation of these cells remains mired in controversy, including severe restrictions on their use in research endeavors. As a direct result of these restrictions, far less has been reported about hESC in the decade since their discovery when compared with the volume of discoveries reported in the first decade of mESC investigations. However, many of the ground-breaking techniques that were developed for the research of mESC have had direct application to hESC research, and hepatocyte differentiation protocols developed for mESC have served as a basis for the investigation of the differentiation of hESC down the hepatic lineage [129–132]. The first paper to indicate that hESC were capable of differentiating into the endodermal lineage was presented by Itskovitz–Eldor et al. in 2000 and was supported later in that same year by the findings of Schuldiner et al. who showed the development of endodermal cells in vitro through the treatment of hESC with growth factors identified from studies on mSEC [133,134].

Since their discovery, hESC have always been assumed to be a potential source of hepatocytes for toxicity and tissue engineering applications [135–137]. One of the earliest studies to evaluate the ability of hESC to differentiate into hepatocytes based on previous work with mESC was presented by Haumaitre et al. in 2003. In this study differentiation processes involving a family of HNFs that had been elucidated in the mESC model were tested in the hESC [138]. While demonstrating that HNF1 is directly involved in the hierarchical transcription factor network leading to hepatic maturation, this report suggested the potential to genetically direct a stem cell population toward a desired lineage. Lavon et al. in 2004 showed that an enriched population of hepatocyte-like cells could be developed from hESC that were allowed to spontaneously differentiate and then treated with acidic fibroblast growth factor (aFGF) to create conditions similar to those found in the normal embryonic hepatic milieu [139]. Several additional media supplements have been evaluated for their ability to induce hepatic differentiation in hESC populations including dexamethasone and sodium butyrate. The use of these supplements resulted in the in vitro development of cells that are morphologically similar to hepatocytes that express hepatic proteins [25,140–143]. Cytokines and growth factors that have been evaluated include insulin, aFGF, basic fibroblast growth factor (bFGF), hepatocyte growth factor (HGF), activina A, and oncostatin M (OSM) [25,140–143]. These studies have demonstrated in vitro phenotypic changes, induction of liver-enriched mRNA and secretion of hepatocyte-specific proteins with relatively high efficiency of differentiation, but the absolute yields of differentiated cells in these studies are still quite low.

The principal factor limiting the near-term use of hESC for the evaluation of hepatotoxicity is the limited availability of hESC primarily due to the strict regulations placed on their use in research. These regulations have resulted in a far smaller number of scientists working with heSC versus other stem cell types. In addition these heSC require a great deal of technical expertise to differentiate and even in skilled hands typically result in mixed populations and low yields. When coupled with the general lack of available hESC, the heterogeneous results of spontaneous and induced in vitro differentiation of these cells clearly indicates a need for development of methods to obtain a pure population of hepatocytes in large quantities. These cells are also very technically challenging to work with and do not appear to be easily produced in large quantities; therefore their applicability to HTS for hepatotoxicity appears very limited at this time. A cell source that is easier to work with and is not as politically volatile is needed and adult stem cells may prove to be the answer to this critical shortage. Two potential sources may address this problem namely cells isolated from gestational tissues and from adult mesenchymal stem cells.

8.4.3 Human Gestational Tissues

Cell populations from several tissues associated with gestation yield cells that demonstrate hepatic differentiation characteristics similar to embryonic stem cells; these include umbilical vein or cord blood cells, amnionic cells, and placental cells. Some of the earliest studies to evaluate the hepatic differentiation capacity of human umbilical cord vein stem cells (hUSC) focused on the ability of hUSC to be engrafted in vivo to the liver plate of a NOD/SCID mouse and then transdifferentiate into hepatocyte-like cells [144–146]. Following these reports, Lee et al. demonstrated that hUSC can be differentiated in vitro into a variety of cell types, including, hepatocyte-like cells [147]. Other groups demonstrated that cells with similar plasticity could be derived from human placenta and amnion [76,148–150]. By using cytokine signaling similar to that of previous hESC studies, several groups have shown that hUSC and cells derived from placenta and amnion can proceed down the hepatic lineage [151–156]. These cell populations were only relatively recently discovered and their potential seems limitless, so they represent a promising long-term source of cells for hepatotoxicity screening. These cells are also easier to work with, more abundant, and normally the tissue is discarded following a live birth. Therefore the use of stem cells derived from gestational tissues will likely not encounter the ethical, moral, political, or religious objections commonly associated with the use of embryonic stem cells.

8.4.4 Adult Mesenchymal Stem Cells

MSC refers to cells isolated from an animal that has completed gestation and is physiologically independent of its mother. Theses cells have been found in most tissues but reside in largest numbers within tissues that have a high cellular turnover rate throughout life such as the intestine, epidermis, and bone marrow [157,158]. Bone-marrow mesenchymal stem cells (BMSC) in animals were the first MSC cell types to be evaluated for hepatic differentiation potential. Petersen et al. in 1999 showed that BMSC from rat bone marrow could transdifferentiate from the mesenchymal lineage to an endothelial lineage, ultimately expressing markers consistent with a hepatic cell type [159]. Several other reports have shown that adult stem cells can be differentiated into cells not normally associated with their "committed" state [160]. In 1999, Bjornson et al. demonstrated the conversion, or "fate switch" of neural stem cells in mice into the hematopoietic lineage [161]. This work was advanced into the study of human MSC in 2004 when Lee et al. demonstrated that BMSC had the capacity to differentiate into several cell types including a hepatocyte-like cell type [162]. Several groups have further evaluated the potential of animal and human BMSC for hepatic differentiation both in vitro and in vivo and have found that protocols similar to those used for the differentiation of hESC have generated hepatocyte-like cells [163–168]. In addition Lee et al. also demonstrated that adipose-derived mesenchymal stem (ADMSC) cells had the same differentiation potential as BMSC to develop bone, fat, and cartilage phenotypes, resulting in an evaluation of these ADMSC for hepatic differentiation potential [162].

One of the earliest reports of a pluripotent cell population from adipose tissue came from Zuk et al. in 2002 [169]. They showed that ADMSC had the capacity to differentiate into bone, fat, cartilage, and muscle phenotypes. While this discovery is relatively recent, at least four other studies have confirmed aspects of their findings. Seo et al. showed that ADMSC could be differentiated and would perform isolated hepatic functions, such as LDL uptake, production of ALB, and conversion of ammonia to urea [170]. Talens-Visconti et al. showed that when compared to BMSC, ADMSC have an equivalent ability to differentiate along the hepatic lineage [171]. Banas et al. demonstrated the ability of an enriched population of CD105[+] ADMSC to undergo hepatic differentiation with 60% to 85% efficiency [172]. The cells generated in this study expressed hepatic-specific and selected markers, including ALB and microsomal CYP450 enzymes. The presence of these enzymes involved in drug, sterol, and bile acid metabolism, including CYP7A1, CYP1A1, CYP2C9, CYP3A4, and NADPH-cytochrome P450 reductase, indicate that these cells may have value in in vitro preclinical drug metabolism and toxicity testing [172]. In 2007, Sgodda et al. demonstrated the ability to differentiate ADMSC derived specifically from peritoneal fat into hepatocyte-like cells indicating the presence of ADMSC in different fat populations [173]. All of these studies, while preliminary, highlight the enormous potential of ADMSC as a source of cells for in vitro evaluation of hepatotoxicity.

Of all the cell types currently being evaluated for hepatic differentiation, MSC in general and ADMSC specifically represent the most promising near-term cell sources. Neither one of these human-derived cell sources is encumbered by the legislative and ethical considerations that limit the use of hESC and gestational tissues. Further the tissues from which BMSC and ADMSC are derived are regularly encountered in the clinical environment and are frequently seen as biological waste in that setting. BMSC were discovered first as a consequence of the enormous clinical interest surrounding bone-marrow transplantation for the treatment of hematologic disorders. The procurement of these cells, however, requires an invasive bone-marrow aspiration procedure that can be painful and additionally generate significant clinical complications. In contrast, ADMSC can be derived from healthy donors undergoing common plastic surgery procedures such as abdominoplasty or liposuction. These procedures occur daily and generate a large quantity of otherwise discarded tissue while exposing the donor to no additional risk beyond that typically associated with the elective procedure they have chosen. If ADMSC continue to demonstrate such favorable differentiation characteristics these cells will clearly provide a bountiful and accessible source of adult stem cells with minimal patient discomfort. They will also likely represent the first cell type to demonstrate the enormous potential of stem cell technology in the evaluation of hepatotoxicity of candidate drugs.

8.4.5 Future Directions

The near-term use of stem cell derived hepatocytes for the evaluation of hepatotoxicity will be limited by two principal factors: disagreement concerning the minimum requirement for deriving adult human hepatocytes and technology limitations for the large-scale production of these types of cells. Although there are reports of stem cell-derived hepatocyte-like cells indicating that some selected hepatic functions have been detected, there are nevertheless no reports of complete differentiation of stem cells from any sources to full mature and functional human hepatocytes. In addition, while the studies above report preliminary success in differentiating stem cells of several varieties, attempts to differentiate such pluripotent cells can result in contaminated populations of differentiated cells of other embryonic types including yolk sack cells [8]. During fetal development the yolk sac performs many functions similar to the liver and can express marker genes with a similar profile to hepatocytes, including genetic markers for ALB, α-fetoprotein, and trans-thyretin, without having any certain hepatotoxic predictive capacity. The presence of two cell populations with such similar genetic markers spawned a hunt for a definitive genetic marker of hepatic differentiation. Asahina et al. demonstrated in 2004 that expression of CYP7A1 was a definitive marker of actual hepatic differentiation and could distinguish differentiated hESC from differentiated yolk sac cells [174]. This marker could lead to the enrichment of a densely differentiated cell population. However, it will ultimately be necessary to quantitate the expression of a number of other mature liver enzymes in differentiated hESC and assess functional metabolism with enzyme specific probe substrates to ensure that they compare favorably to the enzyme profile of adult human hepatocytes [174]. Based on maturation-dependent expression patterns, Strom and colleagues [6] suggested that the ratios of CYP's 3A7 to 3A4 and 1A1 to 1A2 should be used as an estimate of the degree of hepatic differentiation within a stem cell population. Since the expression of CYP3A4 and CYP1A2 are favored in mature adult hepatocytes, as each ratio approaches 1, a greater degree of hepatic differentiation is indicated and the resultant cell population would more closely model true hepatotoxicity [6]. Beyond the mere up-regulation of certain gene products, these cells would then have to perform consistently in functional studies when compared to the metabolic activity of comparable CYP450 enzymes found in human primary hepatocytes in vitro and ideally to those present in adult human liver tissue in vivo. A few of the assays that may be especially amenable to the use of stem cell derived hepatocyte-like cells include steatosis, cholestasis, phospholipidosis, mitochondrial toxicity, oxidative stress, and drug metabolism-mediated toxicity (e.g., identification of reactive or toxic metabolites). All of these assays have employed in vitro cultures of primary hepatocytes or cell lines to evaluate conditions of hepatotoxicity with promising predictive success [5,6]. However, in each case the predictive value and ease-of-use of these techniques would be significantly improved with the development of a readily expandable, metabolically competent source of primary human cells. Stem cell derived hepatocytes show promise for providing just such a source of cells.

The application of stem cells with any type for HTS will depend on the development of a consistent ability to differentiate these cells in large quantities. The work to date has been done with cells on a very small scale, less than 1×10^8 in most cases and growth factor concentrations in the ng/ml range. For these cells to advance to a commercially viable state for drug screening, cells will need to be produced in quantities several orders of magnitude larger than those found in a typical in vitro study thus requiring the development of new cell culturing machinery. In addition growth factors will be needed in much larger milligram quantities. While this is currently financially limiting, the cost of purified growth factors will likely decrease through the economy of scale as these technique achieve greater application. Throughout history technologic advances have met challenges such as these; still a larger issue exists (see Section 8.5).

Another breakthrough was announced recently by two teams of scientists independently who reported methods to turn human adult cells into hESC. Thompson and coworkers [175] exposed mammalian somatic (foreskin) cells from a human donor (newborn) to retroviral expressing Oct4, Sox2, NANOG, and Lin28, four transgenes encoding human factors. This group was able to reprogram these adult cells to cells that exhibit normal karyotypes, telomerase activity, and cell surface markers and genes characteristic of pluripotent or embryonic stem cells. At the same time Takahashi and coworkers [176] reported that by overexpressing Oct4, Sox2, Klf4, and c-Myc in human adult fibroblasts, they successfully were able to isolate cells that resemble human embryonic stem cells. Interestingly two of the four genes used by this group were different from those reported by Thompson's team [175]. This significant finding may indicate that there are multiple paths to reprogram the adult cells to behave like embryonic stem cells. It will open the door for important therapeutic applications and for the further understanding and treatment of human diseases. In addition this is a huge breakthrough for the drug industry because the technology is simple and can be reproduced in any laboratory, and specialized cells (cardioymyocytes, hepatocytes, etc. others) may be derived from regular adult cells and not from embryos, thus bypassing the ethical, religious, and political issues that have hindered the use of human embryonic stem cells in bioresearch today. The challenge now is to understand the biology of these human-induced pluripotent stem (iPS) cells (e.g., the mechanisms regulating proliferation, differentiation and reprogramming) and find methods to make these iPS cells useful for drug discovery research and toxicity testing. Although this new technology is now at the very early stages, it is likely that these iPS- and iPS-derived cells will contribute to the field of toxicology with potential for considerable impact over the coming years.

8.5 CONCLUDING REMARKS

Stem cells hold great promise for solving one of the biggest bottlenecks that pharmaceutical and biotech companies encounter today, how to reduce drug attrition rates due to the unacceptable safety profile at the later stages of development. Currently stem cell technology is being implemented in the routine phases of the pharmaceutical pipeline of drug discovery and development. They represent a valuable source of materials for identifying and validating new relevant targets, discovering new drugs, and generating suitable cell-based human models that could be used to improve existing predictive toxicity assays.

The potential use and application of the stem cell technology in toxicology has been discussed here for three important areas of pharmaceutical safety evaluation, namely embryotoxicity, cardiotoxicity, and hepatotoxicity. Although the predictive value of the technology is still limited today in all of these three areas of in vitro toxicity testing, the continuous and rapid technological advances observed in the past few years make these the primary areas for investment, with significant potential impact for research and development. These significant advances have been possible by coupling the stem cell technology with new hi-tech approaches such as "omics," nuclear reprogramming research, RNAi, tissue-engineered devices, high-content screens (HCS), and humanized chimeric animal models. These scientifically relevant approaches make it conceivable that in the near future, human stem cell derived-materials may become the desirable in vitro models for predicting or anticipating toxicity in humans, reducing drug attrition, and ultimately for developing safer drugs.

REFERENCES

1. Lasser K, Allen PD, Woolhandler SJ, et al. Timing of new black box warnings and withdrawals for prescription medications. *JAMA* 2002;287:2215–20.
2. Schuster D, Laggner C, Langer T. Why drugs fail—study on side effects in new chemical entities. *Curr Pharm Des* 2005;11:3545–59.
3. Wysowski DK, Swartz L. Adverse drug event survillance and drug withdrawals in the United States. *Arch Intern Med* 2005;165:1363–9.
4. Dambach DM, Andrews BA, Moulin F. New technologies and screening strategies for hepatotoxicity: use of in vitro models. *Toxicol Pathol* 2005;33: 17–26.
5. Davila JC, Rodrigues RJ, Melchert RB, Acosta D. Predicitive value of in vitro model systems in toxicology. *Ann Rev Pharmacol Toxicol* 1998;38:63–96.
6. Davila JC, Xu JJ, Hoffmaster KA, O'Brien PJ, Strom S. Current in vitro models to study drug-induced liver injury. In Sahu S, ed. *Hepatotoxicity: from genomics to in vitro and in vivo models*. Hoboken, NJ: Wiley, 2007. p. 1–30.
7. Cezar G. Embryonic stem cells: a new avenue to evaluate the effects of chemicals in humans. *Int J Pharm Med* 2006;20:107–14.
8. Davila JC, Cezar GG, Thiede M, Strom S, Miki T, Trosko J. Use and application of stem cells in toxicology. *Tox Sci* 2004;79:214–23.
9. McNeish J. Embryonic stem cells in drug discovery. *Nat Rev Drug Discov* 2004;3:70–80.
10. Poulton CW, Haynes J. Embryonic stem cells as a source of models for drug discovery. *Nat Rev Drug Discov* 2007;6:605–16.

11. Ameen C, Raimund S, Bjorquist P, Lindahl A, Hyllner J, Sartipy P. Human embryonic stem cells: current technologies and emerging industrial applications. *Crit Rev Oncol Hematol* 2008;65:54–80.

12. Mayne J, Ku W, Kennedy S. Informed toxicity assessment in drug discovery: systems-based toxicology. *Curr Opin Drug Discov Dev* 2006;9:75–83.

13. Sartipy P, Bjorquist P, Strehl R, Hyllner J. Pluripotent human stem cells a novel tools in drug discovery and toxicity testing. *I Drugs* 2006;9:702–5.

14. Evans MJ, Kaufmann M. Establishment in culture of pluripotent cells from mouse embryos. *Nature* 1981;292:154–6.

15. Abuin A, Holt KH, Platt KA, Sands AT, Zambrowicz B. Full-speed mammalian genetics: in vivo target validation in the drug discovery process. *Trends Biotechnol* 2002;20:261–8.

16. Allen M, Svensson L, Roach M, Hambor J, McNeish J, Gabel C. Deficiency of the stress kinase p38a results in embryonic lethality: characterization of the kinase dependence of stress responses of enzyme-deficient embryonic stem cells. *J Exp Med* 2000;191:859–70.

17. Harris S. Transgenic knockouts as part of high-throughput, evidence based taget selection and validation strategies. *Drug Discov Today* 2001;6:628–36.

18. Martin GR. Isolation of a pluripotent cell line from early mouse embryos cultured in medium conditioned by teratocarcinoma stem cells. *Proc Natl Acad Sci USA* 1981;78:7634–8.

19. Zambrowicz BP, Sands A. Knockouts of the 100 best-selling drugs—will they model the next 100? *Nat Rev Drug Discov* 203;2:38–51.

20. Genschow E, Spielmann H, Scholz G, Pohl I, Seiler A, Clemann N, et al. Validation of the embryonic stem cell test in the international ECVAM validation study on three in vitro embryotoxicity tests. *ATLA* 2004;32:209–44.

21. Newal DR, Beedles K. The stem cell test: an in vitro assay for teratogenic potential. Results of a blind trial with 25 compounds. *Tox In vitro* 1996;10:229–40.

22. Scholz G, Genschow E, Pohl I, Bremer S, Paparella M, Raabe H, et al. Prevalidation of the embryonic stem cell test (EST)—a new in vitro embryotoxicity test. *Toxicol In vitro* 1999;13:675–81.

23. Scholz G, Pohl I, Genschow E, Klemm M, Spielmann H. Embryotoxicity screening using embryonic stem cells in vitro: correlation to in vivo teratogenicity. *Cells Tiss Org* 1999;165:203–11.

24. Thompson JA, Itskovitz-Eldor J, Shapiro SS, Waknitz MA, Swiergiel JJ, Marshall VS, et al. Embryonic stem cell lines derived from human blastocysts. *Science* 1998;282:1145–7.

25. Lavon N, Benvenistry N. Study of hepatocyte differentiation using embryonic stem cells. *J Cell Biochem* 2005;96:1193–202.

26. Soto-Gutierrez A, Navarro-Alvarez N, Rivas-Carrillo JD, Chen Y. Differentiation of human embryonic stem cells to hepatocytes using deleted variant of HGF and poly-amino-urethane-coated nonwoven polytetrafluoroethylene fabric. *Cell Transpl* 2006;15:335–41.

27. Xu C, Police S, Rao N, et al. Characterization and enrichment cardiomyocytes derived from human embryonic stem cells. *Cir Res* 2002;91:501–8.

28. Leahy A, Xiong JW, Kuhnert F, Stuhlmann H. Use of developmental marker genes to define temporal and spatial patterns of differentiation during embryoid body formation. *J Exp Zool* 1999;284:67–81.

29. Rohwedel J, Guan K, Hegert C, Wobus AM. Embryonic stem cells as an in vitro model for mutagenicity, cytotoxicity and embryotoxicity studies: present state and future prospects. *Toxicol In vitro* 2001;15:741–53.

30. Laschinski G, Vogel R, Spielmann H. Cytotoxicity test using blastocyst-derived euploid embryonal stem cells: a new approach to in vitro teratogenesis screening. *Reprod Toxicol* 1991;5:57–64.

31. Brown NA. Selection of test chemicals for the ECVAM international validation study on in vitro embryotoxicity tests. *ATLA* 2002;30:177–98.

32. Chapin R, Stedman D, Paquette J, Streck R, Kumpf S, Deng S. Struggles for equivalence: In vitro developmental toxicity model evolution in pharmaceuticals in 2006. *Toxicol In vitro* 2007;21:1545–51.

33. Bremer S, Worth AP, Paparella M, Bigot K, Kolossov E, Fleischmann BK, Hescheler J, Balls M. Establishment of an in vitro reporter gene assay for developmental cardiac toxicity. *Toxicol In vitro* 2001;15:215–23.

34. Bigot K, De Lange J, Archer G, Clothier R, Bremer S. The relative semi-quantification of mRNA expression as a useful toxicological endpoint for the identification of embryotoxic/teratogenic substances. *Toxicol In vitro* 1999;13: 619–23.

35. zur Nieden NI, Ruf LJ, Kempka G, Hildebrand H, Ahr H. Molecular markers in embryonic stem cells. *Toxicol In vitro* 2001;15:455–61.

36. zur Nieden NI, Kempka G, Ahr HJ. Molecular multiple endpoint embryonic stem cell test-a possible approach to test for the teratogenic potential of compounds. *Toxicol Appl Pharmacol* 2004;194:257–69.

37. Pellizzer C, Adler S, Corvi R, Hartung T, Bremer S. Monitoring of teratogenic effects in vitro by analysing a selected gene expression pattern. *Toxicol In vitro* 2004;18:325–35.

38. Dvash T, Mayshar Y, Darr H, McElhaney M, Barker D, Yanuka O, et al. Temporal gene expression during differentiation of human embryonic stem cells and embryoid bodies. *Hum Reprod* 2004;19:2875–83.

39. Festag M, Viertel B, Steinberg P, Sehner C. An in vitro embryotoxicity assay based on the disturbance of the differentiation of murine embryonic stem cells into endothelial cells. II: testing of compounds. *Toxicol In vitro* 2007;21: 1631–40.

40. Zhang B, Pan X, Anderson TA. MicroRNA: a new player in stem cells. *J Cell Physiol* 2006;209:266–9.

41. Olson H, Betton G, Robinson D, Thomas K, Monro A, Kolaja G, et al. Concordance of the toxicity of pharmaceuticals in humans and in animals. *Reg Toxicol Pharmacol* 2000;32:56–67.

42. Slordal L, Spigset O. Heart failure induced by no-cardiac drugs. *Drug Saf* 2006;29:567–86.

43. http://www.ich.org.

44. Arrigoni C, Crivori P. Assessment of QT liabilities in drug development. *Cell Biol Toxicol* 2007;23:87–105.

45. Fermini B, Fossa A. The impact of drug-induced QT interval prolongation on drug discovery and development. *Nat Rev Drug Discov* 2003;2:429–47.

46. Hoffmann P, Warner B. Channel inhibition and QT interval prolongation: all there is in drug-induced torsadogenesis? *Toxicol Meth* 2006;53:87–105.

47. Harding SE, Ali NN, Brito-Martins M, et al. The human embryonic stem cell-derived cardiomyocytes as a pharmacological model. *Pharmacol Ther* 2007; 113:341–53.

48. Mitcheson JS, Hancox JC, Levi A. Cultured adult cardiac myocytes: Future applications, culture methods, morpological and electrophysiological properties. *Cardiovas Res* 1998;39:280–300.

49. Piper H, Jacobson S, Schwartz P. Determinants of cardiomyocyte development in long-term primary culture. *J Mol Cell Cardiol* 1998;20:825–35.

50. Beltrami AP, Barlucchi L, Torella D, et al. Adult cardiac stem cells are multipotent and support myocardial regeneration. *Cell Biol Toxicol* 2003;114: 763–76.

51. Urbanek K, Quani F, Giordano T, et al. Intense myocyte formation from cardiac stem cell in human cardiac hyperthrophy. *Proc Natl Acad Sci USA* 2003;100: 10440–5.

52. Urbanek K, Torella D, Sheikh F, et al. Myocardial regeneration by activation of multipotent cardiac stem cells in ischemic heart failure. *Proc Natl Acad Sci USA* 2005;102:8692–7.

53. Bearzi C, Rota M, Hosoda T, et al. Human cardiac stem cells. *Proc Natl Acad Sci USA* 2007;104:14068–73.

54. Chen X, Wilson RM, Kubo H, et al. Adolescent feline heart contains a population of small, proliferative ventricular myocytes with immature physiological properties. *Circ Res* 2007;100:536–44.

55. Linke A, Muller P, Nurzynska D, et al. Stem cells in the dog heart are self-renewing, clonogenic, and multipotent and regenerate infarcted myocardium, improving cardiac function. *Proc Natl Acad Sci USA* 2005;102:8966–71.

56. Matsuura K, Nagai T, Nishigaki N, et al. Adult cardiac Sca-1-positive cells differentiate into beating cardiomyocytes. *J Biol Chem* 2004;279:11384–91.

57. Messina E, Angelis De L, Frati G, et al. Isolation and expansion of adult cardiac stem cells from human and murine heart. *Circ Res* 2004;95:911–21.

58. Laugwitz K, Moretti A, Lam J, et al. Postnatal isl1 cardioblasts enter fully differentated cardiomyocyte lineages. *Nat Biotechnol* 2005;433:647–53.

59. Cai C, Liang X, Shi Y, et al. Isl1 identifies a cardiac progenitor population that proliferates prior to differentation and contributes a majority of cells to the heart. *Dev Cell* 2003;5:877–89.

60. Bobbis S, Jarocha D, Majka M. Mesenchymal stem cells: charateristics and clinical applicaitons. *Folia Histochem Cytobiol* 2003;44:215–30.

61. Makino S, Fukuda K, Miyoshi S, et al. Cardiomyocytes can be generated from marrow stromal cell in vitro. *J Clin Invest* 1999;103:697–705.

62. Rangappa S, Entwistle J, Wechsler A, et al. Cardiomyocyte-mediated contact programs human mesenchymal stem cells to express cardiogenic phenotype. *J Thorac Cardiovasc Surg* 2003;126:124–32.

63. Shim W, Jiang S, Wong P, et al. Ex vivo differentiaiton of human adult bone marrow stem cells into cardiomyocyte-like cells. *Biochem Biophys Res Commun* 2004;324:481–8.

64. Hakuno D, Fukuda K, Makino S, et al. Bone marrow-derived regenerated cardiomyocytes (CMG cells) express functional adrenergic and muscarinic receptors. *Circulation* 2002;105:380–6.

65. Kajstura J, Rota M, Whang B, et al. Bone marrow cells differentiate in cardiac cell lineages after infarction independently of cell fusion. *Cir Res* 2004;96:127–37.

66. Tomita S, Li RK, Weisel RD, et al. Autologous transportation of bone marrow cells improves damaged heart function. *Circulation* 1999;100:II247–56.

67. Collins SD, Baffour R, Waksman R. Cell therapy in myocardial infarction. *Cardiovasc Rvasc Med* 2000;8:43–51.

68. Palpant NJ, Yasuda S, MacDougald O, et al. Non-canonical Wnt signaling enhances differentiation of Sca1+/C-kit adipose-derived murine stromal vascular cells into spontaneously beating cardiac myocytes. *J Mol Cell Cardio* 2007;43:363–70.

69. Planat-Benard V, Menard C, Andre M, et al. Spontaneous cardiomyocyte differentiation from adipose tissue stromal cells. *Circ Res* 2004;94:223–9.

70. Rangappa S, Fen C, Lee E, et al. Transformation of adult mesenchymal stem cells isolated from fatty tissue into cardiomyocytes. *Ann Thorac Surg* 2003;75:775–9.

71. Winitsky SO, Gopal TV, Hassanzadeh S, et al. Adult murine skeletal muscle contains cells that can differentiate into beating cardiomypcytes in vitro. *PLoS Biol* 2005;3:e87.

72. Badorff C, Brandes RP, Popp R, et al. Transdifferentiation of blood-derived human adult endothelial progenitor cells into functionally active cardiomyocytes. *Circulation* 2003;107:1024–32.

73. Bonanno G, Mariotti A, Procoli A, et al. Human cord blood CD133+ cells immunoselected by a clinical-grade apparatus differentiate in vitro into endothelial- and cardiomyocyte-like cells. *Transfusion* 2007;47:280–9.

74. Kadivar M, Khatami S, Mortazavi Y, et al. In vitro cardiomyogenic potential of human umbilical vein-derived mesenchymal stem cells. *Biochem Biophys Res Commun* 2006;340:639–47.

75. Nishiyama N, Miyoshi S, Hidan N, et al. The significant cardiomyogenic potential of human umbilical cord blood-derived mesenchymal stem cells in vitro. *Stem Cells* 2007;10:2006–0662.

76. Miki T, Lehmann T, Cai H, Stolz DB, Strom S. Stem cells characteristics of amniotic epithelial cells. *Stem Cells* 2005;23:1549–59.

77. Okamoto K, Miyoshi S, Toyoda M, et al. Working cardiomyocyte exhibiting plateau action potentials from human placenta-derived extraembryonic mesodermal cells. *Exp Cell Res* 2007;313:2550–62.

78. De Coppi P, Bartsch G, Siddiqui M, et al. Isolation of ammiotic stem cell lines with potential for therapy. *Nat Biotechnol* 2007;25:100–6.

79. Kehat I, Kenyagin-Karsenti D, Snir N, et al. Human embryonic stem cells can differentiate into myocytes with structural and functional properties of cardio-myocytes. *J Clin Invest* 2001;108:407–14.

80. Mummery C, Ward-Van O, Doevendans P, et al. Differentiation of human embryonic stem cells to cardiomyocytes: role of coculture visceral endoderm-like cells. *Circulation* 2003;107:2733–40.

81. Sartiani L, Bettiol E, Stillitano F, et al. Developmental changes in cardiomyocytes differentiated from human embryonic stem cells. *Stem Cells* 2007;25:1136–44.

82. Laflamme MA, Chen KY, Naumova AV, et al. Cardiomyocytes derived from human embryonic stem cells in pro-survival factors enhance function of infarcted rat hearts. *Nat Biotechnol* 2007;25:1015–24.

83. Van Laake LW, Rassier R, Monshouwer-Kloots J, et al. Human embryonic stem cell-derived cardiomyocytes survive and mature in the mouse heart and transiently improve function after myocardial infarction. *Stem Cell Res* 2007;10:1016.

84. Kehat I, Gepstein A, Spira A, et al. High-resolution electrophysiological assessment of human embryonic stem cells derived-cardiomyocytes: a novel in vitro model for the study of conduction. *Cir Res* 2002;91:659–61.

85. Reppel M, Pillekamp F, Brockmeier K, et al. The electrocardiogram of human embryonic stem cell-derived cardiomyocytes. *J Electrocardiol* 2005;38:166–70.

86. Beqqali A, Kloots J, Ward-Van O, et al. Genome-wide transcriptional profiling of human embryonic stem cells differentiating to cardiomyocytes. *Stem Cells* 2006;24:1956–67.

87. Huber I, Itzhaki I, Caspi O, et al. Identification of selection of cardiomyocytes during human embryonic stem cell differentiation. *FASEB* 2007;21:2551–63.

88. Anderson D, Self T, Mellor IR, et al. Transgenic enrichment of cardiomyocytes from human embryonic stem cells. *Mol Ther* 2007;15:2027–36.

89. Zwaka TP, Thompson JA. Homologous recombination in human embryonic stem cells. *Nat Biotechnol* 2003;21:1319–21.

90. Alperin C, Zandstra PW, Woodhouse KA. Engineering cardiac healing using embryonic stem cell-derived cardiac cell seeded constructs. *Front Biosci* 2007;12:3694–712.

91. Feinberg AW, Feigel A, Shevkolyas SS, et al. Muscular thin films for building actuators and power devices. *Science* 2007;317:1366–70.

92. Caspi O, Lesman A, Basevitch Y, et al. Tissue engineering of vascularized cardiac muscle from human embryonic stem cells. *Circ Res* 2007;100:263–72.

93. Shultz LD, Ishikawa F, Greiner DL. Humanized mice in translational biomedical research. *Nat Rev* 2007;7:1121–30.

94. Kehat I, Khimovich L, Caspi O, et al. Electromechanical integration of cardio-myocytes derived from human embryonic stem cells. *Nat Biotechnol* 2004;22:1282–9.

95. Suter L, Babiss LE, Wheeldon E. Toxicogenomics in predictive toxicology in drug development. *Chem Biol* 2004;11:161–71.

96. Farkas D, Tannembaum S. In vitro methods to study chemically-induced hepatotoxicity: a literature review. *Curr Drug Metab* 2005;6:111–25.

97. Grisham JW, Charlton RK, Kaufman DG. In vitro assay of cytotoxicity with cultured liver: accomplishments and possibilities. *Environ Health Perspect* 1978;25: 161–71.

98. Zimmerman HJ. *Hepatotoxicity: the adverse effects of drugs and other chemicals on the liver*. Philadelphia: Lippincott Williams Wilkins, 1999.

99. Zimmerman HJ. *Drug-induced liver disease. Clin Liver Dis* 2000;4:73–96.

100. Dambach DM, Andrews BA, Moulin F. New technologies and screening strategies for hepatotoxicity: use of in vitro models. *Toxicol Pathol* 2005;33:17–26.

101. Martin GR. Isolation of a pluripotent cell line from early mouse embryos cultured in medium conditioned by teratocarcinoma stem cells. *Proc Natl Acad Sci USA* 1981;78:7634–8.

102. Evans MJ, Kaufman MH. Establishment in culture of pluripotential cells from mouse embryos. *Nature* 1981;292:154–6.

103. Scherer CA, Chen J, Nachabeh A, Hopkins N, Ruley HE. Transcriptional specificity of the pluripotent embryonic stem cell. *Cell Growth Differ* 1996;7: 1393–401.

104. Beddington RS, Robertson EJ. An assessment of the developmental potential of embryonic stem cells in the midgestation mouse embryo. *Development* 1989;105: 733–7.

105. Abe K, Niwa H, Iwase K, Takiguchi M, Mori M, Abe SI, et al. Endoderm-specific gene expression in embryonic stem cells differentiated to embryoid bodies. *Exp Cell Res* 1996;229:27–34.

106. Levinson-Dushnik M, Benvenisty N. Involvement of hepatocyte nuclear factor 3 in endoderm differentiation of embryonic stem cells. *Mol Cell Biol* 1997;17: 3817–22.

107. Jones EA, Tosh D, Wilson DI, Lindsay S, Forrester LM. Hepatic differentiation of murine embryonic stem cells. *Exp Cell Res* 2002;272:15–22.

108. Yamada T, Yoshikawa M, Kanda S, Kato Y, Nakajima Y, Ishizaka S, et al. In vitro differentiation of embryonic stem cells into hepatocyte-like cells identified by cellular uptake of indocyanine green. *Stem Cells* 2002;20:146–54.

109. Asahina K, Fujimori H, Shimizu-Saito K, Kumashiro Y, Okamura K, Tanaka Y, et al. Expression of the liver-specific gene Cyp7a1 reveals hepatic differentiation in embryoid bodies derived from mouse embryonic stem cells. *Genes Cells* 2004;9:1297–308.

110. Hamazaki T, Iiboshi Y, Oka M, Papst PJ, Meacham AM, Zon LI, et al. Hepatic maturation in differentiating embryonic stem cells in vitro. *FEBS Lett* 2001;497: 15–9.

111. Kuai XL, Cong XQ, Li XL, Xiao SD. Generation of hepatocytes from cultured mouse embryonic stem cells. *Liver Transpl* 2003;9:1094–9.

112. Kubo A, Shinozaki K, Shannon JM, Kouskoff V, Kennedy M, Woo S, et al. Development of definitive endoderm from embryonic stem cells in culture. *Development* 2004;131:1651–62.

113. Yamamoto H, Quinn G, Asari A, Yamanokuchi H, Teratani T, Terada M, et al. Differentiation of embryonic stem cells into hepatocytes: biological functions and therapeutic application. *Hepatology* 2003;37:983–93.

114. Teratani T, Yamamoto H, Aoyagi K, Sasaki H, Asari A, Quinn G, et al. Direct hepatic fate specification from mouse embryonic stem cells. *Hepatology* 2005;41: 836–46.

115. Yamamoto Y, Teratani T, Yamamoto H, Quinn G, Murata S, Ikeda R, et al. Recapitulation of in vivo gene expression during hepatic differentiation from murine embryonic stem cells. *Hepatology* 2005;42:558–67.

116. Fair JH, Cairns BA, Lapaglia M, Wang J, Meyer AA, Kim H, et al. Induction of hepatic differentiation in embryonic stem cells by co-culture with embryonic cardiac mesoderm. *Surgery* 2003;134:189–96.

117. Hu A, Cai J, Zheng Q, He X, Pan Y, Li L. Hepatic differentiation from embryonic stem cells in vitro. *Chin Med J (Engl)* 2003;116:1893–7.

118. Ishii T, Yasuchika K, Fujii H, Hoppo T, Baba S, Naito M, et al. In vitro differentiation and maturation of mouse embryonic stem cells into hepatocytes. *Exp Cell Res* 2005;309:68–77.

119. Ishizaka S, Ouji Y, Yoshikawa M, Nakatani K. Derivation and characterization of hepatocytes from embryonic stem cells in vitro. *Meth Mol Biol* 2006;330: 387–99.

120. Novik EI, Maguire TJ, Orlova K, Schloss RS, Yarmush ML. Embryoid body-mediated differentiation of mouse embryonic stem cells along a hepatocyte lineage: insights from gene expression profiles. *Tissue Eng* 2006;12:1515–25.

121. Soto-Gutierrez A, Navarro-Alvarez N, Zhao D, Rivas-Carrillo JD, Lebkowski J, Tanaka N, et al. Differentiation of mouse embryonic stem cells to hepatocyte-like cells by co-culture with human liver nonparenchymal cell lines. *Nat Protoc* 2007;2:347–56.

122. Choi D, Oh HJ, Chang UJ, Koo SK, Jiang JX, Hwang SY, et al. In vivo differentiation of mouse embryonic stem cells into hepatocytes. *Cell Transpl* 2002;11: 359–68.

123. Tsutsui M, Ogawa S, Inada Y, Tomioka E, Kamiyoshi A, Tanaka S, et al. Characterization of cytochrome P450 expression in murine embryonic stem cell-derived hepatic tissue system. *Drug Metab Dispos* 2006;34:696–701.

124. Xu JJ, Diaz D, O'Brien PJ. Applications of cytotoxicity assays and pre-lethal mechanistic assays for assessment of human hepatotoxicity potential. *Chem Biol Interact* 2004;150:115–28.

125. Thompson JA, Kalishman J, Golos TG, Durning M, Harris CP, Becker RA, et al. Isolation of a primate embryonic stem cell line. *Proc Natl Acad Sci USA* 1995;92:7844–8.

126. Marshall E. Cell biology: a versatile cell line raises scientific hopes, legal questions. *Science* 1998;282:1014–5.

127. Gearhart J. Cell biology: new potential for human embryonic stem cells. *Science* 1998;282:1061–2.

128. Miller LJ, Bloom FE. Publishing controversial research. *Science* 1998;282: 1045.

129. Hart AH, Hartley L, Ibrahim M, Robb L. Identification, cloning and expression analysis of the pluripotency promoting Nanog genes in mouse and human. *Dev Dyn* 2004;230:187–98.

130. Heins N, Englund MC, Sjoblom C, Dahl U, Tonning A, Bergh C, et al. Derivation, characterization, and differentiation of human embryonic stem cells. *Stem Cells* 2004;22:367–76.

131. Laslett AL, Filipczyk AA, Pera M. Characterization and culture of human embryonic stem cells. *Trends Cardiovasc Med* 2003;13:295–301.

132. Park SP, Lee YJ, Lee KS, Ah-Shin H, Cho H. Establishment of human embryonic stem cell lines from frozen-thawed blastocysts using STO cell feeder layers. *Hum Reprod* 2004;19:676–84.

133. Itskovitz-Eldor J, Schuldiner M, Karsenti D, Eden A, Yanuka O, Amit M, et al. Differentiation of human embryonic stem cells into embryoid bodies compromising the three embryonic germ layers. *Mol Med* 2000;6:88–95.

134. Schuldiner M, Yanuka O, Itskovitz-Eldor J, Melton DA, Benvenisty N. Effects of eight growth factors on the differentiation of cells derived from human embryonic stem cells. *Proc Natl Acad Sci USA* 2000;97:11307–12.

135. Kobayashi N, Okitsu T, Tanaka N. Cell choice for bioartificial livers. *Keio J Med* 2003;52:151–7.

136. Rambhatla L, Chiu CP, Kundu P, Peng Y, Carpenter MK. Generation of hepatocyte-like cells from human embryonic stem cells. *Cell Transpl* 2003;12: 1–11.

137. Sinha G. Cell biology. Human embryonic stem cells may be toxicology's new best friends. *Science* 2005;308:1538.

138. Haumaitre C, Reber M, Cereghini S. Functions of HNF1 family members in differentiation of the visceral endoderm cell lineage. *J Biol Chem* 2003;278: 40933–42.

139. Lavon N, Yanuka O, Benvenisty N. Differentiation and isolation of hepatic-like cells from human embryonic stem cells. *Differentiation* 2004;72:230–8.

140. Chen Y, Soto-Gutierrez A, Navarro-Alvarez N, Rivas-Carrillo JD, Yamatsuji T, Shirakawa Y, et al. Instant hepatic differentiation of human embryonic stem cells using activin A and a deletedvariant of HGF. *Cell Transpl* 2006;15:865–71.

141. Heng BC, Yu H, Yin Y, Lim SC, Cao T. Factors influencing stem cell differentiation into the hepatic lineage in vitro. *J Gastroenterol Hepatol* 2005;20.

142. Schwartz RE, Linehan JL, Painschab MS, Hu WS, Verfaillie CM, Kaufman D. Defined conditions for development of functional hepatic cells from human embryonic stem cells. *Stem Cells Dev* 2005;14:643–55.

143. Tsukada H, Takada T, Shiomi H, Torii R, Tani T. Acidic fibroblast growth factor promotes hepatic differentiation of monkey stem cells. *In vitro Cell Dev Biol* 2006;42:83–8.

144. Newsome PN, Johannessen I, Boyle S, Dalakas E, McAulay KA, Samuel K, et al. Human cord blood-derived cells can differentiate into hepatocytes in the mouse liver with no evidence of cellular fusion. *Gastroenterology* 2003;124: 1891–900.

145. Di Campli C, Piscaglia AC, Pierelli L, Rutella S, Bonanno G, Alison MR, et al. A human umbilical cord stem cell rescue therapy in a murine model of toxic liver injury. *Dig Liver Dis* 2004;36:603–13.

146. Di Campli C, Piscaglia AC, Rutella S, Bonanno G, Vecchio FM, Zocco MA, et al. Improvement of mortality rate and decrease in histologic hepatic injury after human cord blood stem cell infusion in a murine model of hepatotoxicity. *Transpl Proc* 2005;37:2707–10.

147. Lee OK, Kuo TK, Chen WM, Lee KD, Hsieh SL, Chen TH. Isolation of multi-potent mesenchymal stem cells from umbilical cord blood. *Blood* 2004;103:1669–75.

148. Matikainen T, Laine J. Placenta—an alternative source of stem cells. *Toxicol Appl Pharmacol* 2005;207:544–9.

149. McGuckin CP, Forraz N, Baradez MO, Navran S, Zhao J, Urban R, et al. Production of stem cells with embryonic characteristics from human umbilical cord blood. *Cell Prolif* 2005;38:245–55.

150. Saito S, Yokoyama K, Tamagawa T, Ishiwata I. Derivation and induction of the differentiation of animal ES cells as well as human pluripotent stem cells derived from fetal membrane. *Hum Cell* 2005;18:135–41.

151. Hong SH, Gang EJ, Jeong JA, Ahn C, Hwang SH, Yang IH, et al. In vitro differentiation of human umbilical cord blood-derived mesenchymal stem cells into hepatocyte-like cells. *Biochem Biophys Res Commun* 2005;330:1153–61.

152. Kang XQ, Zang WJ, Bao LJ, Li DL, Song TS, Xu XL, et al. Fibroblast growth factor-4 and hepatocyte growth factor induce differentiation of human umbilical cord blood-derived mesenchymal stem cells into hepatocytes. *World J Gastroenterol* 2005;11:7461–5.

153. Kang XQ, Zang WJ, Bao LJ, Li DL, Xu XL, Yu XJ. Differentiating characterization of human umbilical cord blood-derived mesenchymal stem cells in vitro. *Cell Biol Int* 2006;30:569–75.

154. Teramoto K, Asahina K, Kumashiro Y, Kakinuma S, Chinzei R, Shimizu-Saito K, et al. Hepatocyte differentiation from embryonic stem cells and umbilical cord blood cells. *J Hepatobiliary Pancreat Surg* 2005;12:196–202.

155. Chien CC, Yen BL, Lee FK, Lai TH, Chen YC, Chan SH, et al. In vitro differentiation of human placenta-derived multipotent cells into hepatocyte-like cells. *Stem Cells* 2006;24:1759–68.

156. Sun Y, Xiao D, Zhang RS, Cui GH, Wang XH, Chen XG. Formation of human hepatocyte-like cells with different cellular phenotypes by human umbilical cord blood-derived cells in the human-rat chimeras. *Biochem Biophys Res Commun* 2007;357:1160–5.

157. Potten CS, Loeffler M. Stem cells: attributes, cycles, spirals, pitfalls and uncertainties. Lessons for and from the crypt. *Development* 1990;110:1001–20.

158. Schwartz RE, Reyes M, Koodie L, Jiang Y, Blackstad M, Lund T, et al. Multipotent adult progenitor cells from bone marrow differentiate into functional hepatocyte-like cells. *J Clin Invest* 2002;109:1291–302.

159. Petersen BE, Bowen WC, Patrene KD, Mars WM, Sullivan AK, Murase N, et al. Bone marrow as a potential source of hepatic oval cells. *Science* 1999;284: 1168–70.

160. Fuchs E, Segre JA. Stem cells: a new lease on life. *Cell* 2000;100:143–55.

161. Bjornson CR, Rietze RL, Reynolds BA, Magli MC, Vescovi AL. Turning brain into blood: a hematopoietic fate adopted by adult neural stem cells in vivo. *Science* 1999;283:534–7.

162. Lee RH, Kim B, Choi I, Kim H, Choi HS, Suh K, et al. Characterization and expression analysis of mesenchymal stem cells from human bone marrow and adipose tissue. *Cell Physiol Biochem* 2004;14:311–24.

163. Shu SN, Wei L, Wang JH, Zhan YT, Chen HS, Wang Y. Hepatic differentiation capability of rat bone marrow-derived mesenchymal stem cells and hematopoietic stem cells. *World J Gastroenterol* 2004;10:2818–22.

164. Lange C, Bassler P, Lioznov MV, Bruns H, Kluth D, Zander AR, et al. Hepato-cytic gene expression in cultured rat mesenchymal stem cells. *Transpl Proc* 2005;37:276–9.

165. Shimomura T, Yoshida Y, Sakabe T, Ishii K, Gonda K, Murai R, et al. Hepatic differentiation of human bone marrow-derived UE7T-13 cells: effects of cytokines and CCN family gene expression. *Hepatol Res* 2007;37:1068–79.

166. Sato Y, Araki H, Kato J, Nakamura K, Kawano Y, Kobune M, et al. Human mesenchymal stem cells xenografted directly to rat liver are differentiated into human hepatocytes without fusion. *Blood* 2005;106:756–63.

167. Aurich I, Mueller LP, Aurich H, Luetzkendorf J, Tisljar K, Dollinger MM, et al. Functional integration of hepatocytes derived from human mesenchymal stem cells into mouse livers. *Gut* 2007;56:405–15.

168. Oh SH, Witek RP, Bae SH, Zheng D, Jung Y, Piscaglia AC, et al. Bone marrow-derived hepatic oval cells differentiate into hepatocytes in 2-acetylaminofluorene/partial hepatectomy-induced liver regeneration. *Gastroenterology* 2007;132: 1077–87.

169. Zuk PA, Zhu M, Ashjian P, De Ugarte DA, Huang JI, Mizuno H, et al. Human adipose tissue is a source of multipotent stem cells. *Mol Biol Cell* 2002;13: 4279–95.

170. Seo MJ, Suh SY, Bae YC, Jung JS. Differentiation of human adipose stromal cells into hepatic lineage in vitro and in vivo. *Biochem Biophys Res Commun* 2005;328:258–64.

171. Talens-Visconti R, Bonora A, Jover R, Mirabet V, Carbonell F, Castell JV, et al. Hepatogenic differentiation of human mesenchymal stem cells from adipose tissue in comparison with bone marrow mesenchymal stem cells. *World J Gastro-enterol* 2006;12:5834–45.

172. Banas A, Teratani T, Yamamoto Y, Tokuhara M, Takeshita F, Quinn G, et al. Adipose tissue-derived mesenchymal stem cells as a source of human hepato-cytes. *Hepatology* 2007;46:219–28.

173. Sgodda M, Aurich H, Kleist S, Aurich I, Konig S, Dollinger MM, et al. Hepato-cyte differentiation of mesenchymal stem cells from rat peritoneal adipose tissue in vitro and in vivo. *Exp Cell Res* 2007;313:2875–86.

174. Asahina K, Fujimori H, Shimizu-Saito K, Kumashiro Y, Okamura K, Tanaka Y, et al. Expression of the liver-specific gene CYP7A1 reveals hepatic differentiation in embryoid bodies derived from mouse embryonic stem cells. *Genes Cells* 2004;9:1297–308.

175. Yu J, Vodyanik MA, Smuga-Otto K, Antosiewicz-Bourget J, Frane JL, Tian S, et al. Induced pluripotent stem cell lines derived from human somatic cells. *Science* 2007;doi:10.1126.Science 1151526.

176. Takahashi K, Tanabe K, Ohnuki M, Narita M, Ichisaka T, Tomoda K, et al. Induction of pluripotent stem cells from adult human fibroblasts by defined factors. *Cell* 2007;131:1–12.

9

TELEMETRY TECHNOLOGY FOR PRECLINICAL DRUG DISCOVERY AND DEVELOPMENT

YI YANG

Contents

Drug Efficacy, Safety, and Biologics Discovery: Emerging Technologies and Tools,
Edited by Sean Ekins and Jinghai J. Xu
Copyright © 2009 by John Wiley & Sons, Inc.

9.1 OVERVIEW

Telemetry technology, also called radiotelemetry, was first applied by Van Citters's team [1] to remotely monitor the blood pressure from two wild adult male giraffes captured and released near Kiboko, Kenya. The blood pressure monitoring was conducted and compared in the animals' lying position, with their heads on the ground, to their standing erect. Since then further advances in the telemetry technology have made the measurements of the functional changes in cardiovascular, respiratory, central nervous system (CNS), and other systems a simple and routine procedure in drug discovery and development. The significance of telemetry data collection is to allow the normal and pathophysiological variable monitoring to be conducted to investigate the effect of the test articles or medications when animals are conscious and unrestrained, which simulates the clinical setting. In addition to improvement of the quality of data collected with the telemetry method, this is also a significant approach for improving animal welfare by reducing the utilization of animals. Therefore telemetry technology has been increasingly used and continuously expanded to whole animal testing in both efficacy or safety evaluation of a new drug or therapy.

9.2 IN VIVO PHYSIOLOGICAL PARAMETER MONITORING BEFORE TELEMETRY TECHNOLOGY

The major advantage of the telemetry data collection system is to enable the measurements to be performed when the animals are awake and unrestrained. However, such measurements can be particularly challenging to obtain from restrained and/or anesthetized animals. The hemodynamic (heart rate and blood pressure) electrophysiological (ECG intervals) and respiratory (respiratory rate) data collected from restrained animals often suffer from increased blood pressure and heart rate that are much higher than the normal physiological range due to the animals' excitement. The anesthetics used to sedate the animals often cause drug-induced hypotension and respiratory rate or QT interval changes. Without carefully monitoring of blood gas parameters, anesthetics may also cause hypo- or hypercarpnia. Based on our experience with or without telemetry, the heart rate ranged from 90 to 120 beats per minute from conscious telemetered Cynomolgus monkeys with no treatment, to up to 250 beats per minute when the monkey was conscious and restrained. Unwanted artificial interference will mask the test results to a certain degree and can compromise the data integrity and quality. It can also reduce the sensitivity of the testing system for detection of efficacy or side-effect signals, especially when the changes are subtle. As a consequence the disadvantages associated with data collection from restrained and anesthetized animals will certainly make rational data interpretation a challenge. The other negative effects from utilization of restrained animals includes an increase in the inter-animal variability of physiological parameters and potentially cause increased animal usage if it requires increased sample size to offset the larger data variance.

9.3 PRINCIPLES AND COMPONENTS OF THE TELEMETRY SYSTEM

The telemetry physiological data system normally includes (1) the transducer(s) or sensor(s) that can be implanted or attached to the interested area(s) to collect physiological parameter(s), (2) the battery-powered transmitter to emit the signals wirelessly, (3) the receiver(s) that can detect and pick up the sent signals over a range in pre-assigned working radiofrequency, and (4) the data-processing center that can store and analyze the telemetry signals. The implanted transmitter is normally in a watertight stainless steel case with all sensor electronics sealed inside. The transmitter acquires dimension, pressure, core body temperature, and electrocardiography (ECG) from selected lead locations. Figure 9.1 illustrates the major functional devices and working flow of a telemetry system that is often used in a cardiovascular telemetry study with rodents or large animals. The key components of a telemetry data monitoring system are to establish a wireless conversion between the transmission of the physiological data collected and receiving of the data transmitted. Basically telemetry data collection works in a similar way to wireless or mobile phone communications. The transmitter captures physiological signals, and sends them out at a specific radiofrequency to the receiver. The telemetry processing center (normally a computer with installed data analysis software) processes the received physiological signals and converts them into different waveforms for online or offline analysis.

9.4 TELEMETRY TECHNOLOGY IN PRECLINICAL DRUG SAFETY PROFILING AND ASSESSMENT

9.4.1 Telemetry Testing System Validations

The validation of telemetry systems can be divided into two categories. One is to validate the functionalities of a testing system, and the other is to focus on the instrument/system validation. The latter validation is required if the instrument/system is intended to generate study results to support regulatory studies. The major goal of this validation is to establish documented evidence that provides a high degree of assurance that a specific system will consistently function and meet its predetermined specifications and quality attributes, in compliance of 21 CFR part 11 [2]. To accomplish this task, normally a validation team needs to be formed from different functional groups, including potential user representative(s), the information technology (IT) group, and

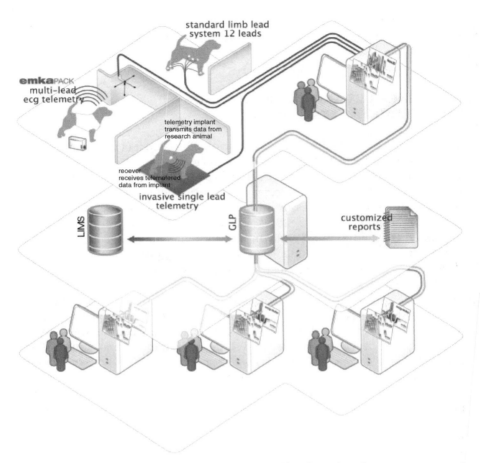

Figure 9.1   Major functional components and working flow of a telemetry system used in a cardiovascular telemetry study with rodent or large animal. (See color insert.)

quality assurance, with active involvement of the vendor technical support. Clearly, identification of user requirements and well-documented instrument, operational, and performance qualifications are required for success.

The purpose of the functional validation is normally to evaluate the testing system (including testing animals)'s sensitivity, specificity, reproducibility, and flexibility in detection and collection of the expected changes. Any practical issues occurring in the validation trail also need to be addressed. The power of the sensitivity to detect the change should be calculated based on the sample size and the variability of the parameters collected. Selection of one or two positive reference compounds at escalating dose levels is the common approach for evaluation of the testing system functionalities [3,4].

9.4.2 Telemetry Applications in the Cardiovascular System

The cardiovascular system is the major physiological system where telemetry technology was first and also is still most frequently used. Probably this is not only because it is relatively easy to apply the telemetry technology in cardiovascular monitoring but also because there is a high demand to monitor the functional parameters of the cardiovascular system as vital signs. In ICH guideline S7A [5] the cardiovascular system is identified as one of the three core batteries (together with CNS and respiratory systems) for safety evaluation of any new drugs. The use of telemetry technology to measure blood pressure, heart rate, core body temperature, and ECG parameters has been well validated in different animal species using different positive reference drugs with well-defined effects on either hemodynamic parameters or ECG intervals. Measurements of systemic arterial blood pressure and heart rate via a chronically implanted telemetric transmitter in unrestrained rats were reported by Guiol et al. [6] who determined that week-to-week variability of systolic, diastolic, and mean arterial pressures, and heart rate was found to be minimal over a course of nine weeks. Good reproducibility of cardiovascular response to three successive administrations of sotalol was also described in this study. Furthermore the cardiovascular parameters determined by telemetry were compared to those obtained by direct arterial catheterization and showed a good linear correlation between these two methods. In a cat telemetry model with a catheter implanted into the left femoral artery, no surgical complications occurred. The radiotelemetry catheters were used for an average of 6.5 weeks (range, 5.5 to 9.5 weeks). This technique allowed for long-term monitoring of ambulatory blood pressure and heart rate in the research setting. This methodology is especially useful for studies of the pathophysiology of hypertension and assessment of the efficacy of antihypertensive medications [7].

In accordance with ICH S7A and S7B guidelines [8], one of the tasks of cardiovascular monitoring using the telemetry technique is to identify the prolongation of the heart rate corrected QT interval (QTc) as a surrogate of torsade de pointes, a commonly recognized life-threatening arrhythmia due to delayed ventricular repolarization. Torsadogenic drugs such as cisapride, dofetilide, moxifloxacin, haloperidol, and other pro-arrhythmia drugs are often used to achieve the purpose [9,10]. Based on current pharmaceutical practice, the telemetry models such as dogs and monkeys show low inherent intra-animal variability and high sensitivity to detect small but significant increases in QT/QT(c) interval changes and are generally considered as sensitive models to investigate QT prolongation of novel human pharmaceuticals.

Mice are not commonly used in cardiovascular physiology and electrophysiological studies because of methodological challenges. Initial conventional cardiovascular studies with mice models involved the use of the tail cuff plethysmography method or classical catheterization techniques with a catheter connected to an external pressure transducer. For long-term arterial pressure measurements such studies have been facilitated by the development of telemetry. With the increasing development of transgenic mouse models [11], telemetry technology is now more widely applied in mice. Validation work has also been done to evaluate the use of the telemetry in mice to monitor arterial blood pressure and heart rate recently [12,13]. In contrast, rat is the most frequently used rodent telemetry model in evaluation of efficacy and/or safety profile of cardiovascular system during research and development of new drugs. However, due to fast heart rate in rodents during telemetry data collection, the ECG analysis becomes a challenge.

One of major tasks in cardiovascular telemetry data analysis is to identify an optimal QT correction method to detect and quantify the QTc prolongation in the telemetry-instrumented conscious animal models. Accurate detection of drug-induced QT interval changes is often confounded by concurrent heart rate changes. Application of heart rate correction formulas has been the traditional approach to account for heart rate-induced QT interval changes, and thereby identify the direct effect of the test article on cardiac repolarization. Over- and/or undercorrection of QT intervals for changes in heart rate may lead to misleading conclusions and/or masking of the potential of a drug to prolong the QT interval. This topic is not the focus of this chapter, but a lot of telemetry studies with a variety of pro-arrhythmia reference compounds, in different animal models, have evaluated the approaches in QT interval correction [14–19] and the reader is referred to these.

9.4.3   Telemetry Applications in the Respiratory System

The techniques required to measure respiratory rate, such as plethysmography or pneumotachography, involve moving animals from their natural environments into potentially stressful conditions, which can affect endogenous opioid systems and alter respiration. In addition these methods do not facilitate the long-term measurement of respiratory parameters as the animals cannot remain in the required apparatus for extended periods (e.g., days). Kramer et al. [20] reported that with new software called RespiRATE, a waveform of respiratory rate can also be derived from telemetry blood pressure signals to allow for the continuous measurement of respiratory and cardiovascular parameters of animals in their normal environment and without stress artifacts. A recent approach is to use a pressure-sensitive telemetry jacket worn on test animals to acquire both ECG and respiratory data, but so far the readings from this system only generate indirect respiratory parameters. With the telemetry rat model, To Lewanowitsch et al. [21]

studied the effects of respiratory depressants on respiratory rate and heart rate over four days of treatment with naloxone hydrochloride and naloxone methiodide.

9.4.4 Telemetry Applications in the Central Nervous System

Assessment of proconvulsant risk is an important aspect of CNS safety evaluation, and the electroencephalogram (EEG) is a sensitive technique for identifying pathologic brain activity, and most important, paroxysmal activity. Telemetry technology application to the CNS is mostly focused on monitoring of the EEG spectrum and sleep activity in rats [22–24]. Beig et al. [24] reported a method for simultaneous acquisition of electroencephalogram, heart rate, and arterial blood pressure during seizures in conscious rats after intraperitoneal administration of pentylenetetrazole, with a chronically implanted telemetric device. With the same reference compound, a validation study in telemetry dogs to measure EEG, heart rate, and blood pressure was also conducted. While dogs were placed in slings, the EEG was assessed visually for abnormal activity, and the dogs were also continuously observed for the appearance of overt convulsive activity. All these data show the usefulness of the telemetered dog EEG in safety pharmacology and potential value in anti-seizure efficacy assessment [25]. Combination approaches that integrate EEG and ECG monitoring should reduce animal and test article usage and result in a broader efficacy and safety profile of the test articles. This is especially meaningful since early in drug development the general pharmacologist in the pharmaceutical industry is challenged to generate physiologically relevant data on possible safety liabilities or on secondary therapeutic uses. This calls for efficient use of usually only small supplies of test article.

9.4.5 Other Systems

Applications of telemetry technology have been extended to other physiological function monitoring as well. Telemetry applications have recently been reported in gastrointestinal measurement of intraluminal pressure changes [26,27] and in transit time of intra-ocular pressure monitoring with a telemetry pressure transducer implanted into a rabbit glaucoma model [28].

9.5 PRACTICAL APPROACHES IN TELEMETRY DATA COLLECTION AND ASSESSMENT

9.5.1 Variability with Telemetry Monitoring

While the telemetry technology allows the animals to be monitored in a freely moving and conscious condition mimicking the clinical setting, it also offers the possibility for the animals to "freely" respond to any study-related activities such as blood sampling, clinical observations, and any sound source from the surrounding environment. Furthermore, continued long-term telemetry monitoring invites physiological variance due to circadian change. It can affect hemodynamic and respiratory parameters, the ECG interval, and body temperature [29–33]. For quality data collection and accurate data analysis, a proper procedure is essential to minimize any unnecessary interference, document any interference during the telemetry data collection, and fully understand these variances. Ning et al. [34] have studied the mechanisms of heart rate and blood pressure variability by 24-hour continuous recording of these parameters and their variability spectrum and have related this variability to the activity of the autonomic and central nervous system, which regulates sympathovagal balance and the sympathetic activity. Klumpp et al. [35] tested the influence of housing conditions on hemodynamics during cardiovascular telemetry studies with telemetered dogs and found that the housing arrangement during the study had an effect on the hemodynamics measured. The hemodynamic parameters were best when the dogs were housed with their usual run mate. In this setting they had impressively low average heart rates of about 60 bpm during the entire study, as well as fewer vocalizations. Our experience suggests that when the length of data collection is 24 hours or longer, a pretest baseline and data from the vehicle group can ensure the quality of telemetry data assessment.

9.5.2 Practical Approaches in Telemetry Study Design

A telemetry study can be used for multiple-dose regimens, but most often it is used for acute and single-dose studies to look for functional parameter changes. In most telemetry studies, in-life clinical observations of tested animals (clinical signs, food consumption, and body weight change) are also normally conducted.

As described before, a period (normally 6–24 hours) of pretest telemetry recording is needed for animal selection, and the recording can later be used as a reference baseline if needed. The animals (normally $n = 4$) with normal and quality telemetry signals, together with normal clinical signs and clinical pathological parameters, will be selected for the formal treatment phase. A 4×4 Latin-square crossover paradigm is frequently used in the telemetry cardiovascular and reparatory study. For a telemetry CNS study, a parallel study design can be used. Each of four animals will receive a dose of vehicle and test article at different levels (normally three escalating dose levels) with a minimum washout period between each dose (see Table 9.1). Based on ICH guidelines S7A and S7B, the dose chosen for a safety pharmacology telemetry study is either based on the maximum tolerance dose (MTD) identified from a dose range finding toxicological study or from a dose(s) selection that can achieve a plasma concentration that meaningfully represents a sufficient safety margin if the MTD is unknown.

TABLE 9.1 A 4 × 4 Latin-square Crossover Dose Paradigm and Animal Assignment for a Cardiovascular Telemetry Study

Animal Number	Dosing Schedule of Test Article or Vehicle (mg/kg)			
	Dose 1	Dose 2	Dose 3	Dose 4
1	0	Low	Mid	High
2	Low	Mid	High	0
3	Mid	High	0	Low
4	High	0	Low	Mid

9.5.3 Telemetry Transducer Placement: Intraperitoneal versus Subcutaneous

Intraperitoneal and subcutaneous areas are the most commonly used implantation locations for a telemetry transmitter. For large animals such as dogs and monkeys, the choice of the two implantation positions seems to be mostly related to the user's experience or test center preference. For small animals such as rat, mouse, and gerbil, both locations are still used for transmitter implantation, but a different location may present unique challenges. Based on the author's experience, the subcutaneous method poses less of a challenge to the animal and its subsequent recovery from surgery. Because of the relatively larger size ratio between the currently marketed transmitters and the rodent abdominal cavity, intraperitoneal implantation may cause a higher postsurgery fatality rate, probably because of strangulation of the intestine by the excess lead coiled in the abdomen [36]. In contrast, for the subcutaneous implantation method, the tension on the dermal sutures caused by the presence of the transmitter could be a concern. For both locations, the careful calculation of the length of catheter and lead wires are necessary due to the faster growth ratio in rodents than large animals. Furthermore, based on our experience, the location used to introduce the intra-arterial catheter may affect the implantation surgery success rate. The choice of the surgical implantation approach should be made based on the individuals experience and the animal species used. Continuous improvements to the surgical approach should improve survival rate and increase the potential for robust, long-term use of telemetered animals [11,37].

9.5.4 Invasive versus Noninvasive Telemetry System in Cardiovascular Safety Pharmacology

As well as the invasive (implantation) telemetry system, the noninvasive (jacket) telemetry system has been recently introduced for in vivo telemetry studies. The jacket telemetry system consists of a nonimplanted transmitter that is normally pocketed in a backpack or a jacket and is connected with ECG leads and a host PC. The backpack includes a control unit, Bluetooth radio, and batteries. The control unit digitizes channels of data from the ECG leads and forwards them to the host PC via Bluetooth link. The host PC has a receiving Bluetooth radio and dedicated programs to store, display, and analyze the data. The whole system was successfully tested in animal models and increasingly used in cardiovascular and/or respiratory safety pharmacology evaluations. The noninvasive method has more flexibility and generates result faster. This novel approach has been added as critical tool of early cardiovascular safety screening for new drug development. It can also reduce animal suffering and the number of animal used. However, current noninvasive telemetry systems are only a method capable of collection of blood pressure in a reliable way. The noninvasive jacket ECG telemetry system also tends to generate more signal noise than the implantation telemetry system and may cause signal loss due to a loose contact between the leads and the surface of the skin, as we learned from our experience. Better ECG placement skills and adhesion materials as well as shorter data collection period will minimize the opportunity of the signal loss. When used in monkeys, the animals need to be sedated prior to putting on/removing the telemetry jackets. The nonhuman primates also need proper acclimation prior to any formal data collection to reduce the excitement-induced data contamination. Because of the disadvantages of the jacket telemetry system, invasive (implantation) telemetry system remains today the main data acquisition system used in cardiovascular safety pharmacology assessment for investigational new drug (IND) application.

Telemetry systems allow animals to be monitored under conscious conditions to investigate the safety profile in new drug development. However, it sometimes happens that the evaluation of the system-specific safety margin (e.g., cardiovascular safety margin) is limited because of a severe clinical side effect developed in the tested animals. In that case the anesthetized animal model could still be used to help push the cardiovascular safety margin, and an injectable formulation should be available to support this evaluation.

9.5.5 Other Considerations in Telemetry Technology Applications

While the telemetry technology offers advantages to allow monitoring to be conducted when the animals are awake and unrestrained, it poses technical challenges. The major challenges include the signal originating interference such as muscle tremor and signal transmission interference from electrical appliances nearby. For the noninvasive (jacket) telemetry system, surface ECG leads dislodge and may cause missing signals. Aging may further play a role when examining the effects of compounds on cardiac repolarization, and some studies suggest that age can affect QTc prolongation induced by some IKr blockers [38,39]. Blood pressure signal drifting has also been observed and should be appropriately attended to [40–42].

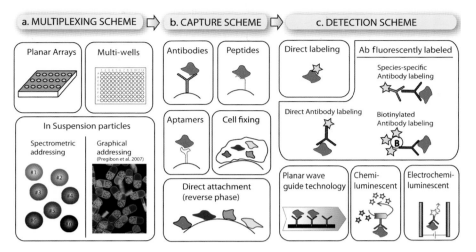

Figure 2.2 The three main characteristics of a high-throughput affinity based assay. (*a*) A multiplexing scheme in which solid supports (e.g., microparticles [35], beads, spots, or wells) obtain a unique identity. (*b*) A capture scheme immobilizes and/or isolates the protein of interest. (*c*) A detection scheme generates a readable output, which is linearly correlated to the amount of the immobilized protein of interest.

Cellular Systems

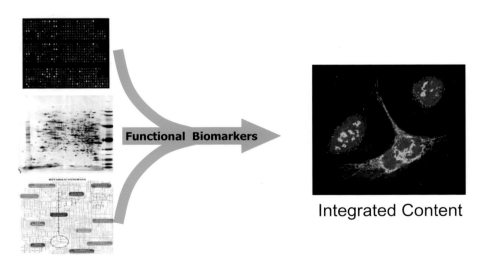

Figure 3.1 Cellular systems biology is the study of the integrated and interacting network of genes, proteins, and metabolic processes that give rise to normal and abnormal conditions. The cell, as the simplest of complex biological systems, exhibits properties in response to external stimulus that are not always anticipated from detailed knowledge of its component parts, or component functions and can be measured and analyzed using panels of fluorescently labeled, functional biomarkers coupled with advanced informatics.

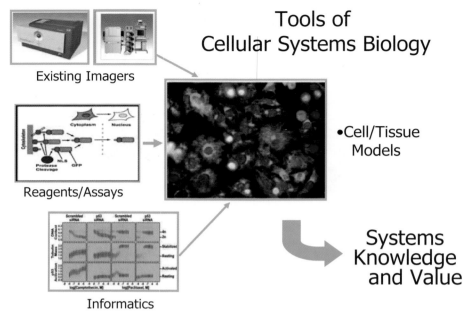

Tools of Cellular Systems Biology

Existing Imagers

Reagents/Assays

• Cell/Tissue Models

Informatics

Systems Knowledge and Value

Figure 3.2 Tools of cellular systems biology. Cells or tissue models are plated in high density 384-well microtiter plates and exposed to treatments. At the end of exposure time the cells are evaluated for 10 or more measurements using panels of fluorescent-based reagents. The 384-well plates are scanned using existing high-content reader instruments with image analysis algorithms. Informatics tools extract contextual information from the multiplex of functional cell features. Databases containing large compound profiles sets can be mined for knowledge.

a.

Building the Generation 1 Classifier for Compound Toxicity

Collection of Compounds

Categorization Based on safety data

Categories: 0 – non-toxic to 4 – highly toxic

0   1   2   3   4

Re-categorized due to limited number of non-toxic compounds

Minimally Toxic   Significant Toxicity

Reference data used to build classifier

Figure 3.4 Constructing the classifier. (See text for full caption.)

b.

Building the Gen 1 Classifier

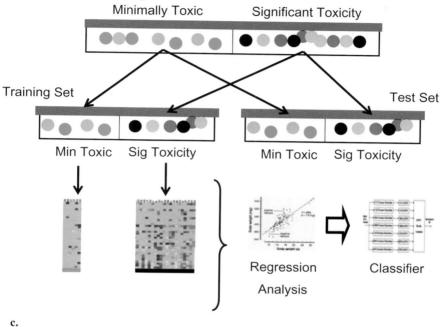

Minimally Toxic   Significant Toxicity

Training Set   Test Set

Min Toxic   Sig Toxicity   Min Toxic   Sig Toxicity

Regression   Classifier

Analysis

c.

Using the Generation 1 Classifier

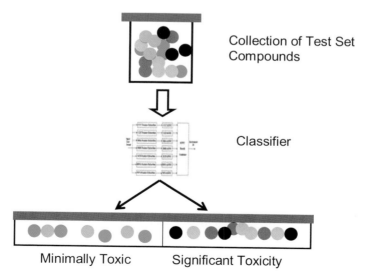

Collection of Test Set
Compounds

Classifier

Minimally Toxic   Significant Toxicity

Figure 3.4 *Continued*

Classifier output of training and test set of compounds building the algorithm

Cmpd	Score	Sig Toxic	Min Toxic
W11	1.00	•	
Y30	0.85	•	
O3	0.82	•	
F84	0.78	•	
R90	0.76	•	
T42	0.74	•	
A55	0.73	•	
A85	0.71	•	
U28	0.71	•	
E7	0.70	•	
C77	0.69	•	
N6	0.69	•	
L38	0.67	•	
Z12	0.67	•	
N16	0.67	•	
I78	0.65	•	
S23	0.63	•	
B4	0.63	•	
W61	0.61	•	
T63	0.60	•	
O45	0.60	•	
L75	0.60	•	
V27	0.60		•
L65	0.60	•	
S13	0.60	•	
B74	0.60	•	
Y10	0.58	•	
F34	0.57	•	

Cmpd	Score	Sig Toxic	Min Toxic
A29	0.53	•	
W91	0.53		•
Y50	0.53	•	
X49	0.53	•	
R50	0.53	•	
R40	0.53		•
O53	0.53		•
Z22	0.53	•	
D61	0.53	•	
G1	0.53		•
H35	0.53		•
D11	0.53	•	
B54	0.53	•	
D51	0.53	•	
E62	0.53	•	
S63	0.53	•	
Z82	0.53	•	
P70	0.53	•	
D71	0.53	•	
G61	0.53	•	
B64	0.53	•	
W81	0.53	•	
T2	0.53	•	
Z42	0.53	•	
O93	0.51		•
K59	0.51	•	
A75	0.51	•	
H27	0.50		•

Cmpd	Score	Sig Toxic	Min Toxic
H85	0.50		•
C67	0.49	•	
T72	0.48	•	
M26	0.48	•	
E72	0.47	•	
J27	0.46	•	
K32	0.45	•	
M36	0.45		•
X39	0.44	•	
I98	0.44		•
F44	0.44		•
F94	0.44		•
T52	0.43		•
B24	0.43	•	
X69	0.43		•
L15	0.43	•	
J37	0.43	•	
H25	0.43		•
U68	0.43		•
U58	0.42	•	
D19	0.42	•	
G18	0.42	•	
I17	0.41		•
Z62	0.41	•	
Y60	0.41	•	
S73	0.40	•	
P20	0.40		•

Figure 3.4 *Continued*

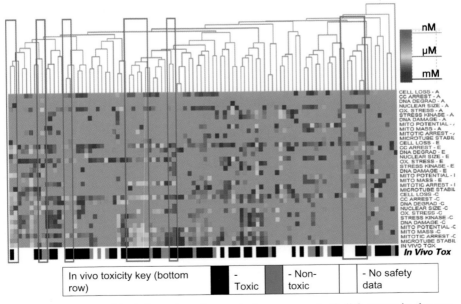

In vivo toxicity key (bottom row)	▮ - Toxic	▮ - Non-toxic	- No safety data

Figure 3.5 Hierarchical clustering of case study compounds. Cell features in the profiles are color coded by AC_{50} value so that red is nM, yellow is μM, and blue is mM concentrations. In vivo results are shown on the bottom axis. Blue rectangles indicate compounds with high degree of in vitro similarity, thus with a high likelihood that they will produce similar responses in vivo. Heat maps are used to identify patterns in response profiles between compounds in large data sets.

a.

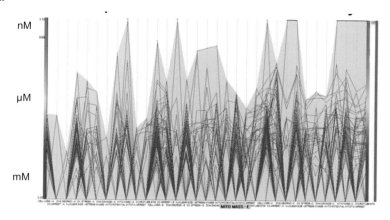

b.

Unknowns I17 (blue) and I98 (gray) with high similarity to Terfenadine (red)

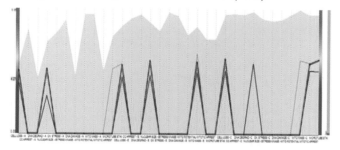

Unknown H25 with high similarity to Etoposide

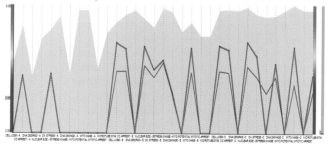

Figure 3.6 Application of Pearson's correlation plot similarity analysis. (*a*) The universe of all compounds plotted as cell features against magnitude of the response. The lines represent individual compounds, with the gray background showing the maximum value of feature responses for all compounds in the first-generation database. (*b*) Test compounds I98 and I17 have high similarity to Terfenadine (QT prolongation) while H25 has a nearly identical profile to Etoposide (myleotoxicity). Correlations such as these are used as mechanistic indicators for follow-up investigative toxicology studies.

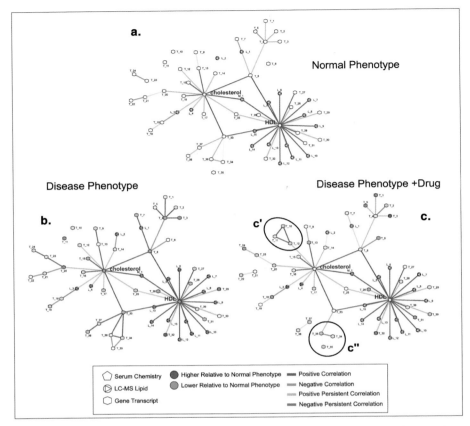

Figure 4.3 Cross-compartment subnetwork constructed from observed changes in a rodent model due to disease and drug administration. The top network (*a*) is the correlation network generated using data from normal phenotype animals. The left network (*b*) is the corresponding network for the disease phenotype group. The right network (*c*) is the corresponding network for a disease phenotype group administered the therapeutic compound. Node positions are fixed to compare identical analytes in the three treatment groups. Apart from imposing inclusion criteria that analytes be either one or two correlation links away from either serum cholesterol or serum HDL, each network was generated in an unsupervised manner. Except for the two serum clinical chemistry nodes, cholesterol and HDL, all nodes represent analytes in adipose tissue. Node colors in networks *b* and *c* reflect concentration levels relative to the baseline normal phenotype state (*a*). "Persistent correlations," (edges colored gold or blue) are unchanged across these three states. Highlighted in network *c* are two areas of interest, namely *c″*, a group of three analytes among which the disease induces correlations that are in turn reverted by drug administration, and *c′*, a group of another three analytes among which the drug induces correlations that were not observed in either the normal phenotype or the disease phenotype. All correlations shown are based on Pearson product–moment correlation metrics. Analytes have been de-identified except for serum cholesterol and serum HDL.

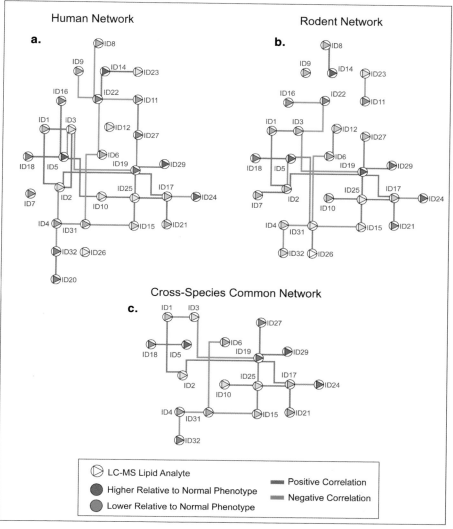

Figure 4.4 Correlation subnetworks constructed from molecular profiling measurements in a rodent model of disease and the human disease condition. Network *a* represents the correlation network in the human disease, and network *b* represents the correlation network in the rodent model. Network *c* is the intersection of networks *a* and *b*; it is a candidate network biomarker of disease common to both species. The spatial coordinates of all nodes are fixed across networks for clarity. Each node is a distinct lipid as measured by liquid chromatography and mass spectrometry (LC-MS). Node colors represent analyte concentration relative to the normal healthy phenotype of each species (normal phenotype networks not shown). Each network was generated in an unsupervised manner solely from the LC-MS lipid molecular profiling data. All network edges represent correlations based on Pearson product–moment correlation metrics. Analytes have been de-identified.

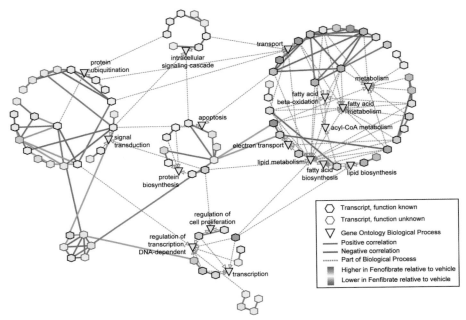

Figure 4.10 Gene Ontology Biological process database traversal on top of a rat skeletal muscle correlation network. Red and green edges denote correlations shared between fenofibrate and a novel PPARα agonist. Dotted lines denote inclusion in a particular biological process node (triangle), and node color indicates direction of transcript abundance change between fenofibrate and a vehicle group. Transcripts that are either unidentified or poorly characterized have a blue border.

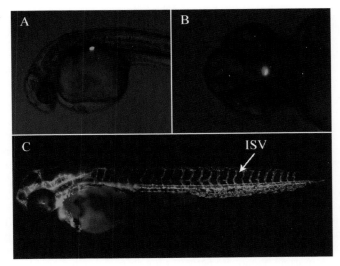

Figure 5.1 Representative transgenic zebrafish lines. (*A*) Insulin:gfp transgenic line, 30 hpf; (*B*) pomc:gfp and prol:rfp double transgenic line, 36 hpf (the pituitary is labeled with both GFP and RFP); (*C*) flk1:gfp transgenic line, 48 hpf. The white arrow points an ISV.

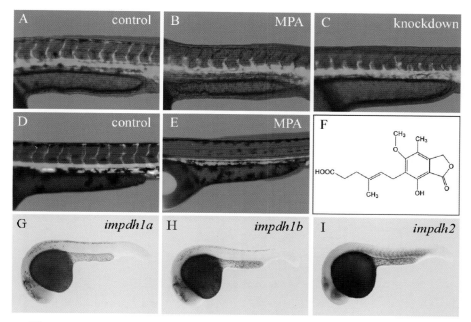

Figure 5.3 MPA inhibits angiogenesis in zebrafish. (See text for full caption.)

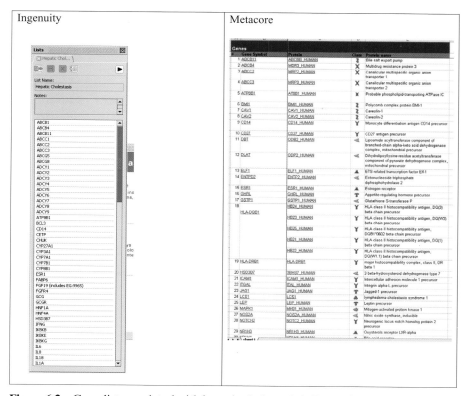

Figure 6.2 Gene list associated with hepatic cholestasis in Ingenuity Pathway Analysis and MetaCore version 4.5.

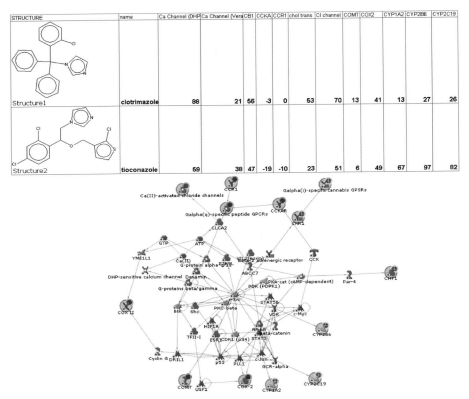

STRUCTURE	name	Ca Channel (DHP)	Ca Channel (Vera)	CB1	CCKA	CCR1	chol trans	Cl channel	COMT	COX2	CYP1A2	CYP2B6	CYP2C19
Structure1	clotrimazole	88	21	56	-3	0	53	70	13	41	13	27	26
Structure2	tioconazole	59	38	47	-19	-10	23	51	6	49	67	97	82

Figure 6.4 High-throughput data analysis on a net work using data for two molecules from Fliri et al. [79].

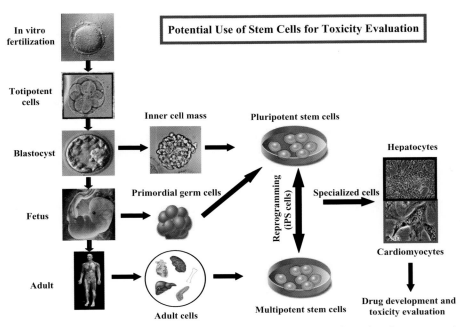

Figure 8.1 Origin and establishment of human stem cells for drug development and toxicity evaluation. (See text for full caption.)

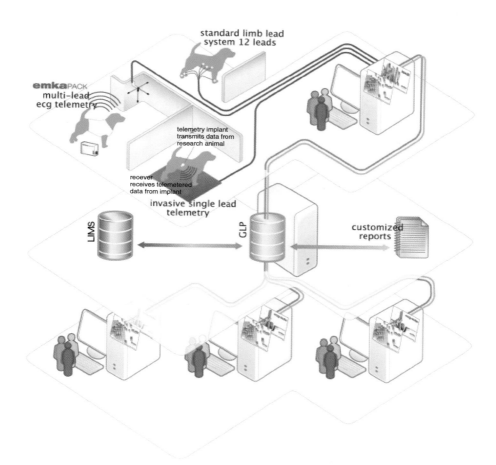

Figure 9.1 Major functional components and working flow of a telemetry system used in a cardiovascular telemetry study with rodent or large animal.

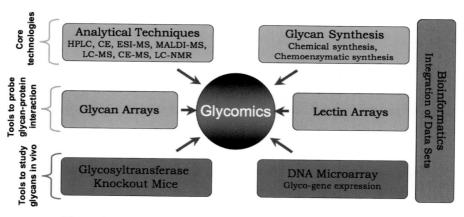

Figure 11.1 Tools and technologies used in glycomics research.

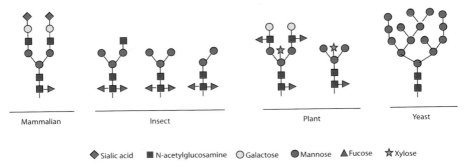

Figure 11.2 Typical structures of *N*-glycans present on recombinant proteins produced in mammalian, insect, plant, and yeast cell systems.

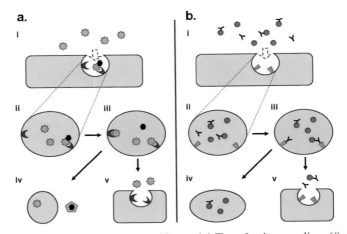

Figure 12.1 Endocytotic recycling machinery. (*a*) Transferrin recycling. (*i*) At neutral pH, transferrin (orange) bound to iron (black) has affinity for the transferrin receptor (purple); unbound (apo-) transferrin must passively diffuse into the forming endosome (*ii*). (*iii*) When the endosome acidifies, iron loses affinity for transferrin while apotransferrin gains affinity for the receptor. (*iv*) Free (nonrescued) transferrin is shuttled to a lysosome and degraded; iron is processed by the cell using other machinery such as ferritin (yellow). (*v*) Receptor-bound apotransferrin is exported to the cell surface where it loses affinity for the receptor at neutral pH. (*b*) IgG recycling. (*i*) At neutral pH, IgG ("*Y*") and target (red) molecules (and the complex of the two) have no affinity for the FcRn receptor (green), and must passively diffuse into the forming endosome (*ii*). (*iii*) When the endosome acidifies, IgG gains affinity for FcRn and may (either free or in complex with the target) bind FcRn. (*iv*) Non–receptor-bound endosome components are moved to a lysosome and destroyed. (*v*) Receptor-bound IgG and complex are returned to the cell surface and released at neutral pH. Note that for both (*a*) and (*b*), the efficiency of recycling of transferrin/IgG is much more efficient than shown here, leading to the lengthy observed half-lives for these proteins.

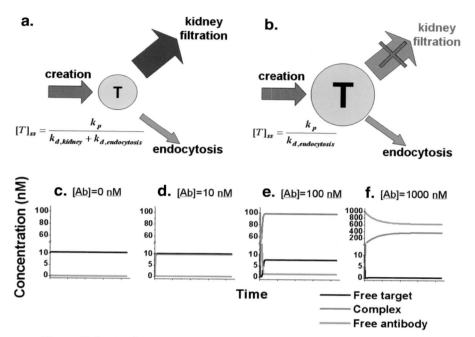

Figure 12.2 Antibody–target complex buildup. (See text for full caption.)

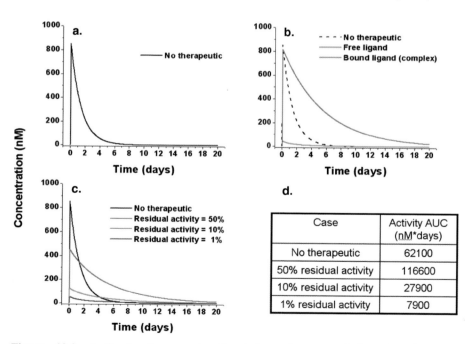

Figure 12.3 Antibody therapeutic directed against acutely-introduced target. (See text for full caption.)

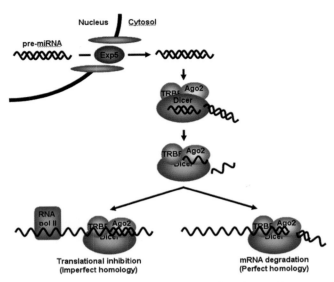

Figure 13.1 Schematic representation of the RNAi pathway. Exogenously administered siRNA or dsRNA produced by viral infection incorporate into the processing pathway at different steps to affect cellular signaling and gene expression. Ago2—argonaute 2; TRBP—tar-binding protein.

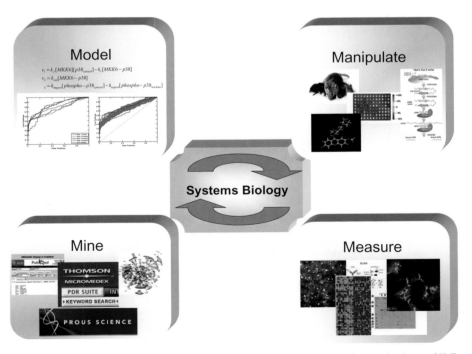

Figure 14.1 Schematic of the model, mine, measure, and manipulate (4M) paradigm.

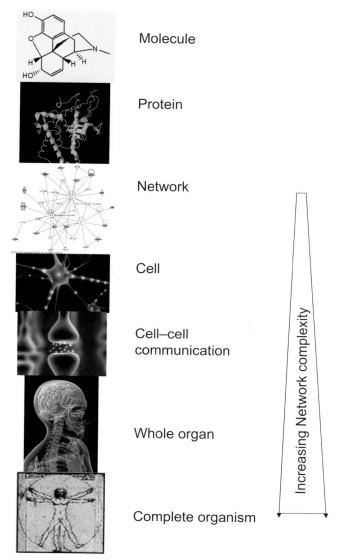

Figure 14.2 Schematic of the different levels at which models can be generated and the influence of networks.

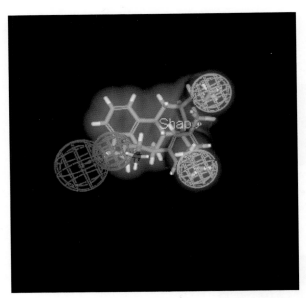

Figure 14.3 A shape feature HIPHOP pharmacophore model (Discovery Studio 2.0 Catalyst, Accelrys, San Diego, CA) of pergolide and norfenfluramine. Purple sphere = hydrogen bond donor, blue spheres = hydrophobic features, gray shape = van der Waals surface around pergolide.

9.6 FUTURE APPLICATIONS OF TELEMETRY SYSTEMS IN DRUG DISCOVERY AND DEVELOPMENT

Combination approaches with telemetry monitoring of multiple physiological systems simultaneously is a current trend. The immediate benefits include reducing animal numbers and amount of test compound. Such an approach is useful for obtaining an early safety readout for potential drug development candidates, as well as for detecting possible secondary therapeutic actions of a drug [43]. Current telemetry data systems are mostly limited to one-way data transfer; however, bidirectional data transfer can increase the capability and feasibility to diagnose tip clot formation, recharging the battery, and delivery of medications. Recently telemetry technology has been applied to state-of-the-art wireless endoscope capsule system to delivery real-time and bidirectional data transfer [44]. Telemetry technology has also recently been used to generate high tier cardiovascular function data such as cardiac output and left ventricular injection.

9.7 CONCLUSION

The use of a telemetry system that is implanted in the body for physiological monitoring in new drug discovery and development was presented in this chapter. With an implantable or noninvasive device, telemetry technology offers the possibility to observe physiological activity of animals in a conscious, free moving state, and the monitored physiological parameters can be displayed in real time that is close to a clinical setting, which is impossible by conventional methods. This new approach to physiological study offers great promise for drug efficacy and safety profiling and assessment. The telemetry technologies promote the potential for robust, long-term use of telemetered animals in drug discovery and development.

REFERENCES

1. Van Citters RL, Franklin DL. Telemetry of blood pressure in free-ranging animals via an intravascular gauge. *J Appl Physiol* 1966;21(5):1633–6.
2. USFDA. Title 21 Code of Federal Regulations (21 CFR Part 11) Electronic Records; Electronic Signatures. http://www.fda.gov/ora/compliance_ref/part11/
3. Truett AA, West DB. Validation of a radiotelemetry system for continuous blood pressure and heart rate monitoring in dogs. *Lab Anim Sky* 1995;45(3):299–302.
4. Gelzer AR, Ball HA. Validation of a telemetry system for measurement of blood pressure, electrocardiogram and locomotor activity in beagle dogs. *Clin Exp Hypertens* 1997;19(7):1135–60.
5. ICH guidance for industry. *S7A Safety pharmacology studies for human pharmaceuticals*. http://www.fda.gov/Cber/gdlns/ichs7a071201.htm

6. Guiol C, Ledoussal C, Surgé JM. A radiotelemetry system for chronic measurement of blood pressure and heart rate in the unrestrained rat validation of the method. *J Pharmacol Toxicol Meth* 1992;28(2):99–105.

7. Miller RH, Smeak DD, Lehmkuhl LB, Brown SA, DiBartola SP. Radiotelemetry catheter implantation: surgical technique and results in cats. *Contemp Top Lab Anim Sci* 2000;39(2):34–9.

8. ICH S7B Guideline. *Step 2 revision. The nonclinical evaluation of the potential for delayed ventricular repolarization (QT interval prolongation) by human pharmaceuticals.* http://www.fda.gov/cder/guidance/5533dft.htm

9. Kijtawornrat A, Ozkanlar Y, Keene BW, Roche BM, Hamlin DM, Hamlin RL. Assessment of drug-induced QT interval prolongation in conscious rabbits. *J Pharmacol Toxicol Meth* 2006;53(2):168–73.

10. Chaves AA, Zingaro GJ, Yordy MA, Bustard KA, O'Sullivan S, Galijatovic-Idrizbegovic A, et al. A highly sensitive canine telemetry model for detection of QT interval prolongation: studies with moxifloxacin, haloperidol and MK-499. *J Pharmacol Toxicol Meth* 2007;24:103–14.

11. Butz GM, Davisson RL. Long-term telemetric measurement of cardiovascular parameters in awake mice: a physiological genomics tool. *Physiol Genomics* 2001;5(2):89–97.

12. Carlson SH, Wyss JM. Long-term telemetric recording of arterial pressure and heart rate in mice fed basal and high NaCl diets. *Hypertension* 2000;35(2):E1–5.

13. Somody L, Fagette S, Frutoso J, Gharib C, Blanquie JP, Gharib T, Thierion D, Gauquelin G. Cardiovascular adaptations to parabolic flight in rats: a radiotelemetry feasibility study. *J Gravit Physiol* 1997;4(2):P43–4.

14. Toyoshima S, Kanno A, Kitayama T, Sekiya K, Nakai K, Haruna M, et al. QT PRODACT: in vivo QT assay in the conscious dog for assessing the potential for QT interval prolongation by human pharmaceuticals. *J Pharmacol Sci* 2005;99(5):459–71.

15. Shiotani M, Harada T, Abe J, Sawada Y, Hashimoto K, Hamada Y, Horii I. Practical application of guinea pig telemetry system for QT evaluation. *J Toxicol Sci* 2005;30(3):239–47.

16. King A, Bailie M, Olivier NB. Magnitude of error introduced by application of heart rate correction formulas to the canine QT interval. *Ann Noninvasive Electrocardiol* 2006;11(4):289–98.

17. Shiotani M, Harada T, Abe J, Hamada Y, Horii I. Methodological validation of an existing telemetry system for QT evaluation in conscious guinea pigs. *J Pharmacol Toxicol Meth* 2007;55(1):27–34.

18. Ollerstam A, Persson AH, Visser SA, Fredriksson JM, Forsberg T, Nilsson LB, et al. A novel approach to data processing of the QT interval response in the conscious telemetered beagle dog. *J Pharmacol Toxicol Meth* 2007;55(1):35–48.

19. Miyazaki H, Watanabe H, Kitayama T, Nishida M, Nishi Y, Sekiya K, et al. QT PRODACT: sensitivity and specificity of the canine telemetry assay for detecting drug-induced QT interval prolongation. *J Pharmacol Sci* 2005;99(5):523–9.

20. Kramer K, Grimbergen JA, Van der Gracht L, Van Iperen DJ, Jonker RJ, Bast A. The use of telemetry to record electrocardiogram and heart rate in freely swimming rats. *Meth Find Exp Clin Pharmacol* 1995;17(2):107–12.

21. Lewanowitsch T, White JM, Irvine RJ. Use of radiotelemetry to evaluate respiratory depression produced by chronic methadone administration. *Eur J Pharmacol* 2004;26;484(2–3):303–10.

22. Tang X, Yang L, Sanford LD. Sleep and EEG spectra in rats recorded via telemetry during surgical recovery. *Sleep* 2007;1;30(8):1057–61.

23. Stephenson R, Liao KS, Hamrahi H, Horner RL. Circadian rhythms and sleep have additive effects on respiration in the rat. *J Physiol* 2001;536(Pt 1):225–35.

24. Beig MI, Bhagat N, Talwar A, Chandra R, Fahim M, Katyal A. Simultaneous recording of electroencephalogram and blood pressure in conscious telemetered rats during ictal state. *J Pharmacol Toxicol Meth* 2007;56(1):51–7.

25. Dürmüller N, Guillaume P, Lacroix P, Porsolt RD, Moser P. The use of the dog electroencephalogram (EEG) in safety pharmacology to evaluate proconvulsant risk. *J Pharmacol Toxicol Meth* 2007;56(2):234–8.

26. Wang L, Hammond P, Johannesson E, Boon Tang T, Astaras A, Cumming S, et al. An on-chip programmable instrumentation microsystem for gastrointestinal telemetry applications. *Conf Proc IEEE Eng Med Biol Soc* 2004;3:2109–12.

27. Zhang WQ, Yan GZ, Ye DD, Chen CW. Simultaneous assessment of the intraluminal pressure and transit time of the colon using a telemetry technique. *Physiol Meas* 2007;28(2):141–8.

28. Cooper RL, Beale DG, Grose GC, Constable IJ. Aspects of continual monitoring of intra-ocular pressure by radiotelemetry. *Aust J Ophthalmol* 1980;8(2):193–4.

29. Seifert EL, Mortola JP. Circadian pattern of ventilation during acute and chronic hypercapnia in conscious adult rats. *Am J Physiol Regul Integr Comp Physiol* 2002;282(1):R244–51.

30. Seifert EL, Mortola JP. The circadian pattern of breathing in conscious adult rats. *Respir Physiol* 2002;129(3):297–305.

31. Gauvin DV, Tilley LP, Smith FW Jr, Baird TJ. Electrocardiogram, hemodynamics, and core body temperatures of the normal freely moving laboratory beagle dog by remote radiotelemetry. *J Pharmacol Toxicol Meth* 2006;53(2):128–39.

32. Soloviev MV, Hamlin RL, Shellhammer LJ, Barrett RM, Wally RA, Birchmeier PA, et al. Variations in hemodynamic parameters and ECG in healthy, conscious, freely moving telemetrized beagle dogs. *Cardiovasc Toxicol* 2006;6(1):51–62.

33. Mortola JP. Correlations between the circadian patterns of body temperature, metabolism and breathing in rats. *Respir Physiol Neurobiol* 2007;155(2):137–46.

34. Ning G, Bai Y, Wang X, Yu F, Zheng X. New approaches to physiological study by telemetry technology. *Conf Proc IEEE Eng Med Biol Soc* 2005;6:6654–7.

35. Klumpp A, Trautmann T, Markert M, Guth B. Optimizing the experimental environment for dog telemetry studies. *J Pharmacol Toxicol Meth* 2006;54(2):141–9.

36. Moons CP, Hermans K, Remie R, Duchateau L, Odberg FO. Intraperitoneal versus subcutaneous telemetry devices in young Mongolian gerbils (*Meriones unguiculatus*). *Lab Anim* 2007;41(2):262–9.

37. Provan G, Stanton A, Sutton A, Rankin-Burkart A, Laycock SK. Development of a surgical approach for telemetering guinea pigs as a model for screening QT interval effects.

38. Mittelstadt SW, Adams NA, Spruell RD. Age-dependent effects on cisapride-induced QTc prolongation in the isolated guinea pig heart. *J Pharmacol Toxicol Meth* 2006;54(2):159–63.

39. Shiotani M, Harada T, Abe J, Hamada Y, Horii I. Aging-related changes of QT and RR intervals in conscious guinea pigs. *J Pharmacol Toxicol Meth* 2008;57(1): 23–9.

40. Brockway BP, Mills PA, Azar SH. A new method for continuous chronic measurement and recording of blood pressure, heart rate and activity in the rat via radio-telemetry. *Clin Exp Hypertens A* 1991;13(5):885–95.

41. DePasquale MJ, Ringer LW, Winslow RL, Buchholz RA, Fossa AA. Chronic monitoring of cardiovascular function in the conscious guinea pig using radio-telemetry. *Clin Exp Hypertens* 1994;16(2):245–60.

42. Van Vliet BN, McGuire J, Chafe L, Leonard A, Joshi A, Montani JP. Phenotyping the level of blood pressure by telemetry in mice. *Clin Exp Pharmacol Physiol* 2006;33(11):1007–15.

43. Schierok H, Markert M, Pairet M, Guth B. Continuous assessment of multiple vital physiological functions in conscious freely moving rats using telemetry and a plethysmography system. *J Pharmacol Toxicol Meth* 2000;43(3):211–7.

44. Chi B, Yao J, Han S, Xie X, Li G, Wang Z. Low-power transceiver analog front-end circuits for bidirectional high data rate wireless telemetry in medical endoscopy applications. *IEEE Trans Biomed Eng* 2007;54(7):1291–9.

PART II

BIOLOGICS TECHNOLOGY

10

NANOTECHNOLOGY TO IMPROVE ORAL DRUG DELIVERY

Mayank D. Bhavsar, Shardool Jain, and Mansoor M. Amiji

Contents

Drug Efficacy, Safety, and Biologics Discovery: Emerging Technologies and Tools,
Edited by Sean Ekins and Jinghai J. Xu
Copyright © 2009 by John Wiley & Sons, Inc.

10.1 INTRODUCTION

Nanotechnology, as defined by United States National Nanotechnology Institute, is "the understanding and control of matter at dimensions of roughly 1 to 100 nanometers, where unique phenomena enable novel applications" [1]. "Nano" is one of the most widely used keywords today. Nanotechnology has many applications in fields such as telecommunication, electronics, energy, transportation, and it can also be successfully used in biomedical technologies. "Nanomedicine," a term coined by the US National Institutes of Health through its Roadmap Initiative, is a branch of nanotechnology that refers to "molecular scale medical intervention for the purpose of prevention, diagnosis, and treatment of diseases" [1,2]. The first decade of the twentieth century has seen much advancement in nanotechnology for biomedical applications, including development of pharmaceutical technologies that aid in drug discovery and development. According to the 2005 Nanomarket Report, the nanomedicine market is suggested to generate about $1.7 billion in revenues by 2009, and this is anticipated to increase to $4.8 billion by the year 2012 [3]. Developments in nanotechnology and specifically nanomedicine have the potential to become an essential driving force that can propel the already high-technology-based pharmaceutical drug delivery industry to new limits.

Thus far the pharmaceutical industry has relied heavily on conventional dosage forms comprised of solid or liquid for systemic delivery of therapeutic agents. Neither traditional dosage form always succeeds in addressing issues such as poor solubility, permeability, stability, and site-specific delivery of therapeutic agents for maximum benefit. Based on the limitations of conventional formulations, a significant number of new chemical entities, developed through combinatorial synthesis and high-throughput screening, have had excellent pharmacological properties but have had to be abandoned because of development-related challenges. With many so-called block-buster drugs becoming "off-patent" over recent years, the majority of effort of the pharmaceutical industry has been directed toward development of new generation of formulations of existing therapeutic molecules. The aim is mostly to improve the performance of a drug by altering the disposition and pharmacokinetics and also to enhance patient compliance through a decrease in dosing frequency and limiting side effects. Such strategies have already been shown to help a brand name company retain significant market share of a product in the presence of generic competition.

Additionally a lot of research effort from academe and industry has led to discovery of potent and disease altering therapeutic biomolecules, including proteins, peptides, and nucleic acid-based macromolecules, that cannot be administered using conventional formulations. A combination of the remoteness in accessibility of the drug target inside the affected cells and even in subcellular compartments, lack of adequate permeability through biological membranes, and the high potential for degradation of these newer therapeutic biomolecules have propelled the need for development of effective delivery systems. For instance, the intracellular availability of stable small interfering RNA (siRNA) using specific delivery systems is essential for RNA interference technology to become an effective therapeutic strategy.

Many of the current challenges in pharmaceutical product development can be addressed by advances in nanotechnology. The oral route of administration continues to be desired for a large number of therapeutic compounds, especially those intended for chronic therapy. It is suggested that most nanotechnology research and development funding will be used in the development of oral drug delivery systems [3]. Several companies, including Elan and Baxter, have programs for development of nanoformulations to improve oral bioavailability of already existing drugs. These products are made by either wet grinding (e.g., NanoCrystal® technology) or controlled precipitation and milling (e.g., NanoEdge® technology) of drugs to form nanoparticles. Other examples of nanoplatforms used in drug formulations include polymeric nanoparticles, liposomes, nanoemulsions, micelles, and dendrimers.

10.1.1 Oral Route of Drug Delivery

Noninvasive and patient-controlled administration of therapeutics has proved to be the most favored mode of drug administration in the body, especially for chronic therapy. The oral route of administration continues to be the most common method of drug delivery because of some obvious advantages:

- Noninvasive delivery is known to be the safest route for drug administration
- The gastrointestinal tract provides a large surface area for drug absorption.
- Oral administration can be used for delivery of drugs for both local and systemic effects.
- A variety of liquid, solid, and semisolid drug formulations can be administered via the oral route.
- Multiple administrations of drugs are possible with oral delivery.
- Drugs can be self-administered, eliminating the need for hospital admission and trained personnel.
- Oral delivery ensures patient compliance relative to all other routes.
- The drug manufacture process is economical since it can be easily scaled up for mass production.

Often a quick test to evaluate the oral bioavailability of the new chemical entity is to fill the drug into a hard gelatin capsules along with lactose, as this constitutes the simplest formulation for oral administration. In addition

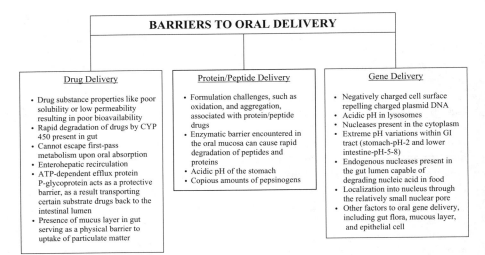

Figure 10.1 Barriers to oral delivery of drugs, protein/peptides, and genes.

to the ease of administration and high patient compliance, the variety of excipients available and relatively lower cost involved in the development of oral dosage forms, favor this route as compared to more invasive approaches.

However, oral formulations are not feasible for a variety of new chemical entities (Figure 10.1). Many of these agents are highly hydrophobic or suffer from stability and permeability constraints, which limit oral bioavailability. Drugs with a narrow therapeutic index are difficult to administer via the oral route. Additionally several dosage forms (crystalline vs. amorphous drug, type of formulation, rates of disintegration and dissolution, etc.) and physiological factors (gastrointestinal [GI] motility, stability in GI fluid, P-glycoprotein efflux, enzymatic degradation, etc.), contribute to poor bioavailability of certain therapeutic molecules upon oral administration.

10.1.2 Anatomical and Physiological Considerations in Oral Delivery

Understanding and exploiting the physiological conditions in the GI tract holds the key to development of a successful oral delivery formulation. In this section the basic anatomy and physiology of the GI tract has been described to understand and explore the opportunities that are available and can be exploited for designing an oral drug delivery system.

The human digestive system is a complex system comprised of many different organs and highly specialized to perform functions like ingestion, digestion, and absorption. The organs of the digestive system are essentially part of two main groups: the gastrointestinal tract or the alimentary canal and the auxiliary structures. The gastrointestinal tract is a long and continuous tube-like structure beginning at the mouth (oral cavity) and continuing further down as the pharynx, esophagus, stomach, small intestine, large intestine, rectum, and finally culminating into the anal canal [4–9]. Almost all the portions of the digestive tract are made up of four basic layers but perform different functions. The four layers of the digestive system include *mucosa*, the innermost lining of the digestive tract consisting principally of epithelial tissue; *submucosa*, primarily a thick layer of connective tissue containing nerves, blood vessels, and glands; *muscularis*, the muscle of the digestive system consisting of two layers of smooth muscles; and *visceral peritoneum*, this tissue is also known as the serosa and is the outermost layer of the tract [4–9].

The oral cavity is lined with the mucous membrane also known as the oral mucosa, and it includes the buccal, sublingual, gingival, palatal, and labial mucosae [10–12]. The oral mucosal surface has variable thickness with buccal mucosa having a thickness of 500 to 800 μm, while the palates, gingivae, and floor of the mouth measuring 100 to 200 μm [13,14]. From a drug delivery point of view, the buccal and sublingual tissues offer excellent sites for delivery because of the fact that they are more permeable than other mucosal regions of the mouth. The oral mucosal surface is highly vascularized, which allows the drugs diffusing from the oral mucosa direct access to the systemic circulation and can bypass first pass metabolism in liver [10,12]. The permeability of the oral cavity follows the following order: oral mucosa > sublingual > buccal cavity > palatal surface. However, proteins and peptides are very highly susceptible to degradation in the oral cavity because of the presence of an enzymatic barrier in the oral mucosa. In addition to the high vascularization, the cells of the oral mucosa are surrounded by an environment of mucus that is secreted by the mucous membrane and is believed to play a role in bioadhesion of mucoadhesive drug delivery systems [10–13,15]. Following the oral cavity is the esophagus, which ends into the stomach and is not a region of much interest for drug delivery. The stomach consists of the gastric mucosa, which contains many deep glands made up of parietal cells. These cells are responsible for secretion of hydrochloric acid. The major barrier for drug delivery to the stomach is the low pH that exists in the organ because of the secretion of hydrochloric acid; this can lead to ionization of basic drugs, resulting in poor absorption. In addition therapeutic proteins and peptides are degraded very rapidly in the stomach because of the presence of copious amounts of pepsinogen.

The stomach ends into the small intestine, and this orifice is guarded by a pyloric sphincter preventing the re-entry of chyme into the stomach. The small intestine is the most important target organ for oral delivery of therapeutic molecules. The small intestine is further divided into three major parts, which include the duodenum, jejunum, and the ileum. In addition to the general structure, the small intestine also shows the presence of tiny finger like structures called villi, which are made of epithelial tissue and are divided into microvilli, which form the brush border. Throughout the length of the small intestine the mucous membrane is covered by villi. The main function of the small intestine is digestion and absorption of the food that is passed down into it from the stomach. The process of absorption in the small intestine is also assisted by its length and a very large surface area [16–18]. The delivery of the drugs to the small intestine is preferred because drugs typically exhibit maximal absorption from this site compared with other regions of the gastrointestinal tract. The absorption of drugs and particulate delivery systems from the small intestine is believed to occur through gut-associated lymphoid tissue and also from other nonlymphoid tissue [17]. The mucus covered mucosal layer of the small intestine forms a physical barrier to the environment and absorption of drugs [18]. The brush border enzymes also form an enzymatic barrier for absorption of proteins from the small intestine. The other major barrier to drug absorption to the small intestine is the action of ATP-dependent efflux protein P-glycoprotein (P-gp) efflux pump, which is expressed on the membrane of the intestinal epithelial cells. P-gp is part of the protective barrier of the small intestine that limits absorption of potentially toxic substances [19] and can have a significant effect in altering absorption and bioavailability of certain drugs by actively transporting the drug back into the intestinal lumen.

The mucosa of the small intestine contains solitary lymph nodules and aggregated lymph nodules called the Peyer's patches. These are usually oval in shape and occur more frequently in the distal areas of the small intestine and also at the terminal end of the colon. They are comprised of four zones, which are the germinal center, small lymphocytic zone, interfollicular zone, and subepithelial zone. All of these zones are primarily made up of lymphocytes and other antigen-presenting cells like macrophages and dendritic cells. The Peyer's patches are lined above the lymphoid follicles by a membranous layer of epithelial cells called the follicle-associated epithelium, which in turn is composed of absorptive cells, goblet cells, and M cells, and these cells assist the Peyer's patches to transport macromolecules and particulate matter from the GI track into lymphatic/systemic circulation [16]. The physiology of Peyer's patches make them a very important feature of the small intestine as they harbor many immunocompetent cells that can be stimulated by antigenic proteins and genes to generate both humoral and systemic immunity.

The small intestine ends into the large intestine. It is called the large intestine because of the larger diameter of the tract compared to the small intestine. The large intestine is about 1.5 meters in length, beginning at caecum and ending in the rectum and the anal canal. There is a difference between the wall of the large intestine and small intestine. The large intestine shows the presence of simple columnar cells with numerous goblet cells. The goblet cells also secrete mucus that lubricates the colonic content as it passes through the colon. The submucous layer of the large intestine consists of more lymphoid tissue than any other part of the GI tract to provide nonspecific defense against invasion by microbes in the food and the bacterial flora that resides in the gut. Drug delivery to the large intestine via the oral route for local action is a challenging task as the drug carrier system will have to face the rigors of the preceding sections of the GI tract before reaching the desired site of action. Rectal delivery of drugs is an alternative for local action, but it suffers the disadvantage of patient compliance. The mucus layer of the large intestine can take up particles in a particular size range, and this property could be exploited for delivery of drugs to the large intestine [20,21].

10.2 NANOTECHNOLOGY FOR ORAL DELIVERY

The conventional drug delivery systems, including tablet and capsules for oral administration or solution for parenteral administration, may not represent the most efficient way to deliver the drugs [22]. As mentioned earlier, many of the low molecular weight drugs and the new biological molecules (e.g., siRNA) suffer from poor solubility, shorter half-life due to rapid clearance or degradation, poor bioavailability, and potentially toxic side effects due to distribution to nontarget sites [22]. Thus, in order to deliver these new biologics and at the same time improve the efficiency of conventional drugs, it is essential to develop new delivery systems. These systems should aim at improving the efficacy of the drug, minimize side effects and improve patient compliance [22]. Toward this end, research has explored various systems that come under the category of nano-carriers.

One of the major advantages of nanoparticles is that they offer a large surface area because of the nanometer size and they tend to improve the efficiency and bioavailability of the drug by encapsulating and delivering more drug [23]. These systems can be further modified to improve their performance by surface modification of the nanoparticles for specific targeting to a tissue or cell. This aspect of the nanoparticle modification can be certainly advantageous from the oral delivery perspective [23]. Nanoparticle-based delivery systems are also desirable as they exhibit low toxicity and improved patient compliance; they are also more cost effective than conventional drug delivery systems [24,25]. In summary, nanoparticles offer an exciting platform as carriers for their ability to protect the drug/bioactive material from biodegradation.

10.2.1 Polymer and Lipid Nanoparticle Technologies

In the last few decades the advancement in the field of drug delivery has further propelled development of various polymer and lipid based nanosystems for enhanced delivery of therapeutic molecules to the targeted site (Table 10.1). The success and underlying potential of these systems depend on the flexibility of manipulating the polymers (surface modification), small size of the particles, nontoxicity, reproducibility, and high stability [26].

The concept of polymer nanotechnology has started to encompass fields from the pharmaceutical/biotechnology industry to the packaging industry. Polymer nanotechnology implies the use/engineering of appropriate polymer-based nanosystems for intended use. In the field of pharmaceutical sciences, polymer-based nanotechnology has been used for drug, gene, or small/large molecule delivery. The polymeric nanotechnology includes polymeric nanoparticles, polymeric micelles, and functionalized nanoparticles for the delivery of the drugs.

TABLE 10.1   Summary of Polymer-based Nanoparticle Systems Used for Oral Delivery of Drugs, Protein/Peptides, and Genes

Oral Delivery System	Polymer Employed	Size (nm)	Incorporated Active	Reference
Drug delivery	Gliadin	400–500	Carbazole	[128]
	Gliadin	250–400	Amoxicillin	[64]
	Chitosan	50–500	Streptomycin	[67]
	PLGA	200–260	Theophylline in depot tablets	[126]
	PLGA	100–200	Indomethacin	[129]
	Poly(methylvinylether-co-maleic anhydride)	200–250	5-Fluoroudine	[130]
	PLGA	100–200	Vancomycin	[129]
	Polystyrene	50–3000	Iodine-125	[59]
	PLGA	100–200	Valproic acid	[129]
	PLGA	100–200	Phenobarbital	[129]
	PLGA	200–300	Amifostine	[65]
	PLGA	300–400	*H. pylori* lysate	[112]
	Lectin-PLGA	300–400	Rifampicin	[66]
	Lectin-PLGA	300–400	Pyrazinamide	[66]
	PLGA	100–200	Ketoprofen	[129]
	Lectin-PLGA	300–400	Isoniazid	[66]
	Polystyrene nanoparticles coated with poloxamer 188 and 407	60	Fluorescein	[131]
	Polystyrene	100–1000	Fluorescent dye	[20]
	PLGA	300–500	Rolipram	[21,75]
	Poly(methylvinylether-co-maleic anhydride)	200–300	RBITC	[130]

TABLE 10.1 *Continued*

Oral Delivery System	Polymer Employed	Size (nm)	Incorporated Active	Reference
Protein/peptide delivery	PCL, PLGA, PCL-PLGA blend, and PCL-PLGA copolymer	~250	Diptheria toxoid	[132]
	Poly(ethylene glycol-poly(lactic acid)	150–170	Tetanus toxoid	[133]
	PLGA	300–400	*H. pylori* lysate	[112]
	Poly(N-isopropylacrylamide)	148–895	Calcitonin	[14,86,134]
	Poly(N-vinylacetamide)	148–896	Calcitonin	[14,86,134]
	Poly(t-butyl methacrylate)	148–897	Calcitonin	[14,86,134]
	PLGA	200–400	Calcitonin	[104]
	PCL	270–300	Heparin	[105]
	PLGA	250–270		[105]
	Eudragit® RS and RL	250–280		[105]
	Poly(iso-butyl cyanoacrylate)	85	Insulin	[135]
	Polyesters	300–500		[99]
	Poly(methacrylic acid)-g-poly(ethylene glycol)	200–1000		[94]
	Poly(alkylcyanoacrylate)	100–400		[92]
	Chitosan	200–400		[90]
	Poly(isobutylcyanoacrylate)	100–500		[136]
	Poly(acrylicacid)-g-poly(ethylene glycol)	200–100		[94]
	PLGA	>1000		[137]
	Poly(fumaric-*co*-sebacic) anhydride	>1000		[137]
	PLGA	100–200		[129]
	Dextran	150–300		[96]
	PLGA-Hp55	150–180		[98]
	PCL	340–370		[95]
	Poly(methacrylic acid methacrylate)	30–110		[83]
	Hydroxypropyl methylcellulose	50–60		[100]
	Chitosan	150		[138]
	Gelatin	140		[138]
	PLGA	100–200		[129]
	PCL	100–130		[101]
	Eudragit® RS and RL	170–310		[139]
Gene delivery	PLGA	>200	pCMV-lacZ	[140]
	Poly(ethylene oxide)-poly(propylene oxide)	150–190	pCMV-lacZ	[141]
	Chitosan	50–75	DNA	[109]
	Chitosan	100–1000	pCR3Arah2	[110]
	Chitosan	70–150	mEpo gene	[111]

On the other hand, lipid-based formulation in the nanometer range presents an exciting platform for the delivery of highly potent but poorly water soluble drugs. Some of the examples of lipid-based formulations in the nanometer range include liposomes, solid lipid nanoparticles, and lipid emulsions [22]. In the race to develop new compounds via high-throughput screening, many compounds arise from complex structural modifications. Some of these modifications can lead to highly potent lipophilic drugs. Lipid-based formulations are desirable for such molecules because they can enhance the oral bioavailability of the drug by improving the solubility and also enhance permeability, which is another major advantage of lipid-based systems [27,28].

10.2.2 Fundamentals of Polymeric Nanotechnology

The basis in development of nanoparticles lies in Paul Ehrlich's idea of designing a "magic bullet" carrying active molecules in them and being able to target specific sites in the body for their desired therapeutic effects [29]. Depending on the process by which they are prepared, these systems can be classified as nanospheres (nanoparticles) having a dense and solid polymeric network (monolithic matrix) or nanocapsules having a hollow core that is surrounded by a polymeric shell [29,30]. Drug-loaded nanoparticles have been developed for almost every route of administration: nasal, ocular, mucosal, inhalation, oral, transdermal, and parenteral [18,31–36]. Clinically they have found applications for diagnosing and treating a wide range of pathological conditions.

The polymeric nanoparticles can be formulated from both natural and synthetic polymers. Additionally the polymeric material of interest can be made biodegradable or nonbiodegradable. Polymers can be broadly classified into natural and synthetic polymers. Natural polymers include chitosan, gelatin, alginate, hyaluronic acid (HA), starch, and dextran. On the other hand, synthetic polymers include poly(L-lactic acid) (PLA), poly(D,L-lactide-co-glycolide) (PLGA), polyanhydrides, poly(ε-caprolactone), polystyrene, poly(vinyl alcohol), poly(β-amino ester) (PBAE), PLA/PLGA-b-poly(ethylene glycol) (PEG), block copolymers, poly(N-isopropylacrylamide) (PNIPAAm)-based copolymers, poly(β-benzyl-l-aspartate) block copolymer, and poly(trimethylene carbonate) copolymers. The natural and synthetic polymers have their own set of advantages and disadvantages [37–39]. For example, a naturally occurring polymer is often nontoxic and biodegradable, whereas a synthetic polymer can be tailor-made for specific application, having controlled degradation and well-defined physicochemical properties.

There are numerous well defined techniques for the preparation of the polymeric nanoparticles. However, on a broad scale these methods can be attributed to a formulation that either requires polymerization or is directly formed from desolvation of macromolecules or preformed natural or synthetic polymers. The polymerization method can be further classified into emulsion and interfacial polymerization.

Emulsion Polymerization Emulsion polymerization is a very fast process that can be used for the large-scale production of polymeric nanoparticles [40]. The polymerization can be realized either by dissolving the monomer into a continuous phase (organic or aqueous) where the monomer collides with an initiator (ion or radical) or by converting the monomer into an initiating radical by providing high-energy through γ-radiation, ultraviolet radiation, or strong visible light. The emulsion polymerization via the organic continuous phase requires that the monomer be dispersed into an organic phase in which it is insoluble or into an emulsion or microemulsion. Polymeric nanoparticles synthesized by emulsion polymerization in the aqueous continuous phase are more desirable than nanoparticles made from the organic continuous phase as the preparation steps exclude the use of toxic organic solvents, surfactants, or emulsifiers. Polymeric nanoparticles of poly(methylmethacrylate) (PMMA), poly(ethylcyanoacrylate) (PECA), poly(butylcyanoacrylate), and polyacrylamide have been prepared by the emulsion polymerization technique [41]. These polymeric nanoparticles have been known to encapsulate hydrophilic drugs.

Emulsification/Solvent Evaporation Technique Emulsification of the polymer solution in an aqueous phase is followed by evaporation of the polymer solvent [40,42]. This two-step procedure results in polymer precipitation as nanospheres. The drug is dissolved or dispersed into a preformed polymer organic solution containing dichloromethane, chloroform, or ethyl acetate. This mixture is subjected to emulsification in an aqueous medium to make an oil/water emulsion by using emulsifying agents or surfactants. The size of the resulting emulsion can be reduced by high-speed homogenization or sonication. After formation of a stable emulsion, the organic solvent is evaporated by either increasing the temperature/under pressure or constant stirring. Even though other types of emulsions such as water in oil (w/o), water-oil-water (w/o/w), or oil-water-oil (o/w/o) can be formed, oil in water emulsions are preferred as they use water as the nonsolvent. This eliminates the need for recycling, facilitating the washing step and minimizing the agglomeration. Polymers used to formulate nanoparticles via this technique include PLA, PLGA, ethylcellulose (EC), PCL, and poly(β-hydroxybutyrate) (PHB). Drugs that have been encapsulated within the polymer matrix with this process are albumin, tetanus toxoid, testosterone, loperamide, cyclosporine, praziquantel, nucleic acid, and indomethacin.

Solvent Displacement Technique The solvent displacement method is based on the principle of spontaneous emulsification. The polymer is generally dissolved into a water-miscible solvent of intermediate polarity such as ethanol or acetone [40]. The drug to be incorporated is mixed with the polymer in the same phase. This phase is introduced into a stirred aqueous phase containing a surfactant. As the polymer–drug mixture is introduced into the aqueous phase, rapid diffusion of partial polar solvent leads to precipitation of the polymer due to changes in solubility. The precipitation of the polymer in the presence of mechanical stirring results in formation of polymeric nanoparticles. The limiting factor in this approach is the use of the water-miscible solvents that can cause rapid diffusion to produce spontaneous emulsification. For example, both acetone and dichloromethane are used as water-miscible solvents, but dichloromethane increases the mean particle size because the coalescence rate of the formed nanoparticles is not sufficiently high. The polymeric nanoparticles produced by this technique can only be applied to entrapment of lipophilic drugs. Hence the choice of drug/polymer/solvent/ nonsolvent is extremely important in this method. Examples of polymers used for nanoparticle preparation by this technique include PLGA, PLA, PCL, poly(methyl vinyl ether-*co*-maleic anhydride) (PVM/MA). Drugs such as cyclosporine, doxorubicin, paclitaxel, and insulin have been efficiently incorporated within these polymers.

Emulsification/Solvent Diffusion (ESD) Method   In the ESD technique the polymer encapsulating the drug is dissolved in a partially water-soluble solvent such as propylene carbonate and saturated with water so that thermodynamic equilibrium is achieved between the two liquids. The polymer–water-saturated solvent phase is next emulsified in an aqueous solution containing stabilizers in order to precipitate the polymer and form nanoparticles. As a result the solvent diffuses to the outer phase and nanoparticles form. Subsequently, depending on the boiling point, the solvent is removed by filtration or evaporation. High-speed homogenization is not required, and the advantages of employing this technique are high batch-to-batch reproducibility and narrow size distribution. As with the other emulsification techniques, ESD is well suited for encapsulation of lipophilic drugs. Drugs such as doxorubicin, indocyanine, and cyclosporine have been successfully encapsulated into polymers such as PLGA, PLA, gelatin, and sodium-glycolate nanoparticles synthesized via ESD.

Salting-out Technique   The salting-out method is a variation of the emulsification/solvent diffusion method [40,42]. When a water-miscible solvent is added to the aqueous phase containing electrolytes, it results in the separation of the water-miscible solvent, which is known as the salting-out effect. This is the principle applied to produce polymeric nanoparticles. The polymer and the drug are initially dissolved in a water-miscible organic solvent and subsequently emulsified into an aqueous solution containing salting out agents such as electrolytes and colloidal stabilizers. The oil/water emulsion is diluted by adding water to enhance the diffusion of the organic solvent into the aqueous phase, and the result is the formation of nanoparticles. Both the solvent and salting-out agents are then eliminated by cross-flow filtration. This technique enables high-loading efficiency and high-yield for lipophilic drugs. Polymeric nanoparticles of PLA, PMAA, and EC are produced by this process.

Supercritical or Compressed Fluid Technology   The newest method to produce polymeric microparticles and nanoparticles involves the dissolution of the polymer and the drug in a supercritical fluid [40]. The fluid is sprayed into a chamber containing solvent miscible gas, but in which the polymer and the drug are not miscible. The gaseous phase acts as a supercritical fluid (generally supercritical CO_2 gas), and upon spraying, the organic solvent evaporates. Thus the supersaturation of the liquid solution results in the formation of fine, uniform colloidal particles [40,42].

Controlled Complexation   Electrostatic complexation is induced by oppositely charged polymers interacting in aqueous solution, and this can yield stable colloidal dispersions. The interacting polymers could be therapeutically active (e.g., oligonucleotides and plasmid DNA) or may have tailored properties (e.g., pH-sensitivity) [43,44]. A wide variety of charge-bearing polymers have been utilized to manufacture composite nanoparticles with varying physicochemical properties [45–49].

10.2.3   Introduction to Lipid Nanotechnologies

Lipid nanotechnology is another approach for delivering the bioactive molecules to various sites in the GI tract. As mentioned previously, lipid-based formulations are desirable for their ability to encapsulate the lipophilic drug. Liposomal technology was introduced in the mid-1960s by Bangham [50]. Liposomes are mostly made up of phospholipids, and they have proved to be highly biocompatible. They therefore present an interesting prospect for the delivery of drugs, proteins, peptides, and plasmid DNA. However, from the oral delivery perspective, it has been shown that liposomes are not stable within the GI tract but are still desirable because of their ability to encapsulate the lipophilic drug. In order to improve the stability of the liposomes, surface modifications of these colloidal systems has been proposed. Toward this end, use of mucoadhesive polymers and ligands such as lectin has been explored. On the other hand, solid lipid nanoparticles are now also being extensively researched for their properties such as biodegradability, good tolerability, and availability of cost-effective scale-up techniques such as high-pressure homogenization and micro-emulsion technology. This section on lipid nanotechnologies will focus on the surface-modified liposomes. The emphasis will be on the method of preparation and application from the oral drug delivery perspective.

Liposomes comprise amphiphilic molecules of natural or synthetic origin. Either the two hydrocarbon chains are esterified to a glycerol backbone chain (glycerolipids), or they constitute a hydrophobic ceramide moiety that is linked to a hydrophilic head group. The head group can have a phosphate (phospholipids) or a carbohydrate (glycolipids) unit. Some of the examples of biological head groups include zwitterionic phosphatidylcholine (PC), phosphatidylethanolamine (PE), sphingomylein (SM), negatively charged phosphatidic acid (PA), phosphatidylglycerol (PG), phosphatidylserine (PS), phosphatidylinositol (PI), cardiolipin (CL), and monosiagloganglioside (GM1). On the other hand, positively charged amphiphiles of synthetic origin include *N*-[1-(2,3-dioleyloxy)propyl]-*N,N,N*-trimethylammonium (DOTMA), 1-oleoyl-2-[6-[(7-nitro-2-1,3-benzoxadiazol-4-yl)amino]hexanoyl]-3-trimethylammonium propane (DOTAP), and 1,2-dioleoyl-snglycero-3-phosphotidylethanolamine (DOPE). The cationic lipids can interact with negatively charged DNA or oppositely charged biological membranes. The amphiphilic membranous lipids are poorly soluble in water and tend to form bilayers. The resulting structure is a concentric bilayered vesicle enclosing an aqueous volume, and this is what is known as a *liposome*. Liposomes can be characterized as multilamellar vesicles (MLV: 0.1–10 µm) or unilamellar vesicles. The unilamellar vesicles can be further classified into small unilamellar vesicles (SUV: 25–50 nm), large unilamellar vesicles (LUV: 100–500 nm), or giant unilamellar vesicles (GUV: ≥1 µm) [51].

Thin Lipid Film Hydration Method   Multilamellar vesicles (MLVs) were the first liposomal preparation described in the literature to be formed spontaneously [52]. MLVs can be made by readily co-dissolving the desired lipids (including the payload) into an organic solvent. This step is followed by rotary evaporation of the organic solvent under reduced pressure. Subsequently the lipids are hydrated above the lipid phase transition temperature. It is highly desirable to achieve a thin film of the lipids to ensure efficient hydration of the bilayer. The particle size of liposomes achieved via this method is very heterogeneous. Other parameters to be considered are the hydration time and method of re-suspension of the lipids. For example, longer hydration time with gentle shaking results in higher encapsulation of the payload than shorter hydration time with rigorous shaking. Hence, despite identical lipid concentration, composition and aqueous volume, the two formulations of MLV can be different [51,52].

Mechanical Methods   Sonication, extrusion through polycarbonate membrane and microfluidization of MLVs, can result in homogeneous SUVs with radii of around 25 to 50 nm. The sonication can be done via bath or probe sonicator within an inert atmosphere (usually nitrogen). Both the types of sonication methods have their pros and cons. The advantage with the probe sonicator is its ability to cause faster breakdown of the MLVs into SUVs. However, the disadvantage is the possibility of contamination and degradation of the phospholipid from the metal probe. Additionally probe sonication can result in generation of aerosols from the solution containing radioactive, carcinogenic, or infectious excipients in the formulation. Bath sonicators require more time and attention in order to obtain SUVs of very small size. Additionally the temperature of the preparation can be controlled and be maintained above the lipid phase transition temperature [51, 52].

Detergent Removal Methods Another process for the production of unilamellar vesicles involves the removal of the detergent from the phospholipid/detergent mixture. Processes like centrifugation, gel-filtration, or fast controlled dialysis can be employed for the removal of detergent. The vesicles produced via this process have an average diameter of around 100 nm. This process is suitable for entrapping proteins and membrane-bound ligands. Another approach of SUV preparation involves the ethanol injection technique. This process avoids the need of sonication. In this process the lipids dissolved in ethanol are rapidly injected into aqueous buffer. This results in spontaneous formation of a heterogeneous mixture containing MLV, LUV, and SUV. The average vesicle diameter obtained by the ethanol injection method ranges from 30 to 110 nm, depending on lipid concentration [51].

Reverse Evaporation Methods For the formation of large liposomes, the phospholipids are first dissolved in an organic solvent such as diethylether, isopropylether, and chloroform in a 1:1 ratio. The aqueous phase is then added to the phospholipid/solvent mixture. The resulting "water-in-oil" emulsion is sonicated and partially dried to achieve a semisolid gel. The semisolid gel spontaneously forms liposomes upon removal of the residual solvent by continued rotary evaporation under reduced pressure. The vesicles produced via this method range from 0.1 to 1 μm, with up to 50% entrapment. This method is suitable for water-soluble drugs where the aqueous solution of the drug can be injected into the phospholipid/solvent mixture to form a water/oil emulsion [51].

A few other methods for the preparation of liposomes have been described in the literature. The reader interested in learning more about the various other methods for liposomal preparation is referred to [52].

As we mentioned before, stability of the liposomes in the GI tract is the most important limiting factor. The surface modification of the liposomes is an attractive way to enhance the stability of the formulation. Toward this end, polysaccharides such as chitosan, N–O-palmitoylscleroglucan (PSCG), amylopectin, O-palmitoylpullan, and dextran have been used for delivery of peptides and vaccines [53,54]. Additionally coating of liposomes with polymers, such as PEG, ligands such as lectins, and potential of double-liposomes have also been explored.

10.3 POLYMERIC NANOSYSTEMS FOR ORAL DELIVERY

The presence of an absorbing surface on the organs of the gastrointestinal tract makes delivery of therapeutic molecules via the oral route possible. It is a well-known fact that particulate matter can be absorbed by the gastrointestinal tract. The absorption is due to three main mechanisms: (1) translocation of particles across the gastrointestinal wall as intracellular uptake by the absorptive cells of the intestine, (2) paracellular uptake between the cells of the intestinal wall or phagocytic uptake by intestinal macrophages, or (3) uptake by the M cells of the Peyer's patches [16,55–57]. However, the gastro-intestinal tract provides a variety of barriers; which include proteolytic enzymes in the gut lumen and on the brush border membrane, mucus layer, gut flora and epithelial cell lining, to impede the delivery of drugs. Early reports on studies performed by researchers in this area indicate that there are certain essential factors that govern the uptake of particles from the gut. These factors include particle size, physicochemical nature of particles, surface charge, and attachment of uptake enhancers like lectins or poloxamer on the surface of the nanoparticles [58]. After oral administration of nanoparticles they could be (1) directly eliminated in the faeces, (2) adhere to the cells (bioadhesion), and/or (3) undergo oral absorption as a whole. Oral absorption of nanoparticles results in passage across the gastrointestinal barriers and delivery of the payload into the blood, lymph, and other tissues. Jani et al. [59] have shown that particle size plays a major role in uptake. They measured uptake by using radiolabeled polystyrene nanoparticles ranging from 50 nm to 3.0 µm in diameter. From the results of their study, we learn that smaller size particles of 50 nm in diameter showed a 12% uptake by the cells of the small intestine when compared with the 1.0 µm diameter particles, which showed only 1% uptake by the cells of the small intestine. The lower size particles <500 nm were detected in the blood after intestinal uptake, whereas larger size particles >500 nm where not detected in the blood. Also these nanoparticles were detected in other tissues such as the liver and spleen. A low surface charge on the surface of nanoparticles is desirable for good absorption. While Pluronic® or poloxamer (188 and 407) coating on to the surface of 50 nm polystyrene nanoparticles inhibited uptake in the small intestine, a similar coating on the 500 nm polystyrene nanoparticles showed an increased intestinal uptake. There has been yet another report to study the effect of surface modification on uptake of polymeric nanoparticles using ^{14}C-labeled poly(methylmethacrylate) (PMMA), having a mean particle size of 130 nm and coated with polysorbate (Tween®) 80 or poloxamine 908 [60]. These nanoparticles were administered orally to rats, and they were checked for their organ distribution. High radioactivity levels were observed in the stomach contents, with below 5% radioactivity detected in the stomach wall. The highest amount of radioactivity (about 40%) was found in the small intestine, confirming that these coated particles were absorbed in the small intestine.

These studies indicate that polymeric nanoparticles in the appropriate size range can be taken up by the cells of the gastrointestinal tract and that these are well suited for use as an oral drug delivery system. In addition the striking advantage of the nanoparticles is the large surface area that they offer when presented in a biological environment and the flexibility to alter the physico-chemical properties of the core polymer or by surface modification of the nanoparticles.

10.3.1 Illustrative Examples of Polymeric Nanotechnology for Drug Delivery

Polymeric nanoparticulate drug delivery systems have been used for delivery of drugs to organs of the gastrointestinal tract such as stomach, small intestine, and large intestine. Further discussion in this section will focus on various polymeric nanoparticles based drug delivery systems that have been utilized by researchers to overcome the barriers put forth by the gastrointestinal tract to achieve successful drug delivery.

Gastric emptying is one of the many major hurdles to successful delivery of active compounds to the gastric mucosa using conventional delivery systems. These conventional delivery systems do not remain in the stomach for prolonged periods due to them being unable to deliver the drug to the desired site at the effective concentration and in the fully active form. The other major barrier to the delivery of drug is the mucus layer of the gastric mucosa. The primary component of mucus is glycoprotein, which forms a dense condensed and complex microstructure by way of numerous covalent and noncovalent bonds with other mucin molecules. All these issues do not make the stomach a very popular target organ for oral drug delivery. However, the stomach is a target for a few disorders that include infection by *Helicobacter pylori* (*H. pylori*). *H. pylori* has been recognized as a major gastric pathogen responsible for a variety of clinical manifestations including development of gastritis, gastric ulcer, and gastric carcinoma [61].

The microorganism was first isolated by Warren and Marshall in 1982 [62,63] and was recognized to be a gram negative, spiral, urease-producing bacterium. Traditionally orally delivered antibiotics such as amoxicillin and tetracycline have been employed for treatment of this infection, requiring absorption of these drugs into the systemic circulation from the small intestine. However, effective treatment and eradication of *H. pylori* requires site-specific systems that can deliver drugs to the disease area. One way of achieving this is by using mucoadhesive particles that, upon delivery, can successfully adhere onto the gastric mucous layer. Umamaheshwari et al. [64] studied the effectiveness of mucoadhesive nanoparticles prepared from gliadin-bearing amoxicillin for treatment of *H. pylori*. Gliadin is a group of polymorphic proteins extracted from gluten and are soluble in ethanolic solutions. In vivo mucoadhesion capacity was evaluated by oral administration of fluorescent-labeled gliadin nanoparticles. Size-dependent mucoadhesive propensity and specificity were exhibited by gliadin nanoparticles with less than 300 nm particles showing 68% mucoadhesion and 300 nm particles showing 75% and above levels of mucoadhesion. To study in vivo therapeutic efficacy, Mongolian gerbils previously inoculated with human *H. pylori* were administered with amoxicillin-loaded gliadin nanoparticles. These particles were able to show 100% inhibition of *H. pylori* within four hours of administration. However, these nanoparticles were not successful in completely eradicating the *H. pyroli* in vivo. This study showed that amoxicillin-loaded nanoparticles exhibited a longer gastric residence time than the conventional amoxicillin formulation and also that the topical action of amoxicillin on the gastric mucosa plays an important role in the clearance of the bacterium.

The physiological environment existing in the stomach, including its very low pH, does not allow for efficient absorption of basic drugs into the systemic circulation. In one study amifostine was incorporated into PLGA nanoparticles by spray-drying for systemic absorption. Amifostine is an organic thiophosphate prodrug and is dephosphorylated by alkaline phosphatase in the tissue to the active free thiol metabolite. The major drawback of the drug is that it cannot be administered orally in an active form, and when administered systemically, it is rapidly cleared from the body. To overcome this drawback spray-dried PLGA nanoparticles have been investigated for oral delivery [65]. PLGA nanoparticles containing amifostine were administered to mice orally, and tissue distribution was observed for the administered dose. Within 30 minutes post-oral administration the drug was detected in almost all the tissues including blood, brain, spleen, kidney, muscle, and liver.

The small intestine has traditionally been the target organ for drug delivery via the oral route because of the presence of a large absorbing surface area, neutral pH, and opportunity to deliver drugs to the systemic circulation for action at a distant site. Drug substance and drug product development challenges, along with disease physiology (tumor, skin infections), have limited the delivery of therapeutics via the oral route. Nanotechnology-derived drug delivery systems can significantly improve the performance of drugs when administered via the oral route. In an attempt to improve oral bioavailability of antituberculosis drugs, wheat-germ agglutinin lectin-functionalized PLGA nanoparticles were successfully prepared and used to encapsulate isoniazid, rifampicin, and pyrazinamide, the three frontline drugs employed in the treatment of tuberculosis [66]. These PLGA nanoparticles encapsulating the antituberculosis drugs at therapeutic dosage were administered either by oral or aerosol routes for their in vivo drug disposition studies to guinea pigs, which were previously infected with *Mycobacterium tuberculosis* to develop the infection. In this study all three drugs were administered in the free form, namely the non-encapsulated form served as control. Results obtained for the plasma concentration of different drugs suggested that PLGA-nanoparticles helped improve the plasma residence time of different drugs after oral administration. The relative bioavailability of all the drugs except for rifampicin was higher for the orally administered particles when compared to aerosolized nanoparticles and the free drug. Rifampicin was detected for 6 to 7 days in the plasma after oral administration of PLGA-NP when compared to free drug which was detected only for 1 day. Similarly isoniazid and pyrazinamide were maintained for more than 12 days in plasma when compared to a single day for the free drug. The presence of these drugs in the tissues such as liver, lungs, and spleen for a long time favors their application against tuberculosis where infection is largely localized in these tissues. Chemotherapeutic studies revealed that three doses of oral and aerosolized lectin-coated nanoparticles for 15 days could yield undetectable mycobacterial colony forming units when compared to 45 days of oral administration of the free drug to achieve the same results. This study suggests that polymeric nanoparticles could be favorably used for effective treatment of tuberculosis.

There have been very few reports on oral delivery of hydrophilic, cationic drugs by oral administration [67]. Aminoglycosides, polypeptides, proteins, terefenamate, proglumetacin, tiaramide, and apazone are examples of such compounds. Popescu et al. [67] used biodegradable nanoparticles prepared from naturally occurring polymers such as chitosan, dextran sulfate, chondroitin sulfate, and keratin sulfate for oral delivery of highly cationic active compounds that are highly hydrophilic and likely substrates for P-gp. Streptomycin is the best example of this class of drugs, which was loaded into chitosan nanoparticles and tested for in vivo efficacy using *M. tuberculosis* infected mice. Streptomycin was successfully loaded with an encapsulation efficiency of 50% or higher with a minimal drug loading of 30% w/w of polymer. After oral administration of these chitosan nanoparticles in mice a one $\log_{10}$ reduction in colony-forming units of the bacilli was achieved compared to the control group. These results showed that the nanoparticle-based technology can provide a very feasible technology for oral administration of aminoglycoside antibiotics that are inactive via the oral route.

Another report of intestinal delivery of small molecules using polymeric nanoparticles was reported by Jaeghere et al. in 2000 [68]. In their study they used pH-sensitive polymeric nanoparticles made from poly(methacrylic acid-*co*-ethylacrylate) copolymer Eudragit® L100-55. These particles were used for oral delivery of HIV-protease inhibitor (CGP 70726), which is reportedly a very poorly soluble drug. HIV-1 protease inhibitors intervene in a crucial and specific step of the replication cycle of HIV, impairing the processing of viral precursor polypeptides into active functional and structural proteins that are necessary for the maturation of the virus [68–70]. Many different HIV-protease inhibiting agents have been described, with most suffering with problems such as poor solubility and subsequent inadequate oral bioavailability. In this study the authors incorporated CGP 70726 in both nanoparticle and microparticle formulations and compared oral bioavailability of the drug upon oral administration in beagle dogs in both fed and fasted state. The results of this study showed that nanoparticles and microparticles had very similar pharmacokinetic parameters in the both the fed and the fasted state. No significant difference was observed for in C_{max} for nanoparticles (1.62 ± 0.04 fasted, 0.86 ± 0.21 fed) when compared to microparticles (1.59 ± 0.32 fasted, 0.88 ± 0.33 fed). The slightly higher C_{max} observed for microparticles has been attributed to the large specific surface area, but there was very high interindividual variability for this group in both fed and fasted states. It is clear from this study that polymeric nanoparticles offer an attractive platform for improving the bioavailability of drugs that would have otherwise exhibited very limited bioavailability and hence therapeutic efficacy.

Nanotechnology-based drug delivery systems can also be employed for delivery of drug molecules to the large intestine. The large intestine represents the last segment of the gastrointestinal tract and can suffer from two major inflammatory bowel diseases which are ulcerative colitis and Crohn's disease. Very little is known about the pathological mechanisms involved in both the disease [71–74]. Conventionally treatment of these diseases has involved many different approaches with anti- inflammatory drugs and include 5-aminosalicylic acid formulations for mild symptoms, glucocorticoids and immunosuppressive drugs like azathioprine taken along with methotrexate for moderate to severe forms of the disease [75]. The major drawback with these conventional formulations is that they have to be taken at high doses and daily by the oral route, resulting in absorption of these compounds by the small intestine and causing possible strong and highly undesirable side effects [20,21,75].

From a drug delivery point of view, the major barrier to oral delivery for such diseases is the large intestine and stability of drug in the stomach and the small intestine until they reach the disease site. Several strategies have been employed for development of oral delivery systems for transport of drugs to the inflamed sites in the colon, which include sustained release devices such as prodrugs, macroscopic systems such as pH-controlled drug release systems, time-controlled drug release systems, enzyme controlled drug release systems, and microsized delivery forms like microspheres and nanoparticles. One of the best stimuli-responsive drug delivery systems that can be used successfully for local delivery to the colon is enzyme-controlled release systems. Enzyme-controlled release systems make use of the variety of enzymes that are produced by the colonic mucosa to achieve colon-specific drug delivery. These prodrugs and controlled release devices also have the risk of causing adverse side effects which might result from systemic absorption of drug that might occur due to nonspecific delivery of the drug all over the colon [20,21,75–77].

Mucoadhesion is another property of the polymers that could be used for site-specific delivery of the drug to the colon [55]. Polymers like polysaccharides, which include chondroitin sulfate, pectin, dextran and guar gum, have been researched for their use as colon-specific systems [45]. Other polymers bearing a positive charge can also be used successfully for their mucoadhesive properties [78–80]. Chitosan and gelatin are the best examples of such polymers. Chitosan, which is one of the most abundant natural polysaccharides, has also been investigated for development of a colon-specific delivery system because of its well-known mucoadhesive properties; further a study on rats showed that chitosan gets degraded by the cecal and colonic enzymes [61,76,81,82].

Size-dependent bioadhesion of nanoparticles and microparticles in the inflamed colonic mucosa has been demonstrated [20]. Commercially manufactured fluorescent polystyrene particles of different sizes including 100, 1000, and 10,000 nm were used in the study. The experiments were conducted in rats that were rectally treated with hydroalcoholic solution of 2,4,6-trinitroben-zenesulfonic acid (TNBS) for inducing inflammatory bowel disease. Polystyrene particles were administered orally to the rats and were assessed for localization and deposition of the particles in the gastrointestinal tract. The results of this study revealed a size-dependent particle deposition in the gastrointestinal tract of the control group and also in the inflamed tissue. According to the results, lower size particles exhibited a higher incidence of particle deposition in the inflamed tissue with the lowest particle size of 100 nm showing a 6.5-fold increase in percentage particle binding when compared to particle binding of the same size in the healthy control group. The overall distribution of the nanoparticles in the gastrointestinal tract was assessed, and it was found again that 100 nm particles had a higher percentage of localization (38.6%) in the mucus of the inflamed tissue as compared to 31.1% for 1000 nm and only 13.4% for 10,000 nm particles. This study proved that nanoparticles are better localized and deposited by the macrophages of the inflamed tissue and also that size-dependent deposition of particles in the inflamed tissue should be given importance when designing a nanoparticle carrier system for inflammatory bowel disease.

In another study the same group reported on the development of biocompatible and biodegradable PLGA-based nanoparticle system for targeted oral delivery to the inflamed tissues of the colon for patients suffering from inflammatory bowel disease [21]. Two different molecular weights of PLGA (5000 and 20,000) were used to prepare nanoparticles containing rolipram, an anti-inflammatory drug. The emulsification–solvent–evaporation method was used for nanoparticle synthesis to yield sizes of less than 500 nm with an encapsulation efficiency of over 80%. After induction of colonic inflammation using TNBS solution in rats, PLGA nanoparticles were orally administered daily for five days, and the control group received only saline. PLGA nanoparticles controlled drug release, causing a local anti-inflammatory effect, and also proved to be very efficient at decreasing inflammation of the colitis. Interactions of the negatively charged PLGA nanoparticles and the positively charged proteins of the ulcerated tissue showed a further enhancement of binding of these nanoparticles to the inflamed tissue.

All of the above-mentioned examples showcase the use of nanotechnology-based polymeric systems for delivery of drug molecules for either local or systemic effects. The use of such drug delivery systems is not and should not be limited to the use in cases of a handful molecules and disease conditions. This advanced technology can be successfully used for improving the performance of drug molecules in any local or systemic disease. Many clinical situations and conditions demand specialized therapeutics to achieve improved levels of healing. In such situations the requirements are specified by the clinician that forms the basis of product development.

10.3.2   Illustrative Examples of Polymeric Nanotechnology for Oral Macromolecular Delivery

Therapeutic compounds of biotech origin such as proteins, peptides, and nucleic acids are highly unstable in the biological environment in the free form. The physiological conditions such as low pH and high levels of degrading enzymes such as protease and nuclease existing in the intestine present a very hostile environment for delivery of these molecules via the oral route. Much research directed in this area has led to the development of many novel delivery systems for these highly potent molecules. Among them, polymeric nano- and microparticles have emerged as the most successful delivery systems because of their ability to protect these molecules against pH/enzyme-induced degradation and also by prolonging the time of delivery to the mucosal sites [83–87]. These systems have not only been used for delivery of therapeutic and immunogenic proteins/peptides but also for nucleic acid based therapeutics. Although polymeric microparticles have been more popular as delivery devices for immunogenic proteins and peptides, polymeric nanoparticles have been employed to improve the oral bioavailability and performance of therapeutic proteins and peptides upon administration [88,89]. Two of the most extensively researched therapeutic peptide molecules include insulin, an essential enzyme for metabolism of glucose, and cyclosporine, which is an immunosuppressive drug.

Couvreur et al. [84] in 1980 reported the first attempt to deliver insulin via the oral route. In their study insulin was adsorbed on the surface of 200 nm poly(alkylcyanoacrylate) nanoparticles and administered orally to diabetic rats to seek hypoglycemic effects. The investigators did not observe any decrease in glucose level upon oral administration, but good hypoglycemic activity was observed upon subcutaneous administration, suggesting that insulin was getting degraded in the gastrointestinal tract. In another investigation, nanoparticles made from poly(isobutylcyanoacrylate) (PIBCA) loaded with insulin were used for oral delivery [84]. The onset of action was after 2 days of administration, but was seen for 20 days depending on the insulin dose. Administration of these particles orally resulted in a 50% to 60% reduction in blood glucose levels of diabetic rats. These results suggest that PIBCA nanoparticles were not only able to protect the insulin payload from degradation in the gastrointestinal tract, but they were also able to deliver biologically active insulin [85,90,91].

More than a decade after the first report on oral insulin delivery, a patent was issued in 1995 for controlled release of insulin from biodegradable nanoparticles [92]. Insulin was complexed with different polycyanoacrylate monomers at low pH, and nanoparticles were prepared from this complex by an anionic polymerization process. These nanoparticles were dosed orally to rats, and blood glucose levels were monitored over four hours. A considerable decrease in blood glucose levels was observed in the group dosed with insulin-loaded nanoparticles compared to the untreated group.

More reports on the oral delivery of insulin using polymeric nanoparticles have emerged in the current decade. Pan et al. [90] studied the effects of bio-adhesive chitosan nanoparticles for improving the intestinal absorption of insulin in diabetic rats. Chitosan was chosen as the polymer for preparing the delivery system because it exhibits a strong electrostatic interaction with insulin, hence improving the loading efficiency of the polymer. Another reason for choosing chitosan was for its bioadhesive properties for prolonged stay in the gastrointestinal tract, which resulted in prolonged release times for insulin [93]. A dose-dependent decrease in blood glucose levels was observed after oral administration of these 290 nm particles in diabetic rats. Chitosan–insulin nanoparticles showed a higher decrease in blood insulin levels when compared to chitosan–insulin solution, suggesting that they could enhance the intestinal absorption of insulin by promoting protection from gastric clearance and also render longer residence time in the circulation. More recently Foss et al. [94] developed nanospheres from methacrylic acid grafted with poly(ethylene glycol) and also acrylic acid grafted with poly(ethylene glycol) as oral insulin carriers. The results from this study showed that diabetic animals administered with insulin-loaded nanospheres had significantly reduced serum glucose levels with respect to the control animals, and this effect lasted over 6 hours. Many more examples for oral delivery of insulin using polymeric nanoparticles have been reported [95–98].

Another peptide, cyclosporine, has been studied for transport to the gastrointestinal tract using polymeric nanoparticles via the oral route. Cyclosporine is a potent immunosuppressive agent and is widely used for the inhibition of graft rejections in transplant of organs like heart, liver, skin, lungs, kidney, and the like. It is also prescribed in autoimmune disease like rheumatoid arthiritis and Bechet's disease [99]. Currently many different formulations of cyclosporin are being marketed such as Neoral®, oral solution (Novartis), Sandimmune® microemulsion and soft gelatin capsule (Novartis), and SangCyA®, amporphous nanoparticles and oral solution (SangStat Medical Corporation). Although these formulations are available for use in patients, they are plagued by the problem of variable bioavailability, so the patient has to be constantly monitored for blood levels of cyclosporine during the regimen [100]. One of the earlier efforts to improve the bioavailability using nanoparticulate formulation was reported by Dai et al. in 2004 [83]. They used pH-sensitive nanoparticles made from poly(methacrylic acid and methacrylate) copolymer (Eudragit®). In this study the Neoral® formulation was used as a standard to compare oral bioavailability. Nanoparticles exhibited drug entrapment of over 90% for different formulations prepared from different types of Eudragit® systems. Cyclosporin nanoparticles prepared from Eudragit® S100, an anionic polymer, demonstrated the highest relative bioavailability of 132% with respect to Neoral®. Other polymeric nanoparticles also exhibited more than 110% relative bioavailability except for nanoparticles prepared from Eudragit® E100 (CyA-E100), which is a cationic polymer. In vitro release studies of cyclosporine from different nanoparticle preparations showed that all nanoparticle preparations caused pH-specific release of cyclosporine-A at pH 7.4 except for CyA-E100 nanoparticles, which released the whole payload at pH 2.0. This proves that cyclosporine from CyA-E100 nanoparticles was released in the stomach upon oral administration and accounts for its low relative bioavailability with respect to other nanoparticle preparations.

Wang et al. [100] examined hydroxypropyl methylcellulose phthalate (HPMCP) polymer nanoparticles loaded with cyclosporine for oral delivery. HPMCP is a common enteric coating excipient used in the pharmaceutical industry for enteric coating of tablets. It dissolves specifically at a pH of 7.4 and releases the contents in the lower intestine. The investigators used two different cyclosporine nanoparticle preparations made from different molecular weights of the same polymer. Again, a high encapsulation efficiency of over 95% was observed with the nanoparticle preparation due to hydrophobicity of the drug. Cyclosporine nanoparticles made of high molecular weight HPMCP exhibited a relative bioavailability of over 115%, and those made from lower molecular weight exhibited only 82% relative bioavailability against Neoral®. The difference was attributed to the pH-independent property of lower molecular weight polymer, which released the entire payload within the stomach itself, thus inactivating the peptide drug. The results from the studies above indicate that pH-sensitive nanoparticles loaded with cyclosporine can be designed as new carriers that exhibit a better pharmacokinetic profile compared to the currently marketed formulations.

A series of investigations have been directed toward preparation and evaluation of the bioavailability and toxicity profile of cyclosporine-loaded poly(ε-caprolactone) nanoparticles [101,102]. The nanoparticles of roughly 100 nm diameter were prepared by a solvent-evaporation procedure and evaluated for biodistribution, immunosuppressive activity, and nephrotoxicity. Sandimmune® was used as the standard for this investigation in rats following oral administration. A significantly higher tissue (especially kidney) concentration of cyclosporine was achieved with nanoparticle formulations compared to the solution indicating probability of higher nephrotoxicity. However, further toxicological evaluation with kidney function tests indicated no difference in the profiles of the two formulations. In vitro lymphocyte proliferative activity (an indication of immunosuppressive potential) also showed better activity for nanoparticle formulations are comparable doses. The conclusion of the investigation was that the nanoparticle formulations can be effective at a lower dose levels compared to the solution form and thus may help to reduce drug-associated tissue damage.

Cho et al. [103] developed several different oral cyclosporine nanoparticle formulations consisting of one alkanol solvent and a polyoxyalkylene surfactant, and tested them in rats for their bioavailability in comparison to Sandimmune® oral solution. Selected formulations based on these preclinical investigations were further tested for their pharmacokinetic profile in humans. Forty-eight healthy males were chosen and a randomized, double-blinded, three-way crossover study was conducted with the Sandimmune® oral solution as the standard formulation. From the results obtained it was observed that cyclosporine nanoparticles exhibited a C_{max} that was twice as high as those achieved by the Sandimmune® oral solution and the T_{max} was much shorter for cyclosporine nanoparticles compared to the standard. Also the AUC observed for nanoparticle formulations was significantly higher than the standard formulation. Similarly polymeric nanoparticles have also been used for oral delivery of other proteins such as heparin and salmon calcitonin [104–106].

Polymeric nanoparticles have been used as well for delivery of antigenic proteins to the mucosal surfaces present in the gut to generate immunity against pathogenic organisms. Although much research in this area has been done with polymeric microparticles, nanoparticles have proved to be effective carriers of such antigen proteins and peptides. In 2000 Jung et al. developed tetanus toxoid (TT) loaded sulfobutylated poly(vinyl alcohol)-graft PLGA nanoparticles for oral delivery [107]. The nanoparticles were prepared by the solvent displacement technique, and different sizes of nanoparticles were obtained by varying the solvent and co-solvent ratios, resulting in formation of small (~100 nm), medium (~500 nm), and large particles (>1000 nm). Balb/c mice were immunized by oral, nasal, and intraperitoneal administration of TT nanoparticles loaded by adsorption. Certain groups of animals were orally administered with TT-loaded nanoparticles along with a mucosal adjuvant cholera toxin to improve the immunological response. Four to six weeks after immunization serum samples were collected from the immunized animals and assayed for Ig-G and Ig-A antibody titers using ELISA. Groups of animals administered with TT-loaded nanoparticles and cholera toxin showed a 10-fold increase in serum IgG levels compared to oral administration of TT-loaded nanoparticles alone and TT solution in presence and absence of cholera toxin. Similarly the serum IgA response for the group administered with TT-loaded nanoparticles along with cholera toxin showed a more than 10-fold increase when compared to groups orally administered with TT-loaded nanoparticles without mucosal adjuvant and TT solution with and without cholera toxin. Nasal administration of TT-loaded nanoparticles showed generation of lower levels of both IgG and IgA in comparison to the orally administered group. A dose-dependent immune response was also observed in this study with groups administered, with the highest dose (29 μg TT) showing the highest production of IgG and IgA at six weeks after oral immunization compared to lower doses (2.9 and 9.4 μg TT). The results of this study indicate generation of immune response upon oral delivery of antigenic proteins using polymeric nanoparticles.

Polymeric nanoparticles, because of their ability to effectively transport active molecules across the gastrointestinal tract, have been studied as delivery systems for gene therapy and vaccination [41,108]. A range of polycationic polymers including gelatin, chitosan, polylysine, polyarginine, protamine, speramine, spermidine, and polysaccharides could be used to prepare the coacervates of the nucleic acids that result in the formation of discrete nanoparticles.

Roy et al. [109,110] used such coacervates for effective vaccination by the oral route. Chitosan nanoparticles in the size range of 100 to 200 nm were prepared by salting-out technique with the plasmid DNA (pArah2), which encodes for the peanut allergen Arah2. The nanoparticles were orally fed into mice, and the serum and fecal levels of IgG or IgA were measured periodically. High levels of anti–arah2 IgG were observed in the titer of the group that was fed with low molecular weight chitosan nanoparticles housing the plasmid DNA, compared to other groups that were administered with high molecular weight chitosan nanoparticles with or without a booster dose. The mice from all groups were challenged with crude peanut extracts four weeks after the booster dose, and a positive antibody response was detected in groups immunized by DNA nanospheres. These results suggest that chitosan-plasmid DNA nanoparticles delivered through the oral route can modify the immune system in mice and protect against food allergen induced hypersensitivity.

Chen et al. [111] used DNA-complexed with chitosan for transfection of the erythropoietin gene to the intestinal epithelium of mice. Erythropoietin is a glycoprotein that stimulates production of red blood cells. Erythropoietin is used in patients with anemia associated with chronic renal failure and in cancer patients for simulation of erythropoieisis. Chitosan nanoparticles containing plasmid DNA encoding for erythropoietin (mEpo) were administered orally to one group of mice along with other appropriate control dosage forms. Erythropoietin gene expression was determined every two days by measuring the hematocrit of the mice. Mice that were administered with chitosan-loaded mEpo showed a 15% increase in hematocrit over other dosage forms, indicating successful transfection of mEpo gene across the intestinal epithelium. These results suggest that chitosan nanoparticles were able to prevent the mEpo from degradation against DNAses and hence the possibility of using them as gene delivery vehicles via the oral route. In another study nanoparticles prepared from cationic biopolymers (chitin, chitosan, and their derivatives) were proposed to be the carriers for oral administration of bioactive compounds for gene therapy [109]. The nanoparticles with encapsulated plasmid DNA encoding for human coagulation factor IX (pFIX) were prepared. The molecular weight of the cationic biopolymers ranged from 5 to 200 kDa. The nanoparticles in the size range of 100 to 200 nm were generated by the complex coacervation method and were used for oral administration to mice. Human factor IX was detected in the systemic circulation of the mice within 3 days following oral delivery but declined after 14 days. The investigators also demonstrated the bioactivity of the factor IX transgene product in factor IX knockout mice. Haemophilia B is an X-linked bleeding disorder caused by a mutation in the factor IX gene. After orally feeding factor IX transgene-loaded nanoparticles to the knockout mice, the clotting time was reduced from 3.5 to 1.3 minutes, which was comparable with the clotting time of 1 minute observed with wild-type mice. The investigators proposed that the intestinal epithelium was the site of nanoparticle absorption and transfection.

Kim et al. [112] prepared PLGA nanoparticles housing *H. pylori* lysates by the solvent-evaporation method. These nanoparticles were administered orally into mice and antibody induction was assayed in serum and gastrointestinal tract. Serum IgG subclasses were determined by ELISA. The mean antibody titers for serum IgG and gut IgA responses were significantly higher than those of the groups immunized with the soluble antigen alone. Cholera toxin–*H. pylori* (CT—a well-established potent mucosal adjuvant) had a higher antibody titer compared to PLGA–*H. pylori* nanoparticles. The results of this study indicates that PLGA–*H. pylori* nanoparticles could stimulate *H. pylori*–specific mucosal and systemic immune responses in mice and also that nanoparticles can be used for vaccination against *H. pylori*.

10.4 ILLUSTRATIVE EXAMPLES OF LIPOSOMES FOR ORAL DRUG AND GENE DELIVERY

Liposomal formulation for oral delivery is desirable because of their ability to encapsulate hydrophobic or poorly water-soluble drug molecules. Additionally, as liposomes mimic the same organizational setup as the plasma membrane of the living cells, they represent a good platform for drug delivery. Liposomes are also desirable as they are highly biocompatible, biodegradable, and nontoxic in nature [51,113]. Drugs can be characterized as either hydrophilic or hydrophobic. An insight into the liposomal assembly can give information on how a drug of certain nature can be incorporated into liposomes. A liposomal assembly consists of a highly hydrophilic region comprised of an intravesicular aqueous compartment, a hydrophobic region of the bilayer core made up of alkyl chains of constituent lipids, and an amphipathic region represented by vesicular surface made up of polar lipid head groups [113]. That intuition, that a drug of hydrophobic nature will have an affinity toward the bilayer region of the liposome, is based on the simple principle of chemistry that "like dissolves like". Nevertheless, a hydrophilic drug will have an affinity for the intravesicular aqueous compartment and an amphipathic drug can be intercalated into the bilayer, below their critical micelle concentration (CMC) [52,113]. Liposomes also provide an attractive form of drug delivery system because of their ability to deliver the intact payload within the cell and thus bypassing cell level barriers such as P-gp present on the cell surface.

Despite all the above-mentioned advantages the use of liposomes in the oral delivery has been limited because of their instability within the GI tract [114,115] (Table 10.2). Because of the presence of acidic pH, bile salts and hydrolytic enzymes in the GI tract represents a very hostile environment for oral delivery of liposomes. After oral administration, the presence of the lipids in the GI tract leads to the secretion of lipase, which initiates the process of lipolysis in the stomach and in turn results in degradation of not only the liposomal delivery system but also of the encapsulated payload, released from the system much earlier then desired [28]. To overcome these shortcomings

TABLE 10.2   Examples of Liposomal Formulation for Oral Delivery of Therapeutic Molecules

Surface Modifying Entity	Method of Modification	Size (nm)	Incorporated Active and Loading Efficiency	Reference
Submicron size chitosan	Liposomes formed sonicated for longer times to achieve a submicron size. The ssL conjugated with chitosan	300–400	Calcitonin, >90%	[118]
PSCG	Polymer solution mixed with liposomal suspension in 1:2 volumetric ratio and magnetically stirred for 12 hours at a temperature of 50 °C; coated liposomes filtered by gel filtration method	160 ± 3.34	Leuprolide, 37.07 ± 0.04%	[54]
PEG	PEG-derivitized lipid used for the liposomal preparation	306.1*	Human epidermal growth factor, 18.5 ± 1.4%	[119]
WGA lectin	Lectin incorporated into the membrane vesicle by hydrophobic anchor, N-glut PE	191 + 13.62	Insulin, 69.33 ± 4.54%	[120]
Tomato lectin	Lectin incorporated into the membrane vesicle by hydrophobic anchor, N-glut PE	194.1 ± 21.95	Insulin, 82.50 ± 5.57%	[120]
UEA lectin	Lectin incorporated into the membrane vesicle by hydrophobic anchor, N-glut PE	194.1 ± 21.95	Insulin, 39.55 ± 7.28%	[120]

of liposomes, many efforts have been focused on improving the stability of the liposomes within the GI tract. Surface modification of the liposomes is an attractive way to enhance the stability of the formulation in the GI tract Toward this end polysaccharides such as chitosan, N-O-palmitoylscleroglucan (PSCG), amylopectin, O-palmitoylpullan, and dextran have been used for delivery of peptides and vaccines [53,54] (Table 10.2). Additionally surface coating of liposomes with polymers such as polyethylene glycol (PEG), ligands such as lectins, and the drug-delivering potential of double-liposomes and proliposomes have also been explored [49,109,116,117].

As part of surface modifying approach, Takeuchi et al. [118] studied the effectiveness of chitosan-coated liposomes for oral delivery of peptide drugs. The group first evaluated the mucoadhesive and penetrative properties of the submicron-sized chitosan-modified liposomes. The group compared the above-mentioned properties of the submicron chitosan-modified liposomes to the chitosan-modified liposomes, unmodified liposomes, and unmodified submicron-sized liposomes. The multilamellar liposomes comprising of DSPC/DCP/cholesterol incorporated the fluorescent dye and were prepared in 8:2:1 ratio by the thin film hydration method. For the preparation of chitosan-modified liposomes, an aliquot of the liposomal suspension was mixed with the same volume of acetate buffer of chitosan, followed by 1 hour incubation at 10 °C. The liposomes containing 1,1'-dioctadecyl-3,3,3',3'-tetramethylindo-carbocyanine perchlorate (DiI) were administered intragastrically to the rats, and the intestine was removed from rats after 2 hours of oral administration of liposomes. Various parts of the intestine were observed with confocal laser scanning microscopy. They observed that the submicron-sized chitosan-modified liposomes were retained in the GI tract for longer periods of time compared to the chitosan-modified liposomes and other unmodified liposomal formulations. Also the unmodified submicron-sized liposomes were retained in the GI tract for a longer period of time than the unmodified liposomes of larger size. These results indicated that the mucoadhesion and penetrative behavior of the liposomes is dependent on the size and surface modification.

In the next set of experiments, the peptide drug calcitonin was incorporated into the liposomes, followed by surface modification with chitosan. Calcitonin is considered as one of the therapeutic peptides for the treatment of postmenopausal osteoporosis, Paget's disease, and hypercalcemia [117]. Also, before chitosan modification, the liposomal pellet was ultracentrifuged to remove the free calcitonin. The particle sizes of the noncoated liposomes were 4.0 μm, 400 nm, and 200 nm. The particle sizes of the corresponding chitosan-coated liposomes were 4.1 μm, 660.8 nm, and 473.4 nm, respectively. The drug encapsulation efficiency of the liposomes was reported to be greater than 90%. The formulations of calcitonin-loaded chitosan-modified and unmodified liposomes were then administered intragastrically to the male Wistar rats at a dose of 500 IU/Kg. The pharmacologic effects of the various above-mentioned calcitonin-loaded chitosan-modified and unmodified liposmal formulations were evaluated by calculating the area above the blood calcium level. The pharmacologic effect of oral administration of submicron-sized liposomes coated with chitosan was detected up to 120 hours after administration. Additionally the calcitonin submicron-sized unmodified liposomes were also found to alleviate the blood calcium levels. However, the period of reduced calcium levels was much longer in the case of chitosan-modified submicron-sized liposomes. Hence it was concluded that the prolonged pharmacologic effect of calcitonin with submicron-sized chitosan liposomes was attributed to their excellent retentive properties. Also, the noncoated submicron-sized liposome did not show such a prolonged pharmacologic effect. Thus it was concluded that the mucoadhesive property of the submicron-sized chitosan liposome is essential for their long retention time in the intestinal tract.

Li et al. [119] investigated the feasibility of the oral delivery of recombinant human epidermal growth factor (rhEGF) by polyethylene glycol (PEG) modified liposomes. This growth factor is known to inhibit the gastric acid secretion and protect the gastroduodenal mucosa against tissue injury induced by ulcergenic agents. The advantage of "PEGylation" is the ability of the polymer to resist the acidic pH and enzymatic degradation commonly observed in the GI tract. Thus PEG-modification of the liposomes can improve the stability of the liposomes within the GI tract. Two formulations of liposomes were prepared by the thin film hydration method described earlier. The first formulation contained a mixture of PC/cholesterol/DOPE-PEG, and the second formulation contained a mixture of DPPC/cholesterol/DOPE-PEG. After the initial optimization process, the ratio of the PC/cholestrol/DOPE-PEG was 10:5:1, respectively. The same ratio was used in the preparation of the DPPC/cholesterol/DOPE-PEG liposomes. The growth hormone rhEGF was incorporated into the liposomal formulation at a concentration of 0.5 mg/ml. The particle sizes of the PC/Ch/DOPE-PEG and DPPC/Ch/DOPE-PEG were 289.9 and 306.1 nm, respectively. The drug encapsulation efficiency of the PC-liposomes was 15.6%, and that of DPPC/cholesterol/DOPE-PEG was 18.5%. As part of preliminary studies, the bioactivity and permeability of the rhEGF containing liposomal formulations in Caco-2 cells were determined. To determine the bioactivity, the growth-stimulating activity of the rhEGF was determined by the MTT calorimetric assay. The growth stimulating activity of the rhEGF containing liposmal formulations was compared to the rhEGF activity in the solution. The results of the bioactivity assay indicated that the growth activity of the rhEGF in solution was not significantly different from that of rhEGF encapsulated into the liposomal formulations. These results indicated that the rhEGF activity is maintained and the growth factor is stable in the liposomal formulations. In order to measure the permeability of the rhEGF liposomal formulations, the rhEGF solution or liposomes (0.5 ml) were added to the apical side of the Caco-2 cell monolayer, and the incubation medium (1.5 ml) were added to the basolateral side of the monolayer. The monolayers were incubated for a specific period of time at 37°C, and the samples withdrawn from the basolateral side were subjected to quantitative analysis by ELISA in order to determine the concentration of the rhEGF. It was reported that the flux of rhEGF in the PC liposome was not significantly different from the flux of rhEGF in solution. Interestingly, the flux of rhEGF in DPPC liposomes was three times greater than that the flux of rhEGF in solution. This suggested that DPPC liposomes could be used for the improvement of rhEGF transport.

Animal studies were conducted in male Sprague–Dawley (SD) rats. The studies were conducted to determine plasma and gastric ulcer healing effect after oral administration of rhEGF contained in liposomal formulations and solution. The pharmacokinetic parameters such as C_{max}, T_{max}, and AUC_{0-120} clearly indicated that the liposomal formulations were better than the solution. In particular, rhEGF delivered via DPPC-PEG liposomes showed the highest bioavailability than PC-PEG liposomes and the solution. A 2.5-fold increase in the rhEGF bioavailability was observed when DPPC-PEG liposomal formulation was compared to the solution. In comparison, a 1.7-fold increase in the bioavailability of the rhEGF was observed when delivered via PC-liposomes as compared to the solution of rhEGF, upon oral administration. Additionally it was observed that the plasma concentration of rhEGF delivered by liposomal formulations exhibited a double peak after oral administration. It was explained that a plausible reason for such a phenomenon could be the effect of PEG modification on the liposomes. The surface modification must have resulted in delayed gastric emptying. From a therapeutic perspective, the liposomal formulations were also compared to the solution of rhEGF. Toward this end the group decided to conduct a gastric ulcer healing test. Acute gastric ulcer was introduced into the stomach of the male rats by oral administration of ethanol (1 ml). The rats in the control group were given an oral solution of the rhEGF using 400 µg/Kg of the liposomal formulations, and the rats with no treatment were labeled as the normal group. In order to evaluate the degree of gastric mucosal injury, the length of the ulcerated mucosa was measured and the curative ratio was determined. The decline in the ulcer length of the PC-PEG and DPPC-PEG liposomes was 1.3- and 2.5-fold faster in comparison to the solution, respectively, indicating that PC-PEG and DPPC-PEG liposomes were effective in treating acute gastric ulcer.

Last, Zhang et al. [120] studied the design and characterization of the lectin-modified liposomes for the oral delivery of peptide or protein drugs. Lectins are advantageous from the oral delivery perspective as most cell surface proteins and many lipids in the cell membranes of the GI tract are glycosylated, and these glycans act as binding sites for various lectins. Additionally lectins are known to resist acidic pH and enzymatic degradation and can be useful in maintaining stability of the liposomes. Toward this end three types of lectins: wheat germ agglutin (WGA) tomato lectin (TL), and Ulex europaeus agglutin 1 (UEA1) were employed for surface modification of the liposomes. The lectins were first conjugated to N-glutaryl-phosphatidylethanolamine (N-glut-PE) by coupling their amino groups to the carbodoiimide-activated carboxylic groups of the N-glut-PE in a two-step process. The insulin liposomes were prepared by reverse-phase evaporation method, followed by modification with lectin-N-glut-PE conjugates. The particle sizes of the WGA-, TL-, and UEA1-modified insulin liposomes were on average 192 nm. The corresponding drug loading efficiencies were found to be 70% for WGA-, 82.5% for TL-, and 40% for UEA1-modified liposomes. The in vivo studies were conducted on diabetic mice and Sprague–Dawley rats to evaluate the ability of the lectin-modified liposomes in inducing a hypoglycemic effect in both the animal models. It was mentioned that the minimum blood glucose level achieved by the WGA-modified liposomes was 35.4% of the initial blood glucose level in the diabetic mice. The relative pharmacological bioavailabilities of the insulin-loaded liposomes modified with WGA, TL, and UEA1 were 21.40, 15.3%, and 8.9%, respectively. The lectin-modified liposomes were superior to the unmodified liposomes as there was no observable hypoglycemic effect with the oral administration of insulin in unmodified liposomes. In comparison to the subcutaneous injection of the insulin, the relative bioavailability of the WGA-, TL-, and UEA1- modified insulin liposomes in the SD rats were found to be 9.12%, 7.89% and 5.37%, respectively. No significant hypoglycemic effect was observed with the unmodified insulin liposomes.

Apart from the surface modification, other approaches such as pro-liposomes and double liposomes have also been employed to improve the stability of the liposomes in the GI tract. The physiochemical instability of the liposomes in the GI tract is related to the problems such as aggregation, sedimentation, fusion, hydrolysis, and/or oxidation of phospholipids [117]. Techniques such as freeze drying, freezing, and thawing, and chemical polymerization of the liposomes have been employed to overcome these formulation-related challenges. The modifications also have their own drawbacks, since the resulting liposomal formulation can suffer from leakage of the encapsulated drug after re-constitution, oxidation of the drug even in the frozen state, and incomplete polymerization [117].

A pro-liposome is defined as dry, free-flowing particles that spontaneously result in a liposomal formulation upon dispersion into an aqueous medium. In order to protect the pro-liposomes from the harsh environment of the stomach, it has been proposed to encapsulate the dry pro-liposomal formulation into capsules and tablets. In general, pro-liposomes are prepared by penetrating a solution of the drugs and phospholipids in volatile organic solvents into the microporous matrix of the water-soluble carrier particles, followed by the evaporation of the organic solvents [117]. Shah et al. [121] studied the effectiveness of the pro-liposomal formulation for oral delivery of cyclosporine. The pro-liposomes were prepared by spraying a solution of cyclosporine, egg lecithin, and Cremophor EL® in methanol-chloroform mixture onto directly compressible lactose (carrier) in a rotary evaporator. After obtaining a dry, free-flowing proliposomal formulation, the formulation was dispersed in distilled water to form liposomes. The drug-loading efficiency of the resulting liposomal formulation was reported to be about 99%. Also the drug–lipid ratio was considered a significant factor in achieving high drug entrapment efficiency. The in vivo studies were conducted in the male SD rats.

The bioavailability studies were conducted for free drug (cyclosporine) suspension, pro-liposomes derived liposomes, and marketed formulation (Pannium Bioral® microemulsion). The results of the bioavailability studies indicated that the difference in the mean drug concentration of the free drug solution and the pro-liposomal derived formulation was statistically significant ($p < 0.05$, p-value $= 0.032$). Additionally the absorption constant of the liposomal preparation ($k_a = 10.26\,h^{-1}$) was found to be greater than the absorption constants of free drug solution ($k_a = 1.2\,h^{-1}$) and the marketed formulation ($k_a = 2.51\,h^{-1}$). The volume of distribution of the drug was found to be less for the proliposomal derived liposomal formulation ($V_d = 7629.88\,ml/Kg$) than the free drug solution ($V_d = 10{,}971.92\,ml/Kg$) and marketed formulation ($V_d = 9012.07\,ml/Kg$). The study concluded that the pro-liposomal formulation is a stable formulation that can be used to enhance the oral bioavailability of the drugs such as cyclosporine.

Ogue et al. [122] investigated the potential of double liposomes as an oral vaccine carrier. Oral vaccination is desirable for eliciting both mucosal and systemic immune response and is also advantageous from patient compliance point of view. However, the oral vaccination suffers from antigen degradation in gastric pH and hydrolytic enzymes present within the digestive system. As mentioned before, liposomes suffer from the same problem but are desirable for their strong interaction with the macrophages. Thus use of double liposomes is desirable in this scenario. Double liposomes can be defined as liposomes containing small liposomes. It is believed that double liposomes will shield the inner liposomes from degradation within the GI tract until they reach the lower intestine, where the inner liposomes will be eventually be taken up by the M cells. The outer liposomes will be eventually degraded in the process. Three different methods for the preparation of the double liposomes have been mentioned in the literature. These methods are glass bead, glass filtration, and reverse-phase evaporation. In one study the inner liposomes containing the drug ovalbumin (OVA) were prepared by glass bead method, followed by sonication and extrusion. The double liposomes were prepared by both glass bead and reverse-phase evaporation method. The inner liposomes comprised of a mixture of Soy PC/DPPC/cholestrol/sterylamine in a ratio of 7:7:5:4. The outer liposomes comprised of a mixture of DMPC and DMPG at a molar ratio of 10:1. It is also worth mentioning here that the phase transition temperature of the lipids forming the single, inner liposome should be higher than that of lipids forming the outer layer of the double liposomes. The average particle size of the inner liposomes was found to be 236 nm. The drug encapsulation efficiency of the inner liposomes was reported to be 28.8%. The particle size and double-liposome forming efficiency via the glass bead method were reported to be within the range of 1 to 10 μm and 85.1%, respectively. Similarly the particle size and double-liposome forming efficiency via the reverse-phase evaporation method was reported to be in the range of 1 to 5 μm and 94%, respectively. The in vitro studies were conducted to determine the release and the stability of the double-liposomes. Additionally the release and stability profiles of the double liposomes were compared to that of single, inner liposomes. The release and stability of the OVA within the two-model liposomal formulations were carried out with a pepsin solution. From the results it was evident that the OVA release from the double liposomes was significantly less than the release of the OVA from the single liposomes. However, a large amount of OVA was degraded in the stability study. The group mentioned that the presence of lysine in the buffer solution may have had an adverse effect on the lipid bilayer and would have caused destabilization of the lipid bilayers. Also the double liposomes prepared by reverse-phase evaporation method were more effective than double liposomes prepared by glass bead method in suppressing the release of OVA. The in vivo studies were conducted on the female Balb/C mice. The mice were immunized with OVA solution, OVA in single liposomes, and OVA in double liposomes. It was concluded from the in vivo studies that the antibody responses elicited by the oral administration of the OVA in single and double liposomes was higher than that of solution. In particular, double liposomes were most effective in eliciting an antibody response than any other preparation [122].

10.5 TOXICOLOGY AND REGULATORY ISSUES

For any new pharmaceutical, biotechnology product or technology to be tried in the clinic and launched into the market for use in patients, it is necessary to first get approval from the United States Food and Drug Adminstration (US-FDA), which is the major governing/regulatory office. As with other emerging and enabling technologies, nanotechnology poses new questions regarding the adequacy and application of regulatory authorities. To meet the demands and challenges posed by advancements in nanotechnology, the US-FDA has taken parallel measures to enable the continued development of innovative, safe, and effective products that use such nanoscale materials.

Nanotechnology is currently being evaluated under FDA's Critical Path Initiative to keep up with the pace of developments in the pharmaceutical and biotechnology industry. The Nanotechnology Task Force set up by US-FDA in August 2006 submitted a report in July 2007 offering the Task Force's initial findings and recommendations. The report included a synopsis of the state of the science for biological interactions of nanoscale materials, analysis, and recommendations for scientific issues and analysis and recommendations for regulatory policies [123]. To get approval for a nanoparticle-based drug delivery system, the industry has to address the following:

10.5.1 Safety

The nano formulations should be evaluated with respect to toxicological screening, including pharmacology, clinical, and histopathological analysis, with parameters such as absorption, disposition, metabolism, excretion (ADME) in detail, genotoxicity, developmental toxicity, irritation studies, immunotoxicology, and carcinogenicity. The a reduction in the particle size could result in a change in size-specific effects on biological activity of the system [124]. Hence an attempt should be made to address the following issues:

- Investigate in detail the pharmacokinetics and disposition of nanotechnology-based drug delivery systems.
- Investigate biological effects of nanoparticles on cellular and tissue functions.
- Establish ADME profiles for different size of particles, and investigate differences in these parameters for different sized particles.
- Identify potential in vitro/in vivo risks by use of preclinical screening tests.
- Identify potential toxicity issues related to use of nanotechnology-based drug delivery systems with the aid of proteomics and genomics to complement current testing requirements.
- Establish the disposition profile of the nanoparticle in the systemic circulation and also biological (tissue and cellular) effects of these particles if the nanoparticles are able gain access to the systemic circulation from the route of exposure.
- Evaluate the testing methods for different product types to determine whether or how they can be used in assessing the bioavailability of nanoscale materials in humans.

10.5.2 Material Quality and Characterization

As new toxicological risks that derive from novel materials and delivery systems are identified, new tests will be required to ascertain safety and efficacy. Industry and academe need to plan and conduct the research to identify potential risks and to develop adequate characterization methodologies.

- Investigate the effect of the forms in which particles are presented to host, tissues, organs, organelles, and cells.
- Investigate and establish critical physical and chemical properties, including residual solvents, processing variables, impurities, and excipients.
- Design and establish standard tools used for this characterization.
- Design and/or establish validated assays to detect and quantify nanoparticles in tissues, medical products, foods, and processing equipment.
- Establish methodology and experiments to determine long- and short-term stability of nanomaterials.

10.5.3 Environmental Considerations

Along with the investigation of safety of nanotechnology-based drug delivery systems, the environmental impact of such systems is important. This issue requires due consideration when working with this new technology.

- Determine the impact of nanoparticles upon release into the environment following human and animal use.
- Establish methodologies that can identify the nature, and quantify the extent, of nanoparticle release in the environment.
- Investigate the environmental impact on other species (animals, fish, plants, microorganisms).

As the materials and the techniques used to manufacture the novel formulations may not have prior art to refer to (as a standard), there is an additional burden on the pharmaceutical and biotechnology industry to carry out a detailed evaluation of the system to generate a sufficient database for successful industrialization of the product. Some of the industrially relevant criteria include understanding the relationship between the physicochemical properties and product performance, the effect of process and formulation variables on product characteristics, the development of analytical tools and specifications to regulate product quality, accelerated stability testing as per standard protocols to propose a reliable shelf-life, product scale-up to mass production and establishment of manufacturing standards, and development of reference materials/standards as guidelines for quality assurance. Development of validated testing methods/protocols and establishment of reference standards through a thorough and logical process remains the major responsibility of the industry for getting FDA product approval.

10.6 CONCLUSION AND FUTURE OUTLOOK

Industry and academe are witnessing the developments of nanotechnology-based systems to improve drug delivery and are aided to some extent by the private sector as well as the National Institutes of Health and the US-FDA. From the great volume of effort in this field, it is evident that we will be seeing many nanotechnology-based pharmaceutical products in the future. Already a few of nanotechnology-based systems have been launched onto the market and are experiencing great success over their conventional adversaries. For example, Elan's Nanocrystal® Technology has improved the biological performance of many different drugs and has resulted in the products (Rapammune® by Wyeth, Emend® by Merck, TriCor® by Fourier, and Abbott and Megace® by Par) that are today available on the market [124]. Altogether these four products are generating more than $1 billion in revenue. The early market success of nanotechnology-based systems draws attention to the fact that they have the potential to become a market leader in the future. The indications is that the oral formulations will dominate this specialized segment of dosage forms. The chemical/polymer industry has been feeding the drug delivery scientists with a variety of biopolymers having wide range of specialized properties. Nanoparticles made from the biopolymers are likely to dominate the novel drug delivery systems in the oral market because of the cost–benefit ratio, excellent stability, flexibility for industrial production, and the large database available with respect to the regulatory issues addressed earlier. Nanotechnology-based drug delivery system can be potentially combined with tablets, capsules, liquid/dry powders for oral suspension, and soft gelatin formulations [125–127].

The science of pharmaceutical product development is undergoing a transformation from traditional pharmaceutics to a more innovative molecular or nanopharmaceutics. This development is being aided by the US-FDA, which is taking parallel measures to provide continued guidance for the successful development of nanotechnology. The combination of industrial efforts, regulatory guidance, and the cutting-edge research of academe that is being pursued for nanotechnology-based drug delivery systems will provide the future direction for this exciting new technology with potential to improve drug performance as well as the quality of life.

REFERENCES

1. Zhang L, Gu F, Chan J, Wang A, Langer RS, Farokhzad O. Nanoparticles in medicine: Therapeutic applications and developments. *Clin Pharmacol Therapeut* 2007; doi: 10.1038/sj.clpt.6100400.

2. NIH Road map. http://nihroadmap.nih.gov/nanomedicine/index.asp

3. Nanoenabled Drug Delivery Systems Markets. *Impact of nanotechnology in drug delivery: global developments, market analysis and future prospects*. Nanomarkets, December, 2004.

4. Ganong W. *Regulation of Gastrointestinal Function. Review of Medical Physiology*. Norwalk, CT: Appleton and Lange, 2003, p. 444–67.

5. McClintic JR. *The digestive system: basic anatomy and physiology of the human body*. New York, John Wiley & Sons, Inc., 1980, p. 566–94.

6. Solomon E. *The digestive system: human anatomy and physiology*. Philadelphia: Saunders, 1992, pp. 209–28.

7. Tate P, Seeley R, Stephens T. *The digestive system: human body*. St. Louis: Mosby, p. 261–77.

8. Tortora G, Anagnostakos N. *Principles of anatomy and physiology*. New York: Harper and Row, 1978.

9. Wilson K, Waugh A. *The digestive system: anatomy and physiology system*. New York: Churchill Livingston, 1996, p. 279–335.

10. Collins LDC. The surface area of the adult human mouth and thickness of the salivary film covering the teeth and oral mucosa. *J Dent Res* 1987;66:1300–2.

11. Shojaei A. Buccal mucosa as a route for systemic drug delivery: a review. *J Pharm Pharmaceut Sci* 1998;1:15–30.

12. Zhang H, Zhang J, Streisand JB. Oral mucosal drug delivery: clinical pharmaco-kinetics and therapeutic applications. *Clin Pharmacokinet* 2002;41:661–80.

13. Harris D, Robinson J. Drug delivery via the mucous membranes of the oral cavity. *J Pharmaceut Sci* 1992;81:1–10.

14. Sakuma S, Hayashi M, Akashi M. Design of nanoparticles composed of graft copolymers for oral peptide delivery. *Adv Drug Deliv Rev* 2001;47:21–37.

15. Gandhi R, Robinson J. Oral cavity as a site for bioadhesive drug delivery. *Adv Drug Deliv Rev* 1994;13:43–74.

16. Florence AT. Particulate delivery: the challenge of the oral route. *Drugs Pharmaceut Sci* 1993;61:65–107.

17. Friend DR. Drug delivery to the small intestine. *Curr Gastroenterol Rep* 2004;6: 371–6.

18. Jung T, Kamm W, Breitenbach A, Kaiserling E, Xiao JX, Kissel T. Biodegradable nanoparticles for oral delivery of peptides: is there a role for polymers to affect mucosal uptake? *Eur J Pharm Biopharm* 2000;50:147–60.

19. Florence AH, Hillery A, Hussain N, Jani P. Nanoparticles as carriers for oral peptide absorption: studies on particle uptake and fate. *J Control Release* 1995;36:39–46.

20. Lamprecht A, Schafer U, Lehr CM. Size-dependent bioadhesion of micro- and nanoparticulate carriers to the inflamed colonic mucosa. *Pharm Res* 2001;18: 788–93.

21. Lamprecht A, Ubrich N, Yamamoto H, Schafer U, Takeuchi H, Maincent P, et al. Biodegradable nanoparticles for targeted drug delivery in treatment of inflammatory bowel disease. *J Pharmacol Exp Ther* 2001;299:775–81.

22. Rawat M, Singh D, Saraf S, Saraf S. Nanocarriers: promising vehicle for bioactive drugs. *Biol Pharmaceut Bull* 2006;29:1790–8.

23. Anne des Rieux, Fievez V, Garinot M, Schneider YJ, Préat V. Nanoparticles as potential oral delivery systems of proteins and vaccines: a mechanistic approach. *J Control Release* 2006;116:1–27.

24. Quintanar-Guerrero D, Allemann E, Fessi H, Doelker E. Preparation techniques and mechanisms of formation of biodegradable nanoparticles from preformed polymers. *Drug Dev Indust Pharm* 1998;24:1113–28.

25. Emerich DF, Thanos CG. The pinpoint promise of nanoparticle-based drug delivery and molecular diagnosis. *Biomol Eng* 2006;23:171–84.

26. Nahar M, Dutta T, Murugesan S, Asthana A, Mishra D, Rajkumar V, et al. Functional polymeric nanoparticles: an efficient and promising tool for active delivery of bioactives. *Crit Revi Therapeut Drug Carrier Sys* 2006;23:259–318.

27. Prabhu S, Ortega M, Ma C. Novel lipid-based formulations enhancing the in vitro dissolution and permeability characteristics of a poorly water-soluble model drug, piroxicam. *Int J Pharmaceut* 2005;301:209–16.

28. Porter CJ, Trevaskis NL, Charman WN. Lipids and lipid-based formulations: optimizing the oral delivery of lipophilic drugs. *Nat Rev* 2007;6:231–48.

29. Quintanar-Guerrero D, Alleman E, Fessi H, Doelker E. Preparation techniques and mechanisms of formation of biodegradable nanoparticles from preformed polymers. *Drug Dev Indust Pharm* 1998;24:1113–28.

30. Solaro R. *Nanostructured polymeric systems in targeted release of proteic drugs and in tissue engineering.* China-EU Forum on Nanosized Technology. Beijng: China-EU Forum, 2002. p. 225–44.

31. Panyam J, Labhasetwar V. Biodegradable nanoparticles for drug and gene delivery to cells and tissue. *Adv Drug Deliv Rev* 2003;55:329–47.

32. Alonso MJ. Polymeric nanoparticles: new systems for improving ocular bioavailability of drugs. *Arch Soc Esp Oftalmol* 2001;76:453–4.

33. Prego C, Garcia M, Torres D, Alonso MJ. Transmucosal macromolecular drug delivery. *J Control Release* 2005;101:151–62.

34. Shim J, Seok Kang H, Park WS, Han SH, Kim J, Chang IS. Transdermal delivery of mixnoxidil with block copolymer nanoparticles. *J Control Release* 2004;97: 477–84.

35. Videira MA, Botelho MF, Santos AC, Gouveia LF, De Lima JJ, Almeida AJ. Lymphatic uptake of pulmonary delivered radiolabelled solid lipid nanoparticles. *J Drug Target* 2002;10:607–13.

36. Vila A, Sanchez A, Evora C, Soriano I, Vila Jato JL, Alonso MJ. PEG-PLA nanoparticles as carriers for nasal vaccine delivery. *J Aerosol Med* 2004;17: 174–85.

37. Brannon-Peppas L. Polymers in controlled drug delivery. *Med Plast Biomat Mag* 1997;34. http://www.devicelink.com/mpb/archive/97/11/003.html

38. Majeti RK. Nano and microparticles as controlled drug delivery devices. *J Pharm Pharmaceut Sci* 2000;3:234–58.

39. Kashyap N, Modi S, Jain JP, Bala I, Hariharan S, R B, et al. Polymers for advanced drug delivery. *Current Research and Information on Pharmaceutical Science* 2004;5:7–12.

40. Pinto Reis C, Neufeld RJ, Ribeiro AJ, Veiga F. Nanoencapsulation I. Methods for preparation of drug-loaded polymeric nanoparticles. *Nanomedicine* 2006;2: 8–21.

41. Bhavsar MD, Amiji MM. Polyermic nano- and microparticle technologies for oral gene delivery. *Exp Opin Drug Deliv* 2007;4:197–213.

42. Soppimath KS, Aminabhavi TM, Kulkarni AR, Rudzinski WE. Biodegradable polymeric nanoparticles as drug delivery devices. *J Control Release* 2001;70: 1–20.

43. General S, Thunemann AF. pH-sensitive nanoparticles of poly(amino acid) dodecanoate complexes. *Int J Pharm* 2001;230:11–24.

44. Mansouri S, Lavigne P, Corsi K, Benderdour M, Beaumont E, Fernandes JC. Chitosan-DNA nanoparticles as non-viral vectors in gene therapy: strategies to improve transfection efficacy. *Eur J Pharm Biopharm* 2004;57:1–8.

45. Janes KA, Calvo P, Alonso MJ. Polysaccharide colloidal particles as delivery systems for macromolecules. *Adv Drug Deliv Rev* 2001;47:83–97.

46. Thunemann AF, General S. Nanoparticles of a polyelectrolyte-fatty acid complex: carriers for Q10 and triiodothyronine. *J Control Release* 2001;75:237–47.

47. Akiyoshi K, Kobayashi S, Shichibe S, Mix D, Baudys M, Kim SW, et al. Self-assembled hydrogel nanoparticle of cholesterol-bearing pullulan as a carrier of

protein drugs: complexation and stabilization of insulin. *J Control Release* 1998;54:313–20.

48. Sang Yoo H, Gwan Park T. Biodegradable nanoparticles containing protein-fatty acid complexes for oral delivery of salmon calcitonin. *J Pharm Sci* 2004;93: 488–95.

49. Du J, Zhang S, Sun R, Zhang LF, Xiong CD, Peng YX. Novel polyelectrolyte carboxymethyl konjac glucomannan-chitosan nanoparticles for drug delivery. II. Release of albumin in vitro. *J Biomed Mater Res B Appl Biomater* 2005;72: 299–304.

50. Bangham AD, Standish MM, Watkins JC. Diffusion of univalent ions across the lamellae of swollen phospholipids. *J Mol Biol* 1965;13:238–52.

51. Ulrich AS. Biophysical aspects of using liposomes as delivery vehicles. *Biosci Rep* 2002;22:129–50.

52. Szoka F Jr., Papahadjopoulos D. Comparative properties and methods of preparation of lipid vesicles (liposomes). *Ann Rev Biophys Bioeng* 1980;9:467–508.

53. Venkatesan N, Vyas SP. Polysaccharide coated liposomes for oral immunization—development and characterization. *Int J Pharmaceut* 2000;203:169–77.

54. Carafa M, Marianecci C, Annibaldi V, Di Stefano A, Sozio P, Santucci E. Novel O-palmitoylscleroglucan-coated liposomes as drug carriers: development, characterization and interaction with leuprolide. *Int J Pharmaceut* 2006;325:155–62.

55. Ponchel GI, J. Specific and non-specific bioadhesive particulate systems for oral delivery to the gastrointestinal tract. *Adv Drug Deliv Rev* 1998;34:191–219.

56. Florence AT. Issues in oral nanoparticle drug carrier uptake and targeting. *J Drug Target* 2004;12:65–70.

57. Florence AT. The oral absorption of micro- and nanoparticulates: neither exceptional nor unusual. *Pharm Res* 1997;14:259–66.

58. Win KY, Feng SS. Effects of particle size and surface coating on cellular uptake of polymeric nanoparticles for oral delivery of anticancer drugs. *Biomaterials* 2005;26:2713–22.

59. Jani P, Halbert GW, Langridge J, Florence AT. Nanoparticle uptake by the rat gastrointestinal mucosa: quantitation and particle size dependency. *J Pharm Pharmacol* 1990;42:821–6.

60. Araujo L, Sheppard M, Lobenber R, Kreuter J. Uptake of PMMA nanoparticles from the gastrointestinal tract after oral administration to rats: modification of the body distribution after suspension in surfactant solutions and in oil vehicles. *Int J Pharm* 1999;176:209–24.

61. Hejazi R, Amiji M. Stomach-specific anti-H. pylori therapy. I: Preparation and characterization of tetracyline-loaded chitosan microspheres. *Int J Pharm* 2002; 235:87–94.

62. Marshall BJ. Unidentified curved bacilli in gastric epithelium in active chronic gastritis. *Lancet* 1983;1:1273–5.

63. Marshall BJ, Warren JR. Unidentified curved bacilli in the stomach of patients with gastritis and peptic ulceration. *Lancet* 1984;1:1311–5.

64. Umamaheshwari RB, Ramteke S, Jain N. Anti-Helicobacter pylori effect of mucoadhesive nanoparticles bearing amoxicillin in experimental gerbils model. *AAPS PharmSciTech* 2004;5.

65. Pamujula S, Graves RA, Freeman T, Srinivasan V, Bostanian LA, Kishore V, et al. Oral delivery of spray dried PLGA/amifostine nanoparticles. *J Pharm Pharmacol* 2004;56:1119–25.

66. Sharma A, Sharma S, Khuller GK. Lectin-functionalized poly (lactide-co-glycolide) nanoparticles as oral/aerosolized antitubercular drug carriers for treatment of tuberculosis. *J Antimicrob Chemother* 2004;54:761–6.

67. Popescu C, Onyuksel H. Biodegradable nanoparticles incorporating highly hydrophilic positively charged drugs 2004. U.S. Patent 20040247683.

68. De Jaeghere F, Allemann E, Kubel F, Galli B, Cozens R, Doelker E, et al. Oral bioavailability of a poorly water soluble HIV-1 protease inhibitor incorporated into pH-sensitive particles: effect of the particle size and nutritional state. *J Control Release* 2000;68:291–8.

69. Lang M, Roesel J. HIV-1 protease inhibitors: development, status, and potential role in the treatment of AIDS. *Arch Pharm* 1993;326:921–4.

70. Robins T, Plattner J. HIV protease inhibitors: their anti-HIV activity and potential role in treatment. *J AIDS* 1993;6:162–70.

71. Allison MC, Cornwall S, Poulter LW, Dhillon AP, Pounder RE. Macrophage heterogeneity in normal colonic mucosa and in inflammatory bowel disease. *Gut* 1988;29:1531–8.

72. Seldenrijk CA, Drexhage HA, Meuwissen SG, Pals ST, Meijer CJ. Dendritic cells and scavenger macrophages in chronic inflammatory bowel disease. *Gut* 1989;30:484–91.

73. Probert CS, Chott A, Turner JR, Saubermann LJ, Stevens AC, Bodinaku K, et al. Persistent clonal expansions of peripheral blood CD4+ lymphocytes in chronic inflammatory bowel disease. *J Immunol* 1996;157:3183–91.

74. Tabata Y, Inoue Y, Ikada Y. Size effect on systemic and mucosal immune responses induced by oral administration of biodegradable microspheres. *Vaccine* 1996;14:1677–85.

75. Lamprecht A, Stallmach A, Kawashima Y, Lehr C. Carrier systems for the treatment of inflammatory bowel disease. *Drugs Future* 2002;27:961–71.

76. Zhang H, Alsarra IA, Neau SH. An in vitro evaluation of a chitosan-containing multiparticulate system for macromolecule delivery to the colon. *Int J Pharm* 2002;239:197–205.

77. Rodriguez M, Vila-Jato JL, Torres D. Design of a new multiparticulate system for potential site-specific and controlled drug delivery to the colonic region. *J Control Release* 1998;55:67–77.

78. Leung S, Robinson J. The contribution of anionic polymer structural features to mucoadhesion. *J Control Release* 1988;5:223–31.

79. Leung S, Robinson J. Polymer structure features contributing to mucoadhesion: II. *J Control Release* 1990;12:187–94.

80. Park K, Robinson J. Bioadhesive polymers as platforms for oral-controlled drug delivery: method to study bioadhesion. *Int J Pharm* 1984;19:107–27.

81. Hejazi R, Amiji M. Chitosan-based gastrointestinal delivery systems. *J Control Release* 2003;89:151–65.

82. Hejazi R, Amiji M. Stomach-specific anti-H. pylori therapy; part III: effect of chitosan microspheres crosslinking on the gastric residence and local tetracycline concentrations in fasted gerbils. *Int J Pharm* 2004;272:99–108.

83. Dai J, Nagai T, Wang X, Zhang T, Meng M, Zhang Q. pH-sensitive nanoparticles for improving the oral bioavailability of cyclosporine A. *Int J Pharm* 2004;280: 229–40.

84. Couvreur P, Lenaerts V, Kante B, Roland M, Speiser P. Oral and parenteral administration of insulin associated hydrolysable nanoparticles. *Acta Pharm Technol* 1980;26:220–2.

85. Delie F, Blanco-Prieto M. Polymeric particulates to improve oral bioavailability of peptide drugs. *Molecules* 2005;10:65–80.

86. Sakuma S, Suzuki N, Sudo R, Hiwatari K, Kishida A, Akashi M. Optimized chemical structure of nanoparticles as carriers for oral delivery of salmon calcitonin. *Int J Pharm* 2002;239:185–95.

87. Narayani R. Oral delivery of Insulin—making needles needless. *Trends Biomater Artif Organs* 2001;15:12–6.

88. Kreuter J. Nanoparticles and microparticles for drug and vaccine delivery. *J Anat* 1996;189 (Pt3):503–5.

89. Singh M, O'Hagan D. The preparation and characterization of polymeric antigen delivery systems for oral administration. *Adv Drug Deliv Rev* 1998;34:285–304.

90. Pan Y, Li YJ, Zhao HY, Zheng JM, Xu H, Wei G, et al. Bioadhesive polysaccharide in protein delivery system: chitosan nanoparticles improve the intestinal absorption of insulin in vivo. *Int J Pharm* 2002;249:139–47.

91. Damge C, Michel C, Aprahamian M, Couvreur P, Devissaguet J. Nanocapsules as carriers for oral peptide delivery. *J Control Release* 1990;13:233–9.

92. Ramtoola Z. Controlled release biodegradable nanoparticles containing insulin. 1997. U.S. Patent 5641515.

93. Agnihotri SA, Mallikarjuna NN, Aminabhavi TM. Recent advances on chitosan-based micro- and nanoparticles in drug delivery. *J Control Release* 2004; 100:5–28.

94. Foss AC, Goto T, Morishita M, Peppas NA. Development of acrylic-based copolymers for oral insulin delivery. *Eur J Pharm Biopharm* 2004;57:163–9.

95. Damge C, Maincent P, Ubrich N. Oral delivery of insulin associated to polymeric nanoparticles in diabetic rats. *J Control Release* 2007;117:163–70.

96. Chalasani KB, Russell-Jones GJ, Jain AK, Diwan PV, Jain SK. Effective oral delivery of insulin in animal models using vitamin B12-coated dextran nanoparticles. *J Control Release* 2007;122:141–50.

97. Cui F, Shi K, Zhang L, Tao A, Kawashima Y. Biodegradable nanoparticles loaded with insulin-phospholipid complex for oral delivery: preparation, in vitro characterization and in vivo evaluation. *J Control Release* 2006;114:242–50.

98. Cui FD, Tao AJ, Cun DM, Zhang LQ, Shi K. Preparation of insulin loaded PLGA-Hp55 nanoparticles for oral delivery. *J Pharm Sci* 2007;96:421–7.

99. Lee WK, Park JY, Yang EH, Suh H, Kim SH, Chung DS, et al. Investigation of the factors influencing the release rates of cyclosporin A-loaded micro- and nanoparticles prepared by high-pressure homogenizer. *J Control Release* 2002;84: 115–23.

100. Wang XQ, Dai JD, Chen Z, Zhang T, Xia GM, Nagai T, et al. Bioavailability and pharmacokinetics of cyclosporine A-loaded pH-sensitive nanoparticles for oral administration. *J Control Release* 2004;97:421–9.

101. Molpeceres J, Aberturas MR, Guzman M. Biodegradable nanoparticles as a delivery system for cyclosporine: preparation and characterization. *J Microencapsul* 2000;17:599–614.

102. Varela MC, Guzman M, Molpeceres J, del Rosario Aberturas M, Rodriguez-Puyol D, Rodriguez-Puyol M. Cyclosporine-loaded polycaprolactone nanoparticles: immunosuppression and nephrotoxicity in rats. *Eur J Pharm Sci* 2001;12: 471–8.

103. Cho M, Levy R, Pouletty P, Floc'h R, Merle C. Oral cyclosporin formulations. 1997. International Patent WO 97/07787.

104. Yoo H, Park T. Biodegradable nanoparticles containing protein-fatty acid complexes for oral delivery of salmon calcitonin. *J Pharmaceut Sci* 2004;93:488–95.

105. Jiao Y, Ubrich N, Marchand-Arvier M, Vigneron C, Hoffman M, Lecompte T, et al. In vitro and in vivo evaluation of oral heparin-loaded polymeric nanoparticles in rabbits. *Circulation* 2002;105:230–5.

106. Hoffart V, Lamprecht A, Maincent P, Lecompte T, Vigneron C, Ubrich N. Oral bioavailability of a low molecular weight heparin using a polymeric delivery system. *J Control Release* 2006;113:38–42.

107. Jung T, Kamm W, Breitenbach A, Hungerer KD, Hundt E, Kissel T. Tetanus toxoid loaded nanoparticles from sulfobutylated poly(vinyl alcohol)-graft-poly(lactide-co-glycolide): evaluation of antibody response after oral and nasal application in mice. *Pharm Res* 2001;18:352–60.

108. Bhavsar M, Amiji M. Gastrointestinal distribution and in vivo transfection studies with nanoparticles-in-microsphere oral system (NiMOS). *J Control Release* 2007;119:339–48.

109. Leong K, Okoli G, Hottelano G. Compositions for oral gene therapy and methods of using same. 2003. International Patent WO 03/02867 A2.

110. Roy K, Mao HQ, Huang SK, Leong KW. Oral gene delivery with chitosan—DNA nanoparticles generates immunologic protection in a murine model of peanut allergy. *Nat Med* 1999;5:387–91.

111. Chen J, Yang WL, Li G, Qian J, Xue JL, Fu SK, et al. Transfection of mEpo gene to intestinal epithelium in vivo mediated by oral delivery of chitosan-DNA nanoparticles. *World J Gastroenterol* 2004;10:112–6.

112. Kim SY, Doh HJ, Jang MH, Ha YJ, Chung SI, Park HJ. Oral immunization with *Helicobacter pylori*-loaded poly(D,L-lactide-co-glycolide) nanoparticles. *Helicobacter* 1999;4:33–9.

113. Donatella Paolino, Massimo Fresto, Piyush Sinha and Mauro Ferrari. *Drug Delivery Systems*, Encyclopedia of Medical Devices and Instrumentation, 2nd edition, ed. John 6. Webster, John Wiley & Sons, Inc., 2006, p. 437–95.

114. Singh RS, and L. J. W. Past, present, and future technologies for oral delivery of therapeutic proteins. *J Pharmaceut Sci* 2007;97:2397–523.

115. Unger EC, Porter T, Culp W, Labell R, Matsunaga T, Zutshi R. Therapeutic applications of lipid-coated microbubbles. *Adv Drug Deliv Rev* 2004;56: 1291–314.

116. Yamabe K, Kato Y, Onishi H, Machida Y. Potentiality of double liposomes containing salmon calcitonin as an oral dosage form. *J Control Release* 2003; 89:429–36.

117. Song KH, Chung SJ, Shim CK. Preparation and evaluation of proliposomes containing salmon calcitonin. *J Control Release* 2002;84:27–37.

118. Takeuchi H, Matsui Y, Sugihara H, Yamamoto H, Kawashima Y. Effectiveness of submicron-sized, chitosan-coated liposomes in oral administration of peptide drugs. *Int J Pharmaceut* 2005;303:160–70.

119. Li H, Song JH, Park JS, Han K. Polyethylene glycol-coated liposomes for oral delivery of recombinant human epidermal growth factor. *Int J Pharmaceut* 2003;258:11–9.

120. Zhang N, Ping QN, Huang GH, Xu WF. Investigation of lectin-modified insulin liposomes as carriers for oral administration. *Int J Pharmaceut* 2005;294:247–59.

121. Shah NM, Parikh J, Namdeo A, Subramanian N, Bhowmick S. Preparation, characterization and in vivo studies of proliposomes containing Cyclosporine A. *J Nanosci Nanotechnol* 2006;6:2967–73.

122. Ogue S, Takahashi Y, Onishi H, Machida Y. Preparation of double liposomes and their efficiency as an oral vaccine carrier. *Biol Pharmaceut Bull* 2006;29: 1223–8.

123. A report of U.S. Food and Drug Adminstration Nanotechnology Task Force. 2007.

124. http://www.elan.com/drugdelivery/drug_delivery/nanocrystal_technology.asp (Visited: 10/11/2007).

125. Bhavsar MD, Shenoy DB, Amiji MM. Polymeric nanoparticles for delivery in the gastro-intestinal tract. In: Torchilin VP, ed. *Nanoparticulates as drug carriers*. London: Imperial College Press, 2006. p. 609–48.

126. Murakami H, Kobayashi M, Takeuchi H, Kawashima Y. Utilization of poly(D,L-lactide-co-glycolide) nanaoparticles for preparation of mini depot tablets by deirct compression. *J Control Release* 2000;37:29–36.

127. Schmidt C, Bodmeier R. Incorporation of polymeric nanoparticles into solid dosage forms. *J Control Release* 1999;57:115–25.

128. Arangoa MA, Campanero MA, Renedo MJ, Ponchel G, Irache JM. Gliadin nanoparticles as carriers for the oral administration of lipophilic drugs: relationships between bioadhesion and pharmacokinetics. *Pharm Res* 2001;18: 1521–7.

129. Barichello JM, Morishita M, Takayama K, Nagai T. Encapsulation of hydrophilic and lipophilic drugs in PLGA nanoparticles by the nanoprecipitation method. *Drug Dev Indust Pharm* 1999;25:471–6.

130. Arbos P, Campanero MA, Arangoa MA, Renedo MJ, Irache JM. Influence of the surface characteristics of PVM/MA nanoparticles on their bioadhesive properties. *J Control Release* 2003;89:19–30.

131. Hillery A, Florence A. The effect of adsorbed poloxamer 188 and 407 surfactants on the intestinal uptake of 60-nm polystyrene particles after oral administration in the rats. *Int J Pharm* 1996;132:123–30.

132. Singh J, Pandit S, Bramwell VW, Alpar HO. Diphtheria toxoid loaded poly-(epsilon-caprolactone) nanoparticles as mucosal vaccine delivery systems. *Methods* 2006;38:96–105.

133. Tobio M, Sanchez A, Soriano V, Evora C, Vila-Jato J, Alonso M. The role of PEG on the stability in the digestive fluids and in vivo fate of PEG-PLA nanoparticles following oral administration. *Colloids Surf B: Biointerfaces* 2000;18: 315–23.

134. Sakuma S, Sudo R, Suzuki N, Kikuchi H, Akashi M, Ishida Y, et al. Behavior of mucoadhesive nanoparticles having hydrophilic polymeric chains in the intestine. *J Control Release* 2002;81:281–90.

135. Mesiha MS, Sidhom MB, Fasipe B. Oral and subcutaneous absorption of insulin poly(isobutylcyanoacrylate) nanoparticles. *Int J Pharm* 2005;288:289–93.

136. Aboubakar M, Couvreur P, Pinto-Alphandary H, Gouritin BLB, Farinotti R, Puisieux F, et al. Insulin-loaded nanocapsules for oral administration: in vitro and in vivo investigation. *Drug Dev Res* 2000;49:109–17.

137. Carino GP, Jacob JS, Mathiowitz E. Nanosphere based oral insulin delivery. *J Control Release* 2000;65:261–9.

138. El-Shabouri MH. Positively charged nanoparticles for improving the oral bioavailability of cyclosporin-A. *Int J Pharm* 2002;249:101–8.

139. Ubrich N, Schmidt C, Bodmeier R, Hoffman M, Maincent P. Oral evaluation in rabbits of cyclosporin-loaded Eudragit RS or RL nanoparticles. *Int J Pharm* 2005;288:169–75.

140. Dawson M, Krauland E, Wirtz D, Hanes J. Transport of polymeric nanoparticle gene carriers in gastric mucus. *Biotechnol Prog* 2004;20:851–7.

141. Chang SF, Chang HY, Tong YC, Chen SH, Hsaio FC, Lu SC, et al. Nonionic polymeric micelles for oral gene delivery in vivo. *Hum Gene Ther* 2004;15: 481–93.

11

FUNCTIONAL GLYCOMICS AND THE FUTURE OF GLYCOMIC DRUGS

Ram Sasisekharan and Karthik Viswanathan

Contents

11.1 INTRODUCTION

Glycomics is broadly defined as the study of the glycome, which comprises of all the oligosaccharide constituents of a biological system. The glycome includes sugars present in organisms either in a free form or as a conjugate with other biomolecules such as proteins or lipids. Glycomics includes functional characterization of the oligosaccharides present and a comprehensive understanding of their role in the cell physiology via their interactions with proteins. In this postgenomic and postproteomic era, glycomics is often looked upon to explain the complexity of biological systems.

Drug Efficacy, Safety, and Biologics Discovery: Emerging Technologies and Tools,
Edited by Sean Ekins and Jinghai J. Xu
Copyright © 2009 by John Wiley & Sons, Inc.

Most proteins in eukaryotes are modified by posttranslational modification, chief among which is glycosylation. Glycosylation refers to the modification of a protein by the attachment of an oligosaccharide. Protein glycosylation can be classified as either N-linked or O-linked based on the linkage with which the oligosaccharide is attached to the protein [1,2]. In N-linked glycosylation, the glycan moiety is N-glycosidically linked to an asparagine residue on a protein within the consensus sequence Asn-X-Ser/Thr [3]. This posttranslational modification occurs in the secretory pathway and starts with the en bloc transfer of an oligosaccharide to the protein in the endoplasmic reticulum (ER) followed by further processing in the ER and Golgi. O-linked glycosylation involves attachment of an oligosaccharide to a serine or threonine amino acid of a protein [4]. O-linked glycosylation is typically co-translational. These N- and O-linked glycans are branched in nature. Glycosaminoglycans (GAGs) are a class of glycans ubiquitously present on the cell surface and on the cell-extracellular matrix (ECM) interface. These GAGs are polymeric chains of sulfated disaccharide repeat units of a uronic acid linked to a hexosamine [5]. They are predominantly linear in structure and are present either as free polysaccharides or as part of a proteoglycan conjugate. GAGs can be divided into four different classes based on their backbone chemical structure. They are heparan sulfate glycosaminoglycans (HSGAG), chondroitin and dermatan sulfate glycosaminoglycans (CSGAG), keratan sulfate and hyaluronic acid. HSGAGs and CSGAGs are O-linked to proteoglycans and keratan sulfates can be N- on O-linked to the protein. Hyaluronic acid, on the other hand, is present in a free form and not conjugated to a protein [5].

Protein glycosylation has an intracellular and an extracellular role. The intracellular role of the glycosylation includes facilitating the protein folding, sorting and trafficking of glycoproteins to the appropriate cellular compartment [6–9]. Glycans, present as a conjugate on secreted glycoproteins affect their stability, solubility, antigenicity, clearance rate, half-life, and in vivo activity [10,11]. Other than modulating the properties of the lipids and proteins that it is conjugated to, glycans have other important roles in the biological system. Owing to its extensive presence on the cell surface, GAGs along with cell surface glycoproteins interact with a variety of other biological molecules such as cytokines, growth factors, immune receptors, and extracellular enzymes. They are thus involved in anticoagulation [12–14], cell growth and development [15–19], cell signaling and cell–cell interactions [20,21], immune recognition [22–26], host–pathogenesis interactions [27–31], and angiogenesis and tumor growth [32–35].

Despite the critical role that glycans play in diverse biological processes, glycomics has not advanced as much as genomics and proteomics. This is because the study of glycans faces a few fundamental and unique challenges. First, unlike DNA and proteins, the biosynthesis of glycans is a nontemplate-driven process, and its synthesis is governed by a network of enzymes such as glycosyltransferases and glycosidases. This is further complicated by the fact that many of these enzymes are cell-specific and their expression is developmentally regulated [1,2,5,15,36]. The involvement of simultaneous action of multiple enzymes for its biosynthesis makes glycan structures difficult to control by genetic manipulations. Also the synthesis lacks any proofreading mechanism leading to heterogeneity in the glycan structure. Second, these chemically heterogeneous glycan structures are often branched as opposed to DNA and protein structures, which are linear.

The third challenge in the advancement of glycomics has been the lack of availability of enough material. Until recently there were no chemical or chemoenzymatic approaches available to synthesize glycans for study, and researchers have largely depended on material extracted from biological sources that are highly heterogenic and difficult to purify. Fourth, these glycan-protein interactions are multivalent in nature and involve the glycans making multiple contacts with the protein [20,37]. Capturing these avidity effects is often difficult and the correct presentation of glycans becomes critical.

Technological advances in the recent years have helped glycomics research overcome the aforementioned challenges. Two major areas of development have been the use of analytical tools to characterize glycans and chemical and chemoenzymatic techniques for the synthesis of glycans. Glycans and their glycoconjugates have been analyzed using a variety of techniques. These include mass spectrometric (MS) [38–40], capillary electrophoretic (CE) [41,42], high-performance liquid chromatography (HPLC) [43,44], and nuclear magnetic resonance NMR techniques. Among MS techniques the most widely used for glycan characterization are MALDI-MS [45–48] and ESI-MS [49–51]. Each of these techniques has its own limitations and is sometimes not sufficient for complete characterization of glycans as this involves identification of the monosaccharides present, the substitutions on these monosaccharides, and the linkages between the monosaccharides. Glycan identification is further complicated by the presence of isomers among the monosaccharides and the presence of multiple monosaccharide units linked to a single monosaccharide. The need to completely characterize these complex glycans has led to integration of different techniques that combine aspects of separation and analytical measurements. Examples of integration of technologies for complete glycan analysis include capillary liquid chromatography (LC)-MS [52,53], CE-MS [54,55], and LC-NMR [56] techniques. Bioinformatics platforms have successfully enabled the integration of the diverse data from these different techniques [57,58].

The development of novel techniques to synthesize complex glycans has provided a platform for furthering glycomics research. The synthesis of glycans poses unique challenges owing to their branched structure and the presence of monosaccharides in different linkages [59]. Despite these challenges several strategies have been developed over the years for glycan synthesis. These range from purely chemical synthesis to a combination of enzymatic and chemical means for glycan synthesis. Chemical synthesis requires careful choice of hydrogen bond donors, hydrogen bond acceptors, protecting groups, catalysts, and reaction conditions to maintain correct regiochemistry and stereochemistry of the specific linkages [60]. Different chemical synthesis approaches range from traditional solid-phase synthesis [61–64] to a more efficient "one-pot" oligosaccharide synthesis [65]. An alternative to chemical synthesis has been the use of the chemoenzymatic approach. The use of enzymes enables carrying out the glycan synthesis under milder conditions and provides stereo- and regioselectively. Two classes of enzymes are used in glycan synthesis: glycosyltransferases, which add monosaccharides, and glycosidases, which cleave individual monosaccharides from the oligosaccharide chain. An instrument known as the Golgi apparatus has recently been developed to automate the enzymatic reactions of the glycans synthesis [66].

Developments such as these have not only aided glycan analysis [67,68] but also provided a platform to study the interaction of glycans with its binding partners. A major advancement on this front has been the development of glycan arrays. The earliest glycan arrays depended on glycans isolated from natural sources that could not be easily modified [69,70]. In the recent past glycan synthesis methods have been used to synthesize a variety of glycans present on the cell surface [71]. These glycans have been modified with linkers and covalently linked and presented on a variety of surfaces [72–75]. The DNA printing technology has been adapted to print small quantities of a variety of glycans on a surface [76,77]. These glycan arrays have been used to study diverse biological samples such as animal and plant lectins, growth factors, antibodies, serum samples, pathogenic surface proteins, and even whole cells and pathogens [77–79]. Such analyses have led to discovery of new glycan-binding partners and more recently has been used to get a quantitative understanding of the protein–glycan interactions [80].

The field of glycomics has been enriched by advances on the genomics and proteomics fronts. With specially designed "glyco-gene chips" the expression profile of genes relevant to glycan metabolism and glycan-binding partners can be studied [81–83]. These analyses have led to a better understanding of the role of glycans in different biological process and diseases such as cancer. Also the information provided from the glyco-gene microarrays on the simultaneous expression of the glycan biosynthetic enzymes can be correlated with the glycan structures present in the sample. In addition the ability to create transgenic mice with knockouts of specific glycan biosynthesis enzymes has helped further elucidate the biological role of glycans in the context of cellular and whole-organism phenotype. Knockouts of enzymes such as GlcNAc and GalNAc transferases that are involved in the early stages of glycan synthesis show severe abnormalities in their phenotype including embryonic lethality [15]. Transgenic mice containing a knockout of enzymes involved in the later stages of glycan synthesis such as sialyl and fucosyl transferases have provided insight into how the glycan structure mediates cellular function [84–86].

The different methodologies discussed above provide orthogonal data sets. To unravel the role of glycans in biological processes, there needs to be an integration of these data sets (Figure 11.1). Initiatives such as Consortium of

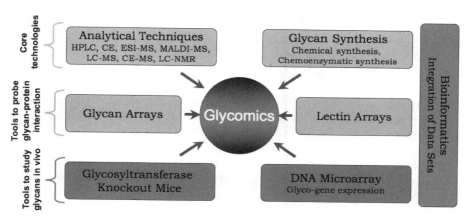

Figure 11.1 Tools and technologies used in glycomics research. (See color insert.)

TABLE 11.1 Examples of Glycan-based Therapeutics

Therapeutic Agent	Clinical Status	Manufacturer
Aransep	Market	Amgen
Cerezyme	Market	Genzyme
Lovenox	Market	Sanofi-aventis
Fragmin	Market	Pfizer
Sepragel	Market	Genzyme
Healon	Market	Pfizer
Precose	Market	Bayer
Aldurazyme	Market	Genzyme
PI-88	Phase II/III	Progen
GCS-100	Phase II	Prospect therapeutics

Functional Glycomics (CFG) and others have established bioinformatics plat-forms to collect, store, and integrate the diverse data sets and disseminate information in a meaningful fashion [87–89].

These advances in our understanding of the biological role of glycans and how they impinge on the various cellular processes have increased our ability to harness them to provide better therapeutics. Over the past few years gly-comics has come to the forefront with many glycan-based therapeutics in various stages of development (Table 11.1). In this chapter we review the role of glycans in drug development and recent advances in glycan-based thera-peutics. The role of glycans in drug development can be classified into (1) glycoprotein therapeutics, (2) unconjugated glycans as therapeutics, and (3) glycans as therapeutic targets. The role of glycans in biomarker discovery is also discussed.

11.2   GLYCOPROTEIN THERAPEUTICS

Many of the drugs on the market or in clinical trials are proteins [90]. Currently there are more than 130 peptides and proteins that are approved [91]. This growing class of protein-based therapeutics includes antibodies, enzymes, cytokines, growth factors, blood clotting factors, and human growth hormones used for treatment of diabetes, anemia, cancer, hepatitis, cardiovascular, and neurological diseases. More than 70% of these therapeutics are glycoproteins and are thus modified by N-linked or O-linked glycosylation [92]. Nevertheless, traditionally little attention has been paid to the glycan component of these glycoproteins. This is in large part due to lack of the technologies to study the role of glycans on these glycoproteins. The lack of homogeneity in the glycans has further confounded our understanding. The technology advances described earlier have facilitated understanding of the role of the glycans in therapeutic glycoproteins. As previously mentioned, the glycan affects the structure, function, stability, and solubility of the protein. In addition, when present as part of a protein therapeutic, the glycan plays a significant role in the therapeutic efficacy of the protein.

Most important, glycosylation affects the pharmacokinetic (PK) behavior of the protein therapeutic. The attached glycans contribute to the mass, charge, and hydrodynamic volume of the protein. In erythropoietin (EPO) the three N-linked glycans contribute upto 40% of the molecular mass [93]. In an experiment with deglycosylated EPO, the absence of glycosylation resulted in no in vivo activity despite having a three-fold increased in vitro activity [94]. Not only the presence but also the nature of glycan attached influence the PK properties. The presence of the negatively charged monosaccharide sialic acid contributes toward the net negative charge of the protein, thereby affecting its PK properties. In the case of erythropoietin, this negative charge improves the in vivo circulating half-life of the protein [95]. Research indicated EPO with tetraantennary sialylated glycans has the greatest potency [96]. In the case of some proteins, the absence of sialic acid from the terminal position results in their being cleared by asialoglycoprotein receptors (ASGPR) present in the liver [97,98]. Also the presence of mannose or GlcNAc at the terminal position causes receptor mediated in vivo clearance of the protein in the reticuloendothelial system [99,100].

Therapeutic glycoproteins are typically produced in recombinant host cell systems. Analyses of glycoproteins thus produced show significant glycan heterogeneity. The heterogeneity is both in the presence or absence of glycans at different glycosylation sites (macroheterogeneity) and in the type of monosaccharides constituting the glycan (microheterogeneity) [1,101]. Macroheterogeneity is caused by a limitation in the availability of dolichol-linked oligosaccharide or by the kinetics of the oligosaccharyltransferase reaction. Microheterogeneity, on the other hand, results from the availability of monosaccharides and the kinetics of processing reactions that take place primarily in the Golgi apparatus. These heterogeneities in glycosylation impede the

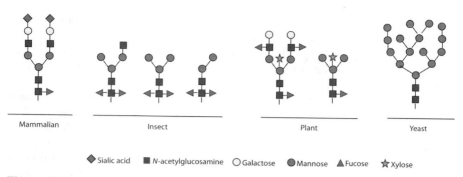

Mammalian Insect Plant Yeast

◆ Sialic acid ■ *N*-acetylglucosamine ○ Galactose ● Mannose ▲ Fucose ☆ Xylose

Figure 11.2 Typical structures of *N*-glycans present on recombinant proteins produced in mammalian, insect, plant, and yeast cell systems. (See color insert.)

development of therapeutic glycoproteins with consistent PK properties [101].

In a manufacturing process the variability in glycosylation is influenced by two major factors: the choice of host cell system (Figure 11.2) used to produce the therapeutic and environmental factors such as cell culture conditions [102–105]. The choice of cell line used is critical, and traditionally recombinant glycoproteins have been synthesized in mammalian cell lines. Mammalian cell lines are capable of carrying out the different posttranslational modifications required for proper expression of the protein and most importantly these cell lines come closest to mimicking human glycosylation. However, even mammalian cell lines such as CHO, BHK, and NS0 do not produce glycoforms identical to those present on human proteins. CHO and BHK typically are unable to produce certain glycan structures found in humans [106], and NS0 is capable of producing potentially immunogenic structures [107]. A major limitation of using mammalian cell lines as a host for producing recombinant proteins is that these cells lines are sensitive to the culture's environment, and the *N*-glycosylation of the recombinant protein produced is affected by fluctuations in pH, changes in the glutamine level, and the availability of nucleotide sugars or their precursors [102–105]. Also, when recombinant proteins are produced with a strong promoter, the glycosylational machinery of the cells is sometimes unable to keep up with the protein synthesis rate. This results in macroheterogeneity with site-occupancy variants.

Different approaches have been taken to overcome these variations in glycosylation of therapeutic proteins. One such approach is to engineer mammalian cell lines such as CHO to overexpress glycosyltransferases. Jenkins et al. [108] engineered sialyltransferase in CHO cells, which led to an improvement in sialylation of expressed interferon gamma without any adverse effect on the cells. In another study Weikert et al. [109] co-expressed galactosyltransferase and sialyltransferase in CHO cells, which led to a more homogeneous glycosylation of the protein. *N*-acetylglucosaminyltransferase III has also been overexpressed in CHO cells to increase the fraction of recombinant protein expressed containing bisecting *N*-acetylglucosamine [109,110]. These efforts not only led to a more uniform glycosylation pattern on the glycoprotein but also modified the pattern of glycosylation to predominantly express the specific desired glycoforms.

Alternative host systems such as yeast, insect, and plant cell lines have been used to produce glycoproteins. These cell lines often produce a high yield of recombinant proteins, but the glycan on these proteins are distinct from those found in humans. Insect cell lines such as Sf9 and *T. ni* generate oligosaccharides that are paucimannosidic, high mannose, or hybrid glycans terminating in *N*-acetylglucosamine [111,112]. Advances in our understanding of glycan-processing pathways combined with improvement in genetic engineering techniques has enabled the creation of engineered cell lines expressing heterologous *N*-glycan-processing enzymes. "Humanizing" these nonmammalian cell lines involved the identification of bottlenecks in the glycan synthesis pathway and complementing it with heterologous glycan synthesis enzymes. Such efforts have resulted in engineered cell lines that perform human-like glycosylation [113].

Similar efforts have been undertaken in yeasts and plant cells where certain undesired genes are knocked out and other genes required for synthesis of appropriate nucleotide sugar or for glycosyltransferase expression engineered into them. Yeasts have been extensively used for recombinant expression of proteins in the industry as they offer the advantages of having the ability to grow on chemically defined media, ease of scale-up, and high yields of protein production. But despite these advantages yeasts are seen as an unattractive system to produce glycoproteins as they typically express high-mannose glycan structures on the proteins, making them therapeutically inefficacious [114]. Again, using genetic manipulations to eliminate expression of undesirable $\alpha(1,6)$-mannosyltransferase activity and expression of heterologous $\alpha(1,2)$-mannosidase along with other glycosyltransferases have resulted in a strain of *Pichia pastoris* that produces glycoproteins with complex-type *N*-glycans [115–117]. The ability to genetically manipulate host systems to produce glycoproteins with desired glycoforms provides a valuable tool for systematically studying the structure–function–activity relationships of the glycans and also enables us to produce designer proteins expressing the optimal glycoforms for a given function.

Another strategy used for producing glycoproteins with specific glycans is the use of in vitro glycosylation techniques. This involves the production of the glycoprotein in a cell system of choice followed by modification of the glycans by the sequential action of specific glycosidases and glycosyltransferases. This technology has been commercialized by Neose Technologies, Inc. and has been used to produce glycoproteins with user-specified glycans [118,119]. The ability to control the glycosylation patterns by appropriate choice of the cell system and the use of metabolic engineering techniques have enabled the synthesis of therapeutics with engineered glycans. Human EPO is an example of a drug that has been engineered to express new glycosylation patterns. EPO stimulates the formation of red blood cells and is used to treat anemia resulting from chronic renal disease, heart failure, or the use of chemotherapeutics in cancer. It is one of the most widely used drugs, with worldwide sales exceeding $6 billion in 2006. A variant of EPO was created by mutating the EPO gene to engineer two additional N-glycosylation sites. The engineered EPO has an increased in vivo activity and duration of action [120, 121].

Glycoengineering has also been used for targeting therapeutic proteins to specific cells and tissues. Different cells express different glycan-binding proteins on their surface, resulting in their having differing affinities for specific glycans. Thus therapeutic proteins expressing specific glycans can be developed for targeting specific cell types. One example of a therapeutic that uses this property of tissue targeting is Glucocerebrosidase (GBA) used for treatment of Gaucher's disease. GBA with terminal mannose residues is used to specifically target the protein to the macrophages in the liver by its binding to mannose-binding lectins. Once in the liver, GBA metabolizes accumulated glucocerebroside [122]. Similarly asialoglycoprotein receptors could be used to target glycoproteins lacking terminal sialic acid to hepatocytes [123].

Glycans can also modulate the biological activity of therapeutic glycoproteins. An example of this is IgG antibodies. The Fc domain of IgG binds to Fc receptors on killer T cells. This interaction is mediated by the N-linked glycans present on the heavy chains of the IgG and is important for antibody-dependent cell cytotoxicity (ADCC) and complement-dependent cytotoxicity (CDC) functions. The affinity of the Fc domain to T-cell Fc receptors can be modulated by controlling the extent of glycosylation. While deglycosylated IgG was found to have very limited ADCC and CDC, the deletion of core fucose and addition of bisecting GlcNAc increased the affinity of IgG to the Fc receptors and thereby ADCC and CDC [124,125].

11.3 GLYCANS AS THERAPEUTICS

Given the role of glycans in modulating the cellular functions, it is not surprising that in addition to their role as conjugates to proteins these glycans have the potential to serve as good therapeutic candidates. Improvement in our understanding of the glycan structure–function–activity relationship has enabled us to harness glycans for direct therapeutic applications.

One of the oldest and most widely used carbohydrate based drug is heparin. Heparin is a highly sulfated glycosaminoglycan and is widely used as an anticoagulant. It acts by forming a ternary complex with thrombin and antithrombin III (AT-III), a serine protease inhibitor. This causes a conformational change of AT-III that enables it to block the action of the serine-proteases thrombin and factor Xa of the coagulation cascade [126]. Heparin for therapeutic use is isolated from the mucosal tissues of pig intestine or bovine lung.

This preparation of heparin is known as unfractionated heparin (UFH), and it is a highly heterogeneous and polydisperse mixture of heparin oligosaccharides, varying both in chain length and composition, having an average molecular weight of 15 kDa. This heterogeneity of heparin affects its therapeutic value as it causes severe side effects, including bleeding, heparin-induced thrombocytopenia, and allergic reactions [127].

In the last decade advances in GAG synthesis and sequencing have lead to better characterization of heparins. The pentasaccharide sequence in heparin responsible for binding to AT-III causes its conformation to change, and it then activates the rapid inhibition of factor Xa. By use of heparin mimetics, the AT-III inhibition of thrombin (factor IIa) is shown to require a longer heparin chain of at least 16 to 18 monosaccharides in addition to the presence of the pentasaccharide motif [14,128]. The identification of the motifs in heparin that bind to the AT-III and modulate the anticoagulant property has lead to the quest for better understanding of the structure–activity relationship of heparins. In the commercially prepared UFH, the pentasaccharide motif makes up only 3% of all chains, and they have an anti-Xa to anti-IIa ratio of approximately 1:1 [129].

To minimize the side effects of heparin and have better predictability of its anticoagulant activity, low molecular weight heparins (LMWH) have been developed by chemical and enzymatic degradation of UFH. Numerous strategies have been employed to create LMWHs, including controlled chemical cleavage, enzymatic digestion, and size fractionation of heparin [130,131]. LMWHs thus generated have an average molecular weight of 4 to 6 kDa and are less polydisperse compared to UFH. Despite still being a heterogenous mixture, these LMWH have largely replaced UFH in clinical applications owing to their better bioavailability, increased in vivo half-life, more predictable anti-coagulant activity, and decreased side effects [132]. LMWHs have an anti-Xa:anti-IIa activity ratio of 1.5:1 and thus have reduced anti-IIa activity compared to UFH, making them ideal for certain clinical applications such as treatment and prevention of deep vein thrombosis but not for arterial thrombosis, where antithrombin activity is required. Also LMWHs differ from one another in their overall efficacy due to differences in their structure [133]. The cloning and characterization of heparin degrading enzymes with different specificities [134–136], advances in sequencing strategies for analysis of heparins [57], and the identification of structures required for anticoagulant activity have enabled rational design of LMWHs. These newer LMWHs are more potent with increased anti-Xa and anti-IIa activity and decreased side effects [137].

HSGAGs are also being evaluated as potential therapeutics to target tumor growth. Tumor development has been associated with changes in cell surface HSGAG [138] and expression of tumor-specific heparanases [139,140]. HSGAG fractions generated by treatment with heparinases I (Hep I) and III (Hep III) have been evaluated for their role in modulating tumor growth. Hep I and Hep III have different substrate specificities and generate fragments that have distinctly different sulfation patterns. While fragments generated by the Hep I cleavage of HSGAG was shown to accelerate tumor growth, Hep III generated HSGAG fragments had inhibitory effects on tumor growth [141]. These Hep III generated fragments are being further characterized and evaluated for use as therapeutics.

Osteoarthritis treatment is another area in which sugars such as CSGAGs and glucosamine sulfate (GS) have been used to provide relief of symptoms [142]. These sugars are considered as a dietary supplement by the US Food and Drug Administration. CSGAGs provide mechanical stiffness to cartilage tissues and enabling joints to function normally [5]. Osteoarthritis causes the degradation of cartilages. There is no clear verdict about the benefits of CSGAG and GS treatment, and further research is needed to study the therapeutic efficacy of these sugars.

Other examples of use of GAGs as therapeutics include hyaluronic acid used in surgical procedures [143]. Sepragels is a product marketed by Genzyme Corporation that contains crosslinked hyaluronic acid. Pfizer's Healon is a formulation containing the high molecular weight fraction of sodium hyaluronate and is used as an aid in ophthalmic surgical procedures. GCS-100 is a polysaccharide derived from citrus pectin that is in clinical trials for tumor treatment [144]. GCS-100 targets the animal lectin galectin-3, a galactoside-binding protein implicated in the inhibition of apoptosis, promotion of angiogenesis, and metastasis. GCS-100, being rich in galactoside residues, interacts with galectin-3 present on tumors and causes caspase activation cascade mediated cell apoptosis [144]. Glycans have also are used for diabetic treatment. Acarbose is a pseudooligosaccharide synthesized by microbes that binds to glucosidases and amylases and reversibly inhibits the activity of these enzymes [145]. Acarbose preferentially binds to α-glucosidase and α-amylase, inhibiting carbohydrate digestion, regulating the absorption of monosaccharides, and thereby controlling blood glucose levels.

Unnatural sugars have also been used as receptor antagonists. Sialic acid analogues oseltamivir (trade name Tamiflu, Roche) and zanamivir (trade name Relenza, GlaxoSmithKline) are neuraminidase inhibitors. These two glycan-based drugs on the market are used for prevention and treatment of influenza [146].

11.4   GLYCANS AS TARGETS FOR THERAPEUTICS AND VACCINES

The ubiquitous presence of glycans on the cell surface and their role in cell signaling and cell–cell interactions makes them ideal targets for therapeutic interventions. These processes are mediated by the interaction of glycans with glycan binding proteins such as enzymes, ligands, growth factors, and cytokines. Until recently it had been difficult to access these physiological glycans to truly identify specific glycan targets and their glycan-binding partners. The use of glycan arrays has enabled identification of glycan specificities of these GBPs. This knowledge has helped develop therapeutics that modulate cell activity by specifically targeting certain glycans. These glycan-binding therapeutics could be used to either promote cell signaling or be used as receptor antagonists that prevent the glycans from interacting with their natural binding partners.

Vaccines and antibodies targeting glycans have been developed over the last few years. A major limitation in the development of glycan-based vaccines has been that glycans, while being mildly antigenic, are rarely immunogenic. That is, even if these glycans are able to elicit antibodies, they are mostly unable to successfully induce T lymphocytes to kill the cells expressing these glycans. A strategy to induce T-cell immunity has been to conjugate the glycan antigen to an immunogenic protein such as keyhole limpet haemocyanin (KLH). KLH is an immunogenic carrier protein, and it increases the immunogenicity of glycans by broadening the spectrum of immunoglobulins produced. Use of such glycoconjugates to vaccinate has improved the effectiveness by increasing the ability to induce both a cell-mediated and a humoral response in humans [147].

Two major areas of application for which glycan-based vaccines are being developed are cancer and infectious diseases. The glycoprofile of cancerous cells is found to be different from normal cells. The cell surface glycans undergo structural changes with the onset of cancer because of the differential expression of glycosyltransferases, which results in overexpression of certain glycoforms, underexpression of other glycoforms, and in some cases, neoexpression of glycans. The property of differential expression of glycans on cancerous cells has been exploited to recruit the immune system to target cancer cells. One of the major challenges in the development of vaccines to target these glycans is the inability of the immune system to challenge the B cells to produce antibodies against these glycans. These glycans found on cancerous cells are often expressed during embryonic development and are sometimes present on normal cells at low levels, resulting in them being perceived as "self" [148]. A major effort has been focused on making the immune system perceive these glycans as foreign and make antibodies against them [149,150]. Glycan-based vaccines for breast, prostate, and ovarian cancer, small-cell and non–small-cell lung carcinoma and malignant melanoma are in different stages of clinical trials [151]. In each of these cases the vaccine targets a single glycan. A more recent approach has been to develop multi-antigenic vaccines. These multi-antigenic vaccines are developed against sets of glycans that are characteristic of a cancer cell type, with the premise being that the presence of multiple antigens would elicit a better immune response than individual antigens [152,153]. In one study in mice with vaccine containing three distinct antigens Globo H, LeY, and Tn, antibodies were generated against each of these glycans [152]. These encouraging results have paved the way for development of other multi-antigenic vaccines with different combinations of glycan antigens.

Vaccines are also being developed to target diseases caused by pathogens that exploit the cell surface glycans. Pathogenic viruses, bacteria, and other microbes have GBPs on their surface. The first step of pathogenesis is typically the attachment of the pathogen's GBP to specific glycan moieties on the host cell surface. The interaction of the pathogen's GBPs with glycans has been studied by a variety of means. Over the last few years the glycan specificity of a variety of pathogens' GBPs has been studied, including those of influenza viruses [154–156], parainfluenza viruses [157], tetanus toxin, and cholera toxin, among others. The identification and synthesis of specific oligosaccharide antigens can help in the development of vaccines against these pathogens. Capsular polysaccharides or their conjugates have been used to develop vaccines against a host of microbial pathogens, including *Haemophilus influenzae* type b (Hib), *Streptococcus pneumoniae*, *Neisseria meningiditis*, *Salmonella typhi*, group B *streptococcus*, and *Staphylococcus aureus* [158]. Another bacterial pathogen, *Bacillus anthracis* (anthrax) has posed the threat of being used as a biological warfare weapon. The anthrax spores have a unique *O*-linked tetrasaccharide on their surface [159], and vaccines are currently being developed using synthetic tetrasaccharide antigens [160]. Vaccines are also being developed against *Plasmodium falciparum*, a parasite-causing malaria. Glycosylinositol phospholipid (GPI) is extensively expressed on the *P. falciparum* cell surface, and it triggers an inflammatory cascade [161]. GPI hexasaccharides have been synthesized and conjugated with immunogenic proteins to be used as vaccines [162]. The identification of glycan specificity of more pathogens along with development of immunogenic conjugates would result in development of many more glycan-based vaccines in the future.

11.5 SUMMARY

Advancement of glycomics has been limited by the lack of appropriate tools to study glycans and their interaction with their binding partners. This has, in large part, precluded it from being fully harnessed for drug development. Technological advances in glycan sequencing and glycan synthesis methodologies in the past few years have helped expand our understanding of the role of glycans in various cellular processes. To date, glycans have been implicated in a diverse set of cellular and pathophysiological processes, including cell growth, development, cell signaling, immune recognition, cancer, angiogenesis, and microbial and viral pathogenesis. The importance of glycosylation in humans is highlighted by the fact that any aberration in the glycosylational machinery can result in severe physical and mental disorders. Changes in the physiological state of the cell often result in disturbing the delicate interplay of glycosyltransferases and glycosidases, which manifests itself by changes in the glycosylation of cellular proteins and lipids.

As these technologies bring the role of glycans to the forefront, the challenge lies in exploiting them for therapeutics. Novel delivery methods are being developed for glycan-based therapeutics. Glycan synthesis by chemical and chemoenzymatic means has facilitated the production of synthetic vaccines. The ability to glycoengineer cell lines provides a means for producing therapeutic glycoproteins with consistent PK properties. With new analytical tools now available to characterize glycans, researchers are identifying diagnostic and prognostic glycan markers for various disease states such as liver cirrhosis [163] and cancer [164,165]. Also research is ongoing to evaluate if the cellular glycans could be used to predict susceptibility to a particular disease. Lectin arrays [166,167] and MS-based analytical techniques [164,165] are being used to screen the sera for disease markers. The identification of these glycan markers could not only provide a means to monitor the health of patients but also could identify novel targets for therapy.

In this post-genomic era, the field of glycomics has contributed to the improvement of current and offered a number of novel therapeutics. While there are already some glycan-based drugs on the market, the nascent field of glycomics promises much more.

ACKNOWLEDGMENT

The authors would like to acknowledge Rahul Raman and Aarthi Chandrasekaran for their helpful suggestions.

REFERENCES

1. Varki A, Cummings R, Esko JD, Freeze H, Hart GW, Marth J. *Essentials of glycobiology*. New York: Cold Spring Harbor Laboratory Press, 1999.

2. Taylor ME, Drickamer K. *Introduction to glycobiology*. Oxford: Oxford University Press, 2003.

3. Kornfeld R, Kornfeld S. Assembly of asparagine-linked oligosaccharides. *Ann Rev Biochem* 1985;54:631–64.

4. Hart GW. Glycosylation. *Curr Opin Cell Biol* 1992;4:1017–23.

5. Sasisekharan R, Raman R, Prabhakar V. Glycomics approach to structure–function relationships of glycosaminoglycans. *Ann Rev Biomed Eng* 2006;8:181–231.

6. Parodi AJ. Protein glucosylation and its role in protein folding. *Ann Rev Biochem* 2000;69:69–93.

7. Parodi AJ. Role of N-oligosaccharide endoplasmic reticulum processing reactions in glycoprotein folding and degradation. *Biochem J* 2000;348(Pt1):1–13.

8. Helenius A, Aebi M. Intracellular functions of N-linked glycans. *Science* 2001;291:2364–9.

9. Helenius A, Aebi M. Roles of N-linked glycans in the endoplasmic reticulum. *Ann Rev Biochem* 2004;73:1019–49.

10. Dwek RA. Biological importance of glycosylation. *Dev Biol Stand* 1998;96:43–7.

11. Varki A. Biological roles of oligosaccharides: all of the theories are correct. *Glycobiology* 1993;3:97–130.

12. Shriver Z, Liu D, Sasisekharan R. Emerging views of heparan sulfate glycosaminoglycan structure/activity relationships modulating dynamic biological functions. *Trends Cardiovasc Med* 2002;12:71–7.

13. Casu B, Guerrini M, Torri G. Structural and conformational aspects of the anticoagulant and anti-thrombotic activity of heparin and dermatan sulfate. *Curr Pharm Des* 2004;10:939–49.

14. Petitou M, van Boeckel CA. A synthetic antithrombin III binding pentasaccharide is now a drug! What comes next? *Angew Chem Int Ed Engl* 2004;43: 3118–33.

15. Lowe JB, Marth JD. A genetic approach to Mammalian glycan function. *Ann Rev Biochem* 2003;72:643–91.

16. Hwang HY, Olson SK, Esko JD, Horvitz HR. Caenorhabditis elegans early embryogenesis and vulval morphogenesis require chondroitin biosynthesis. *Nature* 2003;423:439–43.

17. Inatani M, Irie F, Plump AS, Tessier-Lavigne M, Yamaguchi Y. Mammalian brain morphogenesis and midline axon guidance require heparan sulfate. *Science* 2003;302:1044–6.

18. Lin X. Functions of heparan sulfate proteoglycans in cell signaling during development. *Development* 2004;131:6009–21.

19. Haltiwanger RS, Lowe JB. Role of glycosylation in development. *Ann Rev Biochem* 2004;73:491–537.

20. Collins BE, Paulson JC. Cell surface biology mediated by low affinity multivalent protein-glycan interactions. *Curr Opin Chem Biol* 2004;8:617–25.

21. Crocker PR. Siglecs: sialic-acid-binding immunoglobulin-like lectins in cell–cell interactions and signalling. *Curr Opin Struct Biol* 2002;12:609–15.

22. Kinjo Y, Wu D, Kim G, Xing GW, Poles MA, Ho DD, et al. Recognition of bacterial glycosphingolipids by natural killer T cells. *Nature* 2005;434:520–5.

23. Guo Y, Feinberg H, Conroy E, Mitchell DA, Alvarez R, Blixt O, et al. Structural basis for distinct ligand-binding and targeting properties of the receptors DC-SIGN and DC-SIGNR. *Nat Struct Mol Biol* 2004;11:591–8.

24. Crocker PR. Siglecs in innate immunity. *Curr Opin Pharmacol* 2005;5:431–7.

25. Rudd PM, Elliott T, Cresswell P, Wilson IA, Dwek RA. Glycosylation and the immune system. *Science* 2001;291:2370–6.

26. Rudd PM, Wormald MR, Dwek RA. Sugar-mediated ligand-receptor interactions in the immune system. *Trends Biotechnol* 2004;22:524–30.

27. Chandrasekaran A, Srinivasan A, Raman R, Viswanathan K, Raguram S, Tumpey TM, et al. Glycan topology determines human adaptation of avian H5N1 virus hemagglutinin. *Nat Biotechnol* 2008;26:107–13.

28. Fry EE, Lea SM, Jackson T, Newman JW, Ellard FM, Blakemore WE, et al. The structure and function of a foot-and-mouth disease virus-oligosaccharide receptor complex. *EMBO J* 1999;18:543–54.

29. Liu J, Shriver Z, Pope RM, Thorp SC, Duncan MB, Copeland RJ, et al. Characterization of a heparan sulfate octasaccharide that binds to herpes simplex virus type 1 glycoprotein d. *J Biol Chem* 2002;277:33456–67.

30. Mardberg K, Trybala E, Tufaro F, Bergstrom T. Herpes simplex virus type 1 glycoprotein C is necessary for efficient infection of chondroitin sulfate-expressing gro2C cells. *J Gen Virol* 2002;83:291–300.

31. Shukla D, Liu J, Blaiklock P, Shworak NW, Bai X, Esko JD, et al. A novel role for 3-*O*-sulfated heparan sulfate in herpes simplex virus 1 entry. *Cell* 1999;99: 13–22.

32. Casu B, Guerrini M, Naggi A, Perez M, Torri G, Ribatti D, et al. Short heparin sequences spaced by glycol-split uronate residues are antagonists of fibroblast growth factor 2 and angiogenesis inhibitors. *Biochemistry* 2002;41:10519–28.

33. Iozzo RV, San Antonio JD. Heparan sulfate proteoglycans: heavy hitters in the angiogenesis arena. *J Clin Invest* 2001;108:349–55.

34. Iozzo RV. Basement membrane proteoglycans: from cellar to ceiling. *Nat Rev Mol Cell Biol* 2005;6:646–56.

35. Vlodavsky I, Goldshmidt O, Zcharia E, Atzmon R, Rangini-Guatta Z, Elkin M, et al. Mammalian heparanase: involvement in cancer metastasis, angiogenesis and normal development. *Semin Cancer Biol* 2002;12:121–9.

36. Bishop JR, Schuksz M, Esko JD. Heparan sulphate proteoglycans fine-tune mammalian physiology. *Nature* 2007;446:1030–7.

37. Raman R, Sasisekharan R. Cooperativity in Glycan-Protein Interactions. *Chem Biol* 2007;14:873–4.

38. Dell A, Morris HR. Glycoprotein structure determination by mass spectrometry. *Science* 2001;291:2351–6.

39. Zhang H, Li XJ, Martin DB, Aebersold R. Identification and quantification of *N*-linked glycoproteins using hydrazide chemistry, stable isotope labeling and mass spectrometry. *Nat Biotechnol* 2003;21:660–6.

40. Kaji H, Saito H, Yamauchi Y, Shinkawa T, Taoka M, Hirabayashi J, et al. Lectin affinity capture, isotope-coded tagging and mass spectrometry to identify *N*-linked glycoproteins. *Nat Biotechnol* 2003;21:667–72.

41. Que AH, Mechref Y, Huang Y, Taraszka JA, Clemmer DE, Novotny MV. Coupling capillary electrochromatography with electrospray Fourier transform mass spectrometry for characterizing complex oligosaccharide pools. *Anal Chem* 2003;75:1684–90.

42. Que AH, Novotny MV. Structural characterization of neutral oligosaccharide mixtures through a combination of capillary electrochromatography and ion trap tandem mass spectrometry. *Anal Bioanal Chem* 2003;375:599–608.

43. Tomiya N, Awaya J, Kurono M, Endo S, Arata Y, Takahashi N. Analyses of *N*-linked oligosaccharides using a two-dimensional mapping technique. *Anal Biochem* 1988;171:73–90.

44. Takahashi N, Nakagawa H, Fujikawa K, Kawamura Y, Tomiya N. Three-dimensional elution mapping of pyridylaminated *N*-linked neutral and sialyl oligosaccharides. *Anal Biochem* 1995;226:139–46.

45. Harvey DJ. Matrix-assisted laser desorption/ionisation mass spectrometry of oligosaccharides and glycoconjugates. *J Chromatogr A* 1996;720:429–46.

46. Harvey DJ. Analysis of carbohydrates and glycoconjugates by matrix-assisted laser desorption/ionization mass spectrometry: an update covering the period 1999–2000. *Mass Spectrom Rev* 2006;25:595–662.

47. Kurogochi M, Nishimura S. Structural characterization of *N*-glycopeptides by matrix-dependent selective fragmentation of MALDI-TOF/TOF tandem mass spectrometry. *Anal Chem* 2004;76:6097–101.

48. Wuhrer M, Hokke CH, Deelder AM. Glycopeptide analysis by matrix-assisted laser desorption/ionization tandem time-of-flight mass spectrometry reveals novel features of horseradish peroxidase glycosylation. *Rapid Commun Mass Spectrom* 2004;18:1741–8.

49. Zaia J, Costello CE. Compositional analysis of glycosaminoglycans by electrospray mass spectrometry. *Anal Chem* 2001;73:233–9.

50. Jiang H, Desaire H, Butnev VY, Bousfield GR. Glycoprotein profiling by electrospray mass spectrometry. *J Am Soc Mass Spectrom* 2004;15:750–8.

51. Zaia J. Mass spectrometry of oligosaccharides. *Mass Spectrom Rev* 2004;23: 161–227.

52. Kawasaki N, Itoh S, Ohta M, Hayakawa T. Microanalysis of *N*-linked oligosaccharides in a glycoprotein by capillary liquid chromatography/mass spectrometry and liquid chromatography/tandem mass spectrometry. *Anal Biochem* 2003;316: 15–22.

53. Carr SA, Huddleston MJ, Bean MF. Selective identification and differentiation of *N*- and *O*-linked oligosaccharides in glycoproteins by liquid chromatography-mass spectrometry. *Protein Sci* 1993;2:183–96.

54. Gennaro LA, Delaney J, Vouros P, Harvey DJ, Domon B. Capillary electrophoresis/electrospray ion trap mass spectrometry for the analysis of negatively charged derivatized and underivatized glycans. *Rapid Commun Mass Spectrom* 2002;16:192–200.

55. Campa C, Coslovi A, Flamigni A, Rossi M. Overview on advances in capillary electrophoresis–mass spectrometry of carbohydrates: a tabulated review. *Electrophoresis* 2006;27:2027–50.

56. Manzi AE, Norgard-Sumnicht K, Argade S, Marth JD, van Halbeek H, Varki A. Exploring the glycan repertoire of genetically modified mice by isolation and profiling of the major glycan classes and nano-NMR analysis of glycan mixtures. *Glycobiology* 2000;10:669–89.

57. Venkataraman G, Shriver Z, Raman R, Sasisekharan R. Sequencing complex polysaccharides. *Science* 1999;286:537–42.

58. Guerrini M, Raman R, Venkataraman G, Torri G, Sasisekharan R, Casu B. A novel computational approach to integrate NMR spectroscopy and capillary electrophoresis for structure assignment of heparin and heparan sulfate oligosaccharides. *Glycobiology* 2002;12:713–19.

59. Sears P, Wong CH. Toward automated synthesis of oligosaccharides and glycoproteins. *Science* 2001;291:2344–50.

60. Hanson S, Best M, Bryan MC, Wong CH. Chemoenzymatic synthesis of oligosaccharides and glycoproteins. *Trends Biochem Sci* 2004;29:656–63.

61. Seeberger PH, Haase WC. Solid-phase oligosaccharide synthesis and combinatorial carbohydrate libraries. *Chem Rev* 2000;100:4349–94.

62. Nicolaou KC, Mitchell HJ. Adventures in carbohydrate chemistry: new synthetic technologies, chemical synthesis, molecular design, and chemical. biology. [A list of abbreviations can be found at the end of this article. Telemachos

Charalambous was an inspiring teacher at the Pancyprian Gymnasium, Nicosia, Cyprus.] *Angew Chem Int Ed Engl* 2001;40:1576–624.

63. Liang R, Yan L, Loebach J, Ge M, Uozumi Y, Sekanina K, et al. Parallel synthesis and screening of a solid phase carbohydrate library. *Science* 1996;274:1520–2.

64. Danishefsky SJ, McClure KF, Randolph JT, Ruggeri RB. A strategy for the solid-phase synthesis of oligosaccharides. *Science* 1993;260:1307–9.

65. Zhang Z, Ollmann IR, Ye XS, Wischnat R, Baasov T, Wong CH. Programmable one-pot oligosaccharide synthesis. *J Am Chem Soc* 1999;121:734–53.

66. Nishimura S. Automated glycosynthesizer "Golgi" by mimicking biosynthetic process (in Japanese). *Tanpakushitsu Kakusan Koso* 2003;48:1220–5.

67. Ashline D, Singh S, Hanneman A, Reinhold V. Congruent strategies for carbohydrate sequencing. 1. Mining structural details by MSn. *Anal Chem* 2005;77: 6250–62.

68. Laroy W, Contreras R, Callewaert N. Glycome mapping on DNA sequencing equipment. *Nat Protoc* 2006;1:397–405.

69. Wang D, Liu S, Trummer BJ, Deng C, Wang A. Carbohydrate microarrays for the recognition of cross-reactive molecular markers of microbes and host cells. *Nat Biotechnol* 2002;20:275–81.

70. Fukui S, Feizi T, Galustian C, Lawson AM, Chai W. Oligosaccharide microarrays for high-throughput detection and specificity assignments of carbohydrate-protein interactions. *Nat Biotechnol* 2002;20:1011–17.

71. Blixt O, Razi N. Chemoenzymatic synthesis of glycan libraries. *Meth Enzymol* 2006;415:137–53.

72. Sungjin Park IS. Fabrication of carbohydrate chips for studying protein–carbohydrate interactions. *Angew Chem Int Ed* 2002;41:3180–2.

73. Eddie W. Adams JUDMRBROKDRWPHS. Encoded fiber-optic microsphere arrays for probing protein–carbohydrate Interactions. *Angew Chem Int Ed* 2003; 42:5317–20.

74. Fazio F, Bryan MC, Blixt O, Paulson JC, Wong CH. Synthesis of sugar arrays in microtiter plate. *J Am Chem Soc* 2002;124:14397–402.

75. Houseman BT, Mrksich M. Carbohydrate arrays for the evaluation of protein binding and enzymatic modification. *Chem Biol* 2002;9:443–54.

76. Ratner DM, Adams EW, Su J, O'Keefe BR, Mrksich M, Seeberger PH. Probing protein–carbohydrate interactions with microarrays of synthetic oligosaccharides. *ChemBioChem* 2004;5:379–82.

77. Blixt O, Head S, Mondala T, Scanlan C, Huflejt ME, Alvarez R, et al. Printed covalent glycan array for ligand profiling of diverse glycan binding proteins. *Proc Natl Acad Sci USA* 2004;101:17033–8.

78. Feizi T, Fazio F, Chai W, Wong CH. Carbohydrate microarrays—a new set of technologies at the frontiers of glycomics. *Curr Opin Struct Biol* 2003;13: 637–45.

79. Galanina OE, Mecklenburg M, Nifantiev NE, Pazynina GV, Bovin NV. Glyco-Chip: multiarray for the study of carbohydrate-binding proteins. *Lab Chip* 2003;3:260–5.

80. Srinivasan A, Viswanathan K, Raman R, Chandrasekaran A, Raguram S, Tumpey TM, et al. Quantitative biochemical rationale for differences in transmissibility

of 1918 pandemic influenza A viruses. *Proc Natl Acad Sci USA* 2008;105: 2800–5.

81. Comelli EM, Amado M, Head SR, Paulson JC. Custom microarray for glycobiologists: considerations for glycosyltransferase gene expression profiling. *Biochem Soc Symp* 2002:135–42.

82. Comelli EM, Head SR, Gilmartin T, Whisenant T, Haslam SM, North SJ, et al. A focused microarray approach to functional glycomics: transcriptional regulation of the glycome. *Glycobiology* 2006;16:117–31.

83. Smith FI, Qu Q, Hong SJ, Kim KS, Gilmartin TJ, Head SR. Gene expression profiling of mouse postnatal cerebellar development using oligonucleotide microarrays designed to detect differences in glycoconjugate expression. *Gene Exp Patterns* 2005;5:740–9.

84. Martin LT, Marth JD, Varki A, Varki NM. Genetically altered mice with different sialyltransferase deficiencies show tissue-specific alterations in sialylation and sialic acid 9-*O*-acetylation. *J Biol Chem* 2002;277:32930–8.

85. Homeister JW, Daugherty A, Lowe JB. Alpha(1,3)fucosyltransferases FucT-IV and FucT-VII control susceptibility to atherosclerosis in apolipoprotein E-/- mice. *Arterioscler Thromb Vasc Biol* 2004;24:1897–903.

86. Smithson G, Rogers CE, Smith PL, Scheidegger EP, Petryniak B, Myers JT, et al. Fuc-TVII is required for T helper 1 and T cytotoxic 1 lymphocyte selectin ligand expression and recruitment in inflammation, and together with Fuc-TIV regulates naive T cell trafficking to lymph nodes. *J Exp Med* 2001;194:601–14.

87. Raman R, Raguram S, Venkataraman G, Paulson JC, Sasisekharan R. Glycomics: an integrated systems approach to structure-function relationships of glycans. *Nat Meth* 2005;2:817–24.

88. Raman R, Venkataraman M, Ramakrishnan S, Lang W, Raguram S, Sasisekharan R. Advancing glycomics: implementation strategies at the consortium for functional glycomics. *Glycobiology* 2006;16:82R–90R.

89. von der Lieth CW, Bohne-Lang A, Lohmann KK, Frank M. Bioinformatics for glycomics: status, methods, requirements and perspectives. *Brief Bioinform* 2004;5:164–78.

90. Walsh G. Biopharmaceuticals: recent approvals and likely directions. *Trends Biotechnol* 2005;23:553–8.

91. Leader B, Baca QJ, Golan DE. Protein therapeutics: a summary and pharmacological classification. *Nat Rev Drug Discov* 2008;7:21–39.

92. Sethuraman N, Stadheim TA. Challenges in therapeutic glycoprotein production. *Curr Opin Biotechnol* 2006;17:341–6.

93. Lai PH, Everett R, Wang FF, Arakawa T, Goldwasser E. Structural characterization of human erythropoietin. *J Biol Chem* 1986;261:3116–21.

94. Higuchi M, Oh-eda M, Kuboniwa H, Tomonoh K, Shimonaka Y, Ochi N. Role of sugar chains in the expression of the biological activity of human erythropoietin. *J Biol Chem* 1992;267:7703–9.

95. Macdougall IC. Optimizing the use of erythropoietic agents—pharmacokinetic and pharmacodynamic considerations. *Nephrol Dial Transpl* 2002;17:66–70.

96. Yuen CT, Storring PL, Tiplady RJ, Izquierdo M, Wait R, Gee CK, et al. Relationships between the *N*-glycan structures and biological activities of recombinant

human erythropoietins produced using different culture conditions and purification procedures. *Br J Haematol* 2003;121:511–26.

97. Fukuda MN, Sasaki H, Lopez L, Fukuda M. Survival of recombinant erythropoietin in the circulation: the role of carbohydrates. *Blood* 1989;73:84–9.

98. Stockert RJ. The asialoglycoprotein receptor: relationships between structure, function, and expression. *Physiol Rev* 1995;75:591–609.

99. Schlesinger PH, Rodman JS, Doebber TW, Stahl PD, Lee YC, Stowell CP, et al. The role of extra-hepatic tissues in the receptor-mediated plasma clearance of glycoproteins terminated by mannose or *N*-acetylglucosamine. *Biochem J* 1980;192:597–606.

100. Maynard Y, Baenziger JU. Oligosaccharide specific endocytosis by isolated rat hepatic reticuloendothelial cells. *J Biol Chem* 1981;256:8063–8.

101. Jenkins N, Parekh RB, James DC. Getting the glycosylation right: implications for the biotechnology industry. *Nat Biotechnol* 1996;14:975–81.

102. Goochee CF. Bioprocess factors affecting glycoprotein oligosaccharide structure. *Dev Biol Stand* 1992;76:95–104.

103. Goochee CF, Gramer MJ, Andersen DC, Bahr JB, Rasmussen JR. The oligosaccharides of glycoproteins: bioprocess factors affecting oligosaccharide structure and their effect on glycoprotein properties. *Biotechnology (NY)* 1991;9:1347–55.

104. Goochee CF, Monica T. Environmental effects on protein glycosylation. *Biotechnology (NY)* 1990;8:421–7.

105. Andersen DC, Goochee CF. The effect of cell-culture conditions on the oligosaccharide structures of secreted glycoproteins. *Curr Opin Biotechnol* 1994;5: 546–9.

106. Jenkins N, Curling EM. Glycosylation of recombinant proteins: problems and prospects. *Enzyme Microb Technol* 1994;16:354–64.

107. Bhatia PK, Mukhopadhyay A. Protein glycosylation: implications for in vivo functions and therapeutic applications. *Adv Biochem Eng Biotechnol* 1999;64: 155–201.

108. Jenkins N, Buckberry L, Marc A, Monaco L. Genetic engineering of alpha 2,6-sialyltransferase in recombinant CHO cells. *Biochem Soc Trans* 1998;26:S115.

109. Weikert S, Papac D, Briggs J, Cowfer D, Tom S, Gawlitzek M, et al. Engineering Chinese hamster ovary cells to maximize sialic acid content of recombinant glycoproteins. *Nat Biotechnol* 1999;17:1116–21.

110. Umana P, Jean-Mairet J, Moudry R, Amstutz H, Bailey JE. Engineered glycoforms of an antineuroblastoma IgG1 with optimized antibody-dependent cellular cytotoxic activity. *Nat Biotechnol* 1999;17:176–80.

111. Altmann F, Kornfeld G, Dalik T, Staudacher E, Glossl J. Processing of asparagine-linked oligosaccharides in insect cells. *N*-acetylglucosaminyltransferase I and II activities in cultured lepidopteran cells. *Glycobiology* 1993;3:619–25.

112. Kulakosky PC, Hughes PR, Wood HA. *N*-Linked glycosylation of a baculovirus-expressed recombinant glycoprotein in insect larvae and tissue culture cells. *Glycobiology* 1998;8:741–5.

113. Aumiller JJ, Hollister JR, Jarvis DL. A transgenic insect cell line engineered to produce CMP-sialic acid and sialylated glycoproteins. *Glycobiology* 2003;13: 497–507.

114. Gerngross TU. Advances in the production of human therapeutic proteins in yeasts and filamentous fungi. *Nat Biotechnol* 2004;22:1409–14.

115. Choi BK, Bobrowicz P, Davidson RC, Hamilton SR, Kung DH, Li H, et al. Use of combinatorial genetic libraries to humanize *N*-linked glycosylation in the yeast Pichia pastoris. *Proc Natl Acad Sci USA* 2003;100:5022–7.

116. Hamilton SR, Bobrowicz P, Bobrowicz B, Davidson RC, Li H, Mitchell T, et al. Production of complex human glycoproteins in yeast. *Science* 2003; 301:1244–6.

117. Bobrowicz P, Davidson RC, Li H, Potgieter TI, Nett JH, Hamilton SR, et al. Engineering of an artificial glycosylation pathway blocked in core oligosaccharide assembly in the yeast *Pichia pastoris*: production of complex humanized glyco-proteins with terminal galactose. *Glycobiology* 2004;14:757–66.

118. Johnson KF. Synthesis of oligosaccharides by bacterial enzymes. *Glycoconj J* 1999;16:141–6.

119. Warnock D, Bai X, Autote K, Gonzales J, Kinealy K, Yan B, et al. In vitro galac-tosylation of human IgG at 1 kg scale using recombinant galactosyltransferase. *Biotechnol Bioeng* 2005;92:831–42.

120. Elliott S, Lorenzini T, Asher S, Aoki K, Brankow D, Buck L, et al. Enhancement of therapeutic protein in vivo activities through glycoengineering. *Nat Biotechnol* 2003;21:414–21.

121. Elliott S, Egrie J, Browne J, Lorenzini T, Busse L, Rogers N, et al. Control of rHuEPO biological activity: the role of carbohydrate. *Exp Hematol* 2004;32: 1146–55.

122. Friedman B, Vaddi K, Preston C, Mahon E, Cataldo JR, McPherson JM. A com-parison of the pharmacological properties of carbohydrate remodeled recombi-nant and placental-derived beta-glucocerebrosidase: implications for clinical efficacy in treatment of Gaucher disease. *Blood* 1999;93:2807–16.

123. Cho CS, Kobayashi A, Takei R, Ishihara T, Maruyama A, Akaike T. Receptor-mediated cell modulator delivery to hepatocyte using nanoparticles coated with carbohydrate-carrying polymers. *Biomaterials* 2001;22:45–51.

124. Niwa R, Sakurada M, Kobayashi Y, Uehara A, Matsushima K, Ueda R, et al. Enhanced natural killer cell binding and activation by low-fucose IgG1 antibody results in potent antibody-dependent cellular cytotoxicity induction at lower antigen density. *Clin Cancer Res* 2005;11:2327–36.

125. Shinkawa T, Nakamura K, Yamane N, Shoji-Hosaka E, Kanda Y, Sakurada M, et al. The absence of fucose but not the presence of galactose or bisecting *N*-acetylglucosamine of human IgG1 complex-type oligosaccharides shows the critical role of enhancing antibody-dependent cellular cytotoxicity. *J Biol Chem* 2003;278:3466–73.

126. Capila I, Linhardt RJ. Heparin–protein interactions. *Angew Chem Int Ed Engl* 2002;41:391–412.

127. Baglin TP. Heparin induced thrombocytopenia thrombosis (HIT/T) syndrome: diagnosis and treatment. *J Clin Pathol* 2001;54:272–4.

128. Petitou M, Herault JP, Bernat A, Driguez PA, Duchaussoy P, Lormeau JC, et al. Synthesis of thrombin-inhibiting heparin mimetics without side effects [see com-ments]. *Nature* 1999;398:417–22.

129. Fareed J, Hoppensteadt DA, Bick RL. An update on heparins at the beginning of the new millennium. *Semin Thromb Hemost* 2000;26:5–21.

130. Casu B, Torri G. Structural characterization of low molecular weight heparins. *Semin Thromb Hemost* 1999;25:17–25.

131. Gunay NS, Linhardt RJ. Heparinoids: structure, biological activities and therapeutic applications. *Planta Med* 1999;65:301–6.

132. Hoppensteadt D, Walenga JM, Fareed J, Bick RL. Heparin, low-molecular-weight heparins, and heparin pentasaccharide: basic and clinical differentiation. *Hematol Oncol Clin North Am* 2003;17:313–41.

133. Jeske W, Fareed J. In vitro studies on the biochemistry and pharmacology of low molecular weight heparins. *Semin Thromb Hemost* 1999;25:27–33.

134. Ernst S, Venkataraman G, Winkler S, Godavarti R, Langer R, Cooney CL, et al. Expression in Escherichia coli, purification and characterization of heparinase I from Flavobacterium heparinum. *Biochem J* 1996;315 (Pt 2): 589–97.

135. Ernst S, Langer R, Cooney CL, Sasisekharan R. Enzymatic degradation of glycosaminoglycans. *Crit Rev Biochem Mol Biol* 1995;30:387–444.

136. Pojasek K, Shriver Z, Hu Y, Sasisekharan R. Histidine 295 and histidine 510 are crucial for the enzymatic degradation of heparan sulfate by heparinase III. *Biochemistry* 2000;39:4012–19.

137. Sundaram M, Qi Y, Shriver Z, Liu D, Zhao G, Venkataraman G, et al. Rational design of low-molecular weight heparins with improved in vivo activity. *Proc Natl Acad Sci USA* 2003;100:651–6.

138. Sanderson RD. Heparan sulfate proteoglycans in invasion and metastasis. *Semin Cell Dev Biol* 2001;12:89–98.

139. Hulett MD, Freeman C, Hamdorf BJ, Baker RT, Harris MJ, Parish CR. Cloning of mammalian heparanase, an important enzyme in tumor invasion and metastasis [see comments]. *Nat Med* 1999;5:803–9.

140. Vlodavsky I, Friedmann Y, Elkin M, Aingorn H, Atzmon R, Ishai-Michaeli R, et al. Mammalian heparanase: gene cloning, expression and function in tumor progression and metastasis [see comments]. *Nat Med* 1999;5:793–802.

141. Liu D, Shriver Z, Venkataraman G, El Shabrawi Y, Sasisekharan R. Tumor cell surface heparan sulfate as cryptic promoters or inhibitors of tumor growth and metastasis. *Proc Natl Acad Sci USA* 2002;99:568–73.

142. Gregory PJ, Sperry M, Wilson AF. Dietary supplements for osteoarthritis. *Am Fam Physician* 2008;77:177–84.

143. Chen WYJ, Abatangelo G. Functions of hyaluronan in wound repair. *Wound Repair Regen* 1999;7:79–89.

144. Chauhan D, Li G, Podar K, Hideshima T, Neri P, He D, et al. A novel carbohydrate-based therapeutic GCS-100 overcomes bortezomib resistance and enhances dexamethasone-induced apoptosis in multiple myeloma cells. *Cancer Res* 2005;65:8350–8.

145. Truscheit E, Frommer W, Junge B, Müller L, Schmidt DD, Wingender W. Chemistry and biochemistry of microbial α-glucosidase inhibitors. *Agnew Chem Int Ed Engl* 1981;20:744–61.

146. De Clercq E. Antiviral agents active against influenza A viruses. *Nat Rev Drug Discov* 2006;5:1015–25.

147. Samuel J, Danishefsky JRA. From the laboratory to the clinic: a retrospective on fully synthetic carbohydrate-based anticancer vaccines. *Angew Chem Int Ed* 2000;39:836–63.

148. Speiser DE, Miranda R, Zakarian A, Bachmann MF, McKall-Faienza K, Odermatt B, et al. Self antigens expressed by solid tumors do not efficiently stimulate naive or activated T cells: implications for immunotherapy. *J Exp Med* 1997;186:645–53.

149. Livingston PO. Approaches to augmenting the immunogenicity of melanoma gangliosides: from whole melanoma cells to ganglioside–KLH conjugate vaccines. *Immunol Rev* 1995;145:147–66.

150. Danishefsky SJ, Allen JR. From the laboratory to the clinic: a retrospective on fully synthetic carbohydrate-based anticancer vaccines. [Frequently used abbreviations are listed in the appendix.] *Angew Chem Int Ed Engl* 2000;39:836–63.

151. Dube DH, Bertozzi CR. Glycans in cancer and inflammation—potential for therapeutics and diagnostics. *Nat Rev Drug Discov* 2005;4:477–88.

152. Ragupathi G, Coltart DM, Williams LJ, Koide F, Kagan E, Allen J, et al. On the power of chemical synthesis: immunological evaluation of models for multiantigenic carbohydrate-based cancer vaccines. *Proc Natl Acad Sci USA* 2002;99:13699–704.

153. Livingston P. The unfulfilled promise of melanoma vaccines. *Clin Cancer Res* 2001;7:1837–8.

154. Stevens J, Blixt O, Glaser L, Taubenberger JK, Palese P, Paulson JC, et al. Glycan microarray analysis of the hemagglutinins from modern and pandemic influenza viruses reveals different receptor specificities. *J Mol Biol* 2006;355:1143–55.

155. Stevens J, Blixt O, Paulson JC, Wilson IA. Glycan microarray technologies: tools to survey host specificity of influenza viruses. *Nat Rev Microbiol* 2006;4:857–64.

156. Stevens J, Blixt O, Tumpey TM, Taubenberger JK, Paulson JC, Wilson IA. Structure and receptor specificity of the hemagglutinin from an H5N1 influenza virus. *Science* 2006;312:404–10.

157. Amonsen M, Smith DF, Cummings RD, Air GM. Human parainfluenza viruses hPIV1 and hPIV3 bind oligosaccharides with alpha2-3-linked sialic acids that are distinct from those bound by H5 avian influenza virus hemagglutinin. *J Virol* 2007;81:8341–5.

158. Ada G, Isaacs D. Carbohydrate-protein conjugate vaccines. *Clin Microbiol Infect* 2003;9:79–85.

159. Daubenspeck JM, Zeng H, Chen P, Dong S, Steichen CT, Krishna NR, et al. Novel oligosaccharide side chains of the collagen-like region of BclA, the major glycoprotein of the *Bacillus anthracis* exosporium. *J Biol Chem* 2004;279:30945–53.

160. Werz DB, Seeberger PH. Total synthesis of antigen bacillus anthracis tetrasaccharide—creation of an anthrax vaccine candidate. *Angew Chem Int Ed Engl* 2005;44:6315–18.

161. Berhe S, Schofield L, Schwarz RT, Gerold P. Conservation of structure among glycosylphosphatidylinositol toxins from different geographic isolates of *Plasmodium falciparum*. *Mol Biochem Parasitol* 1999;103:273–8.

162. Schofield L, Hewitt MC, Evans K, Siomos MA, Seeberger PH. Synthetic GPI as a candidate anti-toxic vaccine in a model of malaria. *Nature* 2002;418:785–9.

163. Callewaert N, Van Vlierberghe H, Van Hecke A, Laroy W, Delanghe J, Contreras R. Noninvasive diagnosis of liver cirrhosis using DNA sequencer-based total serum protein glycomics. *Nat Med* 2004;10:429–34.

164. Kirmiz C, Li B, An HJ, Clowers BH, Chew HK, Lam KS, et al. A serum glycomics approach to breast cancer biomarkers. *Mol Cell Proteomics* 2007;6:43–55.

165. An HJ, Miyamoto S, Lancaster KS, Kirmiz C, Li B, Lam KS, et al. Profiling of glycans in serum for the discovery of potential biomarkers for ovarian cancer. *J Proteome Res* 2006;5:1626–35.

166. Kanoelani T. Pilobello LKDSLKM. Development of a lectin microarray for the rapid analysis of protein glycopatterns. *Chembiochem* 2005;6:985–9.

167. Hsu KL, Mahal LK. A lectin microarray approach for the rapid analysis of bacterial glycans. *Nat Protoc* 2006;1:543–9.

12

MODELING EFFICACY AND SAFETY OF ENGINEERED BIOLOGICS

JEFFREY R. CHABOT AND BRUCE GOMES

Contents

12.1 INTRODUCTION

A rapidly growing segment of the pharmaceutical industry is comprised of so-called *biological therapeutics* (or *biologics*). In these therapies the agent molecules are not small, synthetically produced compounds traditionally

Drug Efficacy, Safety, and Biologics Discovery: Emerging Technologies and Tools,
Edited by Sean Ekins and Jinghai J. Xu
Copyright © 2009 by John Wiley & Sons, Inc.

utilized as pharmaceutical agents. The therapeutics are derived instead from naturally occurring biological materials. In some instances, the agents are exactly the same as those occurring in (normal) individuals, and are supplied exogenously to correct for a disease-related deficiency or to confer some other beneficial effect. In other cases, classes of naturally arising molecules provide templates that can be customized to optimize binding properties or other characteristics such as enzymatic activity. There are other therapies that do not closely resemble any particular species but utilize the same building blocks as classes of native factors, for example, nucleotides. Finally, some therapeutic molecules are derived by analogy to natural biomolecules but are altered for improved properties; examples include substituted R-groups that generate nonnatural amino acids and molecules with altered chirality. The growth of biologic therapeutics in recent years has been prodigious, with growth rates from 2001 to 2006 averaging 20% annually (compared to 6–8% for the overall US pharmaceutical market) [1].

Biologics offer a number of advantages over traditional small-molecule therapies. Instead of needing to screen large numbers of synthetic compounds, each of which must be prepared individually, in many cases existing systems can be utilized and manipulated to identify biologic lead material. Some of these processes are not novel; generation of antibodies by challenging animals with non–self-derived factors has been an often-used tool for many years. Other techniques are just emerging for identifying and evolving the properties of biomolecules, but in general, they all take advantage of combinatorial processes that enable the identification of leading candidates from extremely large numbers of other molecules [2,3]. This has the potential to significantly improve the speed with which early stage discovery can progress.

While it is impossible to claim a priori that any exogenously supplied material will not present safety concerns, the scaffolds used for biologics also can lead to improved safety profiles. For example, a humanized antibody generated by grafting specificity-determining residues (only ~7 residues per arm) from the usually nonhuman molecule obtained during screening onto a human IgG scaffold is over 99% homologous to all other IgG molecules in the body [4], and it is therefore highly unlikely to elicit an immunogenic response. The breakdown products of peptide- or nucleotide-based therapeutics are essentially amino acids and nucleic acids. This stands in contrast to small-molecule agents, which need to be carefully screened to identify those that the liver (or other organ/mechanism) will convert into metabolites which also must have an acceptable safety profile.

This chapter will center the discussion on utilizing the tools of systems biology to explore efficacy and safety questions beyond the general features of biologics. This approach utilizes knowledge mining, appropriate experimentation, and mathematical modeling to predict the behavior of biological systems or to explain observed phenomena and offer insight on how to alter them. These tools can be used to gain early insight into how a biologic therapeutic might alter the behavior of a system at the target and organism level.

The process begins with a review of the known relevant biology surrounding the target, often (but not necessarily) including the system or pathway being modulated. (For example, a model of a full signal transduction pathway is unnecessary when the overall response of the organism to the level of stimulant is known, and this "transfer function" may be used as a surrogate for a detailed model of the full system.) Once this model is in place, the action of various biologic agents can be investigated. For example, an antibody that binds the target with a given affinity, or a protease with given binding and catalytic properties, can be introduced into the system. Other properties of the therapeutic agent, such as clearance rates, can be gathered by analysis of typical values for other similar agents; antibodies of a given class tend to be eliminated at similar rates [5,6] (barring significant target-mediated clearances [7,8]). With the inclusion of the proposed therapeutic into the model, various modalities can be compared, ideal or required properties of a chosen modality can also be found, and dosing and/or frequency can be estimated. Potential efficacy or safety concerns can be identified (examples of which will be highlighted later). These predictions can be highly effective when used to inform early-stage decision making to optimize project selection, timeline estimation, and resource allocation.

12.2 PHARMACOKINETIC MODELING

One of the most useful contexts for applying systems biology approaches is the modeling of the dynamics of both the level of therapeutic agents and the body's response to those agents. Historically these time courses are referred to as "pharmacokinetics" and "pharmacodynamics," respectively.

"Pharmacokinetics" refers to the levels of the therapeutic present in the various "compartments" of the body; for an injected circulating biologic often the compartment of interest is the plasma. Some basic features can be applied to pharmacokinetic models of a wide variety of these therapeutics. The next section will deal with modeling the method of delivery, and identification and mathematical description of the route (or routes) of clearance in the system.

Generally, the models utilized for mechanistic pharmacokinetic modeling are comprised of ordinary differential equations (ODEs). These equations, which take the form

$$\frac{d}{dt}[X_i] = f([X_1],[X_2],\ldots,[X_n],k_1,k_2,\ldots,k_p),$$

describe the time course of the concentration of a species X_i. These equations capture the creation, conversion, and destruction of the component species in the model in terms of the concentration of the set of species $\{X_1, \ldots, X_n\}$ and the set of rate constants $\{k_1, \ldots, k_p\}$. Multiple compartments (representing different organs, organelles, cell surface vs. intracellular fluid, etc.) are also allowed, and transfer between these compartments is described similarly using ODEs. A number of software packages exist that allow the user to lay out the framework for a model, set the relevant parameters, simulate a time course, and monitor the levels of any species of interest as well as the fluxes through any reaction.

An important feature to note with these models is that there is no positional dependence; that is, within a "compartment" the system is assumed to be well mixed. In a case where spatial gradients are important (e.g., diffusion of materials within the lens of the eye [9], or therapeutic agent penetration of a tumor mass [10]), partial differential equations (which include variation in position) are employed. These cases can be simulated using finite element modeling approaches, which divide the system into a grid of points and monitor the local concentrations of the species in the model at each point.

12.2.1 Delivery

If intravenous injection is the route of delivery, the concentration within the plasma may be assumed to "jump" in a step increase at the time of delivery. Detailed, finely time-resolved data may actually show some delay in the increase of the therapeutic in the blood as a whole, as it does take some time to get fully mixed with the general circulating plasma pool. However, when considering a model that will simulate days, weeks, or even months of actual time, the few minutes to bring the plasma to well-mixed equilibrium is effectively instantaneous. Other potential delivery mechanisms, such as nasal [11], transdermal [12], subcutaneous [13,14], needle-free injection [15], or oral delivery (often challenging with biologics [16]), require different (and more complicated) approaches.

12.2.2 Clearance

Kidney Filtration   The clearance of substances in the plasma can occur by a variety of mechanisms, some of which can be reasonably approximated. One clearance path, of tremendous significance with small molecules, is via kidney filtration of the plasma. Typically the kidney is perfused by one-fourth of the plasma volume every minute. Filtration occurs as the plasma flows past the glomerulus. Molecules are "sieved" by the glomerulus according to their size (as well as charge and spatial conformation); small molecules readily transfer into the nephron, while larger ones tend to remain in the plasma. In fact, above a threshold around 100 kD, these molecules effectively never partition into the kidney. Table 12.1 (from [17] and [18]) shows the molecular weight and measured glomerular sieving coefficient θ for a list of proteins. The value of θ is not strictly monotonically decreasing as molecular weight increases. If these proteins were purely spherical in shape, with no charge character to their surfaces, θ would be expected to smoothly decline with molecular weight; instead varying degrees of spatial extension and

TABLE 12.1 Glomerular Sieving Coefficients θ for Various Proteins of Given Molecular Size

Protein	Molecular Weight (kD)	Sieving Coefficient θ
Insulin	5.7	0.9
Cytochrome C	12.3	0.9
Lysozyme	14.4	0.8
Myoglobin	19.6	0.794
Ovomucoid	28	0.18
Ovalbumin	43	0.2
Hemoglobin	64	0.046
HAS	69	0.00066
Neutral HAS	70	0.0065
IgG	150	0.00016

Source: From [17,18].

charge largely cause the deviations seen. The sieving coefficient is additionally dependent on the volume flow rate through the kidney; for individuals with significantly altered renal blood flow, this may be an important factor to consider. One publication describes this [17] and includes an analysis of how molecular size and glomerular flow rate combine to produce an effective value for θ.

A potential complication when modeling kidney filtration is the reabsorption of molecules (e.g., glucose) into the plasma that can occur within other parts of the nephron such as the proximal tubule; this can lead to longer half-lives even if glomerular filtration is efficient [19]. If the experimental results do not agree with a model using this approach for representing kidney filtration, reabsorption should be considered (and tested, if possible). Note that filtered molecules may be unstable in the urine (e.g., the activation peptide from carboxypeptidase B (CAPAP) [20]), so measuring the intact levels excreted may not be reflective of the amount filtered. Also the nephron can produce and secrete peptides or other biomolecules into the urine (e.g., adrenomedullin [21]); hence various potential sources of the molecule studied in collected samples may need to be considered.

Additionally, biomolecules have the potential to bind to other, larger proteins. In this case the clearance of the complex depends on the combined sizes of the two proteins, so it may be much slower. For example, human growth hormone (hGH) has a molecular weight of 22 kD, which would give an expected half-life of about 1.5 hours. However, in the plasma, hGH is largely bound to a much larger protein (~60 kD) to form a complex with molecular weight of roughly 82 kD [22] that approaches the limits of kidney filtration and consequently has a much longer half-life (via the kidney route). Such details can easily be included in a mechanistic model of pharmacokinetics.

A half-life implies a first-order decay (with a total flux rate proportional to the amount of the species present) that is characterized by a single first-order rate constant. This constant is given by

$$k = \frac{\ln(2)}{t_{1/2}}.$$

This parameter can then be employed in an ODE model to represent kidney elimination of the filtered species.

Proteolysis   Another clearance route for proteins arises from proteolysis. (If the therapeutic is based on nucleic acids as opposed to amino acids, the action of nucleases can be similarly described.) One or more of the endogenous proteases may cleave the protein of interest, effectively removing it from consideration. If the half-life of the protein in plasma is known, this can be converted into a first-order decay reaction as before. To separate this phenomenon from kidney filtration, proteolytic rates may be measured ex vivo, using plasma collected from the species to be modeled [23]. This allows for translation of this part of the model between species.

Once again, attention must be paid to the various configurations the protein of interest can take, when in certain complexes, or in certain compartments, proteolysis may be enhanced or limited. For example, insulin-like growth factor (IGF) has a half-life (when free) of less than 10 minutes; when in complex with one of several IGF binding proteins and acid-labile subunit (ALS), this half-life grows to 12 hours [24]. An example of a compartment-specific protease is the serine protease neurotrypsin precursor (formerly BSSP-3), which is confined to the brain [25].

Fluid Phase Endocytosis   A third route for clearance of plasma-residing molecules is fluid phase endocytosis [26]. In this process, cells of the endothelium effectively sample small volumes of plasma. This usually happens indiscriminately, meaning that the process does not target particular molecules in the plasma but rather engulfs a mix of factors with concentrations matching the rest of the plasma. The pH within the endocytotic vesicle (endosome) is lowered by the action of proton pumps. At this lower pH certain mechanisms may become active for "rescuing" some of the contents of the endosome. For example, the iron-binding protein transferrin has negligible affinity for its receptor in its apo (non-iron-bound) configuration at neutral pH, but binds avidly ($K_d = 13\,\text{nM}$) at endosomal pH [27,28] (see Figure 12.1a). Once these (and other) sorting steps have taken place, the "rescued" components are exported back to the plasma membrane. Once at the extracellular pH, these factors typically lose their affinity for the membrane-bound machinery and are released. The nonrescued components may be shuttled to a late endosome and eventually a lysosome for degradation at a more acidic pH [29,30]. Fluid phase endocytosis results in a half-life of about one to three days in humans

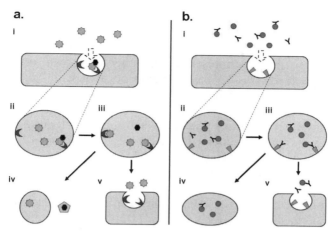

Figure 12.1   Endocytotic recycling machinery. (*a*) Transferrin recycling. (*i*) At neutral pH, transferrin (orange) bound to iron (black) has affinity for the transferrin receptor (purple); unbound (apo-) transferrin must passively diffuse into the forming endosome (*ii*). (*iii*) When the endosome acidifies, iron loses affinity for transferrin while apotransferrin gains affinity for the receptor. (*iv*) Free (nonrescued) transferrin is shuttled to a lysosome and degraded; iron is processed by the cell using other machinery such as ferritin (yellow). (*v*) Receptor-bound apotransferrin is exported to the cell surface where it loses affinity for the receptor at neutral pH. (*b*) IgG recycling. (*i*) At neutral pH, IgG ("*Y*") and target (red) molecules (and the complex of the two) have no affinity for the FcRn receptor (green), and must passively diffuse into the forming endosome (*ii*). (*iii*) When the endosome acidifies, IgG gains affinity for FcRn and may (either free or in complex with the target) bind FcRn. (*iv*) Non–receptor-bound endosome components are moved to a lysosome and destroyed. (*v*) Receptor-bound IgG and complex are returned to the cell surface and released at neutral pH. Note that for both (*a*) and (*b*), the efficiency of recycling of transferrin/IgG is much more efficient than shown here, leading to the lengthy observed half-lives for these proteins. (See color insert.)

for plasma factors that are not actively rescued and recycled using machinery such as that described above [31].

Other Routes for Clearance   Other methods may exist for elimination of therapeutic molecules; if these are known, they can be explicitly included. If, on the other hand, they are unknown, they may sometimes still be effectively represented in an ODE model. A molecule cleared by a number of first-order processes will display an exponential decay, as if it was cleared by a single first-order process. The half-lives of all of the individual processes are connected to the overall half-life by the following formula:

$$\frac{1}{t_{1,2;overall}} = \frac{1}{t_{1/2;proteolysis}} + \frac{1}{t_{1/2;kidney}} + \frac{1}{t_{1/2;endocytosis}} + \frac{1}{t_{1/2;other}}.$$

Note that the final half-life $t_{1/2;overall}$ will be less than any one of the other half-lives, which makes intuitive sense. Given this formula, if the overall half life is known from measurements in some in vivo model, a rate constant for a first-order decay process representing the other "unknown" routes for clearance can be derived. This approach should be used with caution, as these routes may be altered under different, unanticipated situations and the resulting model then offers limited guidance on improving the therapeutic. Nonetheless, it may help recapture the behavior of the system and give a first estimate for what may be expected under different conditions.

An example of a protein class eliminated via "other routes" is IgG. These molecules are too big to be eliminated by the kidney and are mostly resistant to proteolysis. Additionally IgG have a recycling machinery to rescue them from fluid phase endocytosis. At the acidic pH of the endosome, the Fc domain of IgG gains affinity for the FcRn receptor, which returns the IgG to circulation [32] (see Figure 12.1*b*). Experimentally, IgG molecules are found to have a three-week half-life [33] (Table 12.2). A good explanation for the three week half-life comes from failure of the FcRn to rescue the IgG from fluid phase endocytosis [31]. Usually this machinery is successful in preserving the IgG, but a finite chance exists that the recycling will fail for an individual molecule during an endocytosis cycle. The failure rate coupled to the rate of endocytosis gives the three-week half-life. The clearance of IgG can be modeled simply by ascribing a single, first-order decay process with a time constant giving a three-week half-life. This comes at the cost of losing the mechanistic detail that could enable alteration the half-life by modulating the FcRn machinery, but it will suffice if that is not a concern.

Using these general principles, it is possible to generate a model that reasonably describes the pharmacokinetics of many biologic therapeutics. Of course, there are exceptions. The target may mediate some clearance, in proportion to the amount of therapeutic/target complex. The therapeutic may be effectively sequestered within a different "compartment"; for example, it may bind to cells or tissues within another organ and be cleared or slowly released back into the plasma from this reservoir. In any case, a consideration of the biology specifically relevant to the target must take priority with respect to

TABLE 12.2 "Typical" Time Scales of Clearance

Process	Typical Half-life	Reference
Kidney filtration	Size dependent; 40 minutes (<20 kD)→∞ (>100 kD)	[40]
Fluid phase endocytosis	1–3 days (no recycling mechanism)	[31]
IgG clearance	3 weeks (subtype dependent)	[33,79]
Proteolysis	Target/protease dependent	
Target-mediated clearance	Target/mechanism dependent	

the hypotheses used to generate a model. In general, however, the previously described concepts can form a workable initial chassis on which to develop a more informed description of the pharmacokinetics of a particular therapeutic.

12.3 PHARMACODYNAMIC MODELING

With respect to the pharmacodynamics of a particular therapeutic and target, it is more difficult to make general statements. If the target is a receptor present at a constant level, the percentage bound can be calculated using the levels of therapeutic determined in the pharmacokinetic modeling, and the amount free may be input to an experimentally measured transfer function to estimate the therapeutic impact. If the target is a circulating factor, the model may become more complicated as the therapeutic may interfere with natural clearance mechanisms. If the target can complex with other factors (e.g., forming heterodimers), the degree to which this process can occur while bound to the therapeutic needs to be assessed. If the target transfers between "compartments" (e.g., by crossing the blood–brain barrier), the impact of the therapeutic on the rate of transition needs to be considered. In all cases the particulars of the interactions of the therapeutic at the molecular level need to be determined or estimated. An effective pharmacodynamic model will codify and utilize the relevant biology of the target to generate predictions of the efficacy of the proposed therapy.

12.4 ANTIBODY-BASED THERAPIES

Exogenous antibody therapies comprise an important category of biotherapeutics [34,35]. These are of great interest to the pharmaceutical industry because typically there are low safety concerns with antibody use (not precluding the possibility of target-linked toxicities). They can be engineered to have excellent affinity and specificity for their targets, mirroring the properties of the body's own immune system to recognize and efficiently neutralize specific immunogenic targets by the generation of endogenous antibodies. There are numerous established practices for screening, maturation, and production of antibodies that can speed the early discovery process through the identification of lead material [36]. Antibodies have long half-lives that can lead to a reduced frequency of dosing [37]; this can also lead to certain safety concerns, as will be discussed later. Because antibodies require injection for delivery (at this time, there is no orally bioavailable antibody therapy) infrequent dosing represents a desirable improvement and can significantly improve the attractiveness of the therapy as well as patient compliance. These therapies are also typically non-immunogenic, as long as the antibodies are significantly or fully humanized and expressed in an appropriate format [38,39]. A number of antibody therapies are on the market currently. The targets of these antibodies include receptors (e.g., Zenapax® [Roche] for CD25, Erbitux® [ImClone/Bristol Myers Squibb] for EGFR) as well as soluble proteins (e.g., Xolair® [Genentech/Novartis] for IgE, Remicade® [Centocor] for TNFα). Because antibodies do not generally penetrate the cell surface, their targets are usually restricted to the extracellular space.

It is possible to do simple but practically useful pharmacokinetic modeling of antibodies directed against a target of choice. An illustrative example of a target for antibody therapy is a small protein (e.g., a signaling peptide or hormone). Small proteins are very often cleared in a rapid fashion by filtration in the kidney. The smallest proteins cleared predominantly by the kidney have half-lives approaching 40 minutes [40]. However, once the size of the target exceeds about 70 kD, filtration by the kidney is tremendously restricted to the point where its contribution to overall clearance is negligible. In the case of an antibody (with a mass of ~150 kD), which binds very stably to a short peptide, a peptide with a mass of 4 kD is effectively converted into a 154 kD protein. The size of this complex will severely restrict its renal clearance. Consequently, if the small target is expressed with a rate not altered by some biological feedback mechanism, then the rate of generation of target is fixed, but the removal has been slowed. The result is a buildup of total target (the sum of free plus complexed with antibody) present in the system (see Figure 12.2a–b).

In the presence of a high-affinity antibody at a sufficiently high concentration, the target will be almost completely in complex with the antibody. If the target is completely inactive in complex, its buildup will have no adverse effect. Practically speaking, however, two concerns arise. First, the buildup of this complex can lead to issues with the dosing of the therapeutic. To allow for full binding of the target, the antibody must be dosed at or above the projected complex buildup concentration (see Figure 12.2c–f). The second concern is related to the residual activity of the complex. Under ideal conditions, the target–antibody complex would have no potential for interacting with the target's natural partners (receptors, etc.). Practically, however, it is a real concern that the complex may possess some (reduced but nonzero) residual activity. For example, suppose the antibody-binding epitope lies outside the active site of the target but that it is still able to reduce the potency of the target through steric hindrance of interactions to 2% of its original efficacy. Coupled with a hundred-fold buildup, a 2% residual activity implies that the overall target activity would be increased by a factor of two. In one dramatic case [41] the residual activity of the complex buildup proved to be the downfall of an anti-rheumatoid arthritis therapy.

In addition to reduced renal clearance, another factor leading to the long lifetime of exogenous antibodies and antibody-ligand complexes is the circumvention of fluid phase endocytosis. This clearance process by cells of the vasculature would normally lead to the destruction of circulating proteins on the time scale of one to three days [31]. The FcRn machinery, which serves to

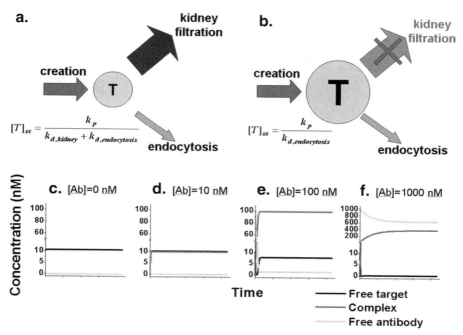

Figure 12.2 Antibody–target complex buildup. (*a, b*) Steady state level of a continuously produced (rate k_p) target T in the presence (*a*) or absence (*b*) of fast kidney filtration (rate $k_{d,kidney}$) and in the presence of slow fluid phase endocytosis (rate $k_{d,endocytosis}$). The formula giving the steady state concentration [T_{ss}] as a function of these rates is shown. In the absence of kidney filtration, the resulting target concentration is significantly increased. (*c–f*) Free target (black), target–antibody complex (red), and free antibody (green) levels for a target normally with 10 nM concentration and 40 minute half-life (i.e., filtered by the kidney). In the presence of 0.1 nM affinity antibody at 10 nM (*d*), 100 nM (*e*), and 1000 nM (*f*), the level of free target is reduced, and the level of target–antibody complex climbs. Note that even when dosed at 100 nM (10 times the starting concentration of target), the entire antibody supply is bound into the complex and a significant amount of target remains unbound. The target is not effectively fully bound until the antibody is dosed above the maximum complex buildup level (thus making the level of target the limiting concentration). Note: In these simulations, the antibody clearance is taken to be zero (total antibody is fixed). (See color insert.)

recycle IgG molecules and prolong their lifetimes, may also reduce the efficiency of endocytosis for clearing the target when in complex with the IgG. If the target does not dissociate from the antibody in the endosome, the FcRn will rescue the target as well as the IgG, leading to a prolongation of the lifetime of the target beyond the one to three days expected for soluble but non–kidney-filterable targets.

Pharmacokinetic modeling indicates that the buildup of this complex may be a concern. The model may be utilized to identify possible solutions. One possible solution might be to take an antibody and modulate the affinity of the Fc region for the FcRn receptor under endosomic pH. Alteration of antibody half-life by altering FcRn binding has previously been reported [42]. By lowering this affinity, the frequency with which the antigen is recycled can be reduced. This lowered affinity can be codified into the pharmacokinetic model. The predictions of this modified model do include a reduced complex buildup, but at the cost of a reduced half-life for the therapeutic (arising from the concomitantly reduced recycling of the antibody). The consequence of this would be a higher frequency dosing regimen.

A more extreme strategy to ameliorate complex buildup is to completely truncate the Fc region of the antibody, leaving the Fab2 region (the branched antigen-binding end of the antibody). This strategy should not alter antigen binding, but completely eliminate the recycling of the therapeutic via the FcRn machinery [43]. The target–antibody complex can now be removed with 100% efficiency by fluid phase endocytosis with the time scale of one to three days (instead of up to three weeks with full IgG). This can lead to a drop of about an order of magnitude in built-up complex. Again, this comes at the cost of more frequent dosing. As Fab2 therapeutics are usually generated by enzymatic cleavage of full IgG molecules (and consequently possess an even greater cost of goods than traditionally produced antibodies), the increase in expense to frequently dose with these fragments can be prohibitive. An alternative strategy for lowering complex buildup should be sought.

Another possibility besides Fab2s would be to produce just the very tip of the antibody (the part that actually binds the ligand); this region is called the V_H (variable heavy) domain on the heavy chain of the antibody, and the V_L (variable light) domain on the light chain. These two domains can be converted into a single peptide referred to as single chain variable fragment (ScFv) and expressed in a high-yield system [44]. These are significantly less expensive to manufacture than full IgG molecules and can therefore represent significant savings on cost of goods. However, these short antibody fragments are sufficiently small (20–30 kD) that they can be efficiently cleared by kidney filtration [45], so the avoidance of complex buildup is only achieved at the expense of requiring injections daily or even more frequently.

In order to make the use of ScFv's more feasible, techniques to avoid of kidney filtration must be identified. One frequent solution employed when increased molecular weight is needed is PEGylation. Adding a polymer of ethylene glycol has been shown in many cases to produce biologically well-tolerated molecules with the advantages (or disadvantages, in some instances) of increased size [46,47]. By PEGylating ScFv's and raising their molecular weight above the effective kidney filtration size limit, the therapeutic half-life can be raised [45]. Once again, however, the buildup of the complex is a consideration. A potential issue also exists when employing PEGylation. An attenuation of the potency of PEGylated therapeutic molecules has been reported [48,49], which may arise from the polymer "wrapping around" the therapeutic or otherwise sterically hindering its ability to interact with its target. If this strategy enables the maintenance of a significant increase in concentration by prolonging the half-life, a similarly significant decrease in potency may effectively eliminate any gains achieved.

An additional concern with PEGylation is "syringability." At high concentrations and large PEG sizes, PEGylation can cause a dramatic increase in viscosity, to the extent that injection through a reasonably sized hypodermic needle becomes impractical. One strategy to mitigate this difficulty involves the utilization of multiarm or "dendronized" PEG molecules for conjugation [50]. These polymers allow for the conjugation of a number of therapeutic agents, lowering the overall number of conjugate molecules needed in order to achieve the same effective therapeutic dose.

Another possible solution to the antibody dilemma is the fusion of antibodies to other proteins (either wholly or with their appropriate functional domains). An ideal antibody-based therapy would combine the rapid destruction of the target with efficient recycling of the therapeutic. Antibodies already possess sufficient recycling; the problem is the lack of rapid target destruction (thus leading to the complex buildup). If an appropriate fusion protein could be developed, a long-lasting therapy with less complex buildup would result. One possible approach might be to fuse functional domains of other proteins to the variable (i.e., antigen-binding) region of antibodies. One such candidate for fusion to antibodies that has been gaining in popularity is transferrin [51]. As discussed in Section 12.2.2, this iron-binding protein is efficiently recycled by its receptor. In addition, when complexed to iron in the plasma, it is very rapidly bound to a surface receptor, actively endocytosed, and (following iron unloading in the acidic endosomal environment) recycled to the plasma [27]. Compared to normal antibodies, a binding domain fused with transferrin should lead to more rapid uptake of the therapeutic/target complex. This greater endocytosis frequency, coupled with a finite chance of destroying the target per endocytosis event, translates to a more rapid overall clearance of the target. This makes the fusion protein/transferrin receptor/endosome system effectively behave catalytically, where over time a single therapeutic molecule could remove a number of the target molecules. This increased turnover would result in a lower complex buildup without necessarily shortening the lifetime of the therapeutic.

A final comment on the use of antibody (or antibody-based derivative) therapies: the concern about complex buildup for soluble factors is only relevant for continuously produced targets (and worst for small, rapidly cleared ligands). A therapeutic target may originate from an acute injury, trauma, or environmental factor such as stroke, heart attack, or poisoning (see Figure 12.3). In these instances there is a single bolus of target, and the total level (free plus bound) will not exceed that initial level. However, the average lifetime of a target molecule may still be significantly prolonged. This results in a larger "area under the curve" for the target, which is actually the sum of two curves representing free and bound target. An effect versus time curve can be generated if the activity of the bound target is known. If the target acts imme-

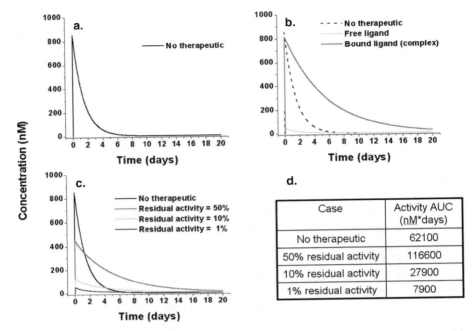

Figure 12.3 Antibody therapeutic directed against acutely-introduced target. (*a*) Time course of target level in the absence of treatment. Target is introduced at $t = 0$ at a level of $1\,\mu M$, and is assumed to clear by fluid phase endocytosis (with $t_{1/2} = 1$ day). (*b*) Time course of target in the presence of $1\,\mu M$ IgG (affinity = $10\,nM$). Bound ligand/IgG complex is shown in red (with a clearance time $t_{1/2} = 5$ days), and free ligand is shown in green. The same curve as in (*a*) is shown as a dashed line for reference. (*c*) Time courses of total target activity. The sum of the free ligand and the activity of the bound complex (the product of residual activity and complex level) is shown for various residual activities (50%, 10%, 1%). (*d*) Area-under-the-curve values for curves shown in (*c*). A therapy leaving 50% residual activity represents approximately a twofold worsening of integrated target activity, 10% residual activity represents only a twofold improvement, and 1% residual activity results is about a 10-fold therapeutic advantage. (See color insert.)

diately, and has no cumulative effect over time, an antibody therapy is an excellent approach if it serves to even partially reduce the activity of the target. The peak of the target effect curve is necessarily lower in the presence of even mildly inactivating, moderate affinity antibody than in its absence. In contrast, if the target's biological impact is cumulative, then the area under the target effect curve is the relevant quantity. The area under the treatment curve may significantly exceed the area under the no-treatment curve if the complex retains significant activity. In general, if the fold increase in half-life is less than the fold decrease in complex activity, a therapeutic benefit will be realized for all patients.

12.5 APTAMER-BASED THERAPIES

The next category of biotherapeutics to be considered is aptamers. An excellent overall review of aptamer technology and comparison to antibodies can be found in a recent review [52]. Aptamers are short oligonucleotide sequences, similar to RNA or DNA. However, the sequence of an aptamer is not selected to code for any peptide or to interact with genetic material (as for siRNA). Rather, the sequence is chosen because it possesses the property of binding to a target of interest (e.g., an active domain of a disease-linked factor). The advantages of using aptamers instead of antibodies are twofold. First, it is very easy to pan for sequences with affinity for the target. From a "soup" of random sequences, those that adhere to an immobilized target can be extracted and amplified using polymerase chain reaction procedures. Additionally the number of different sequences used during the first rounds of screening can be 10^5 times higher than when panning for antibodies using techniques such as phage display [53]. The second advantage comes from a cost-of-goods standpoint: aptamers are considerably less expensive to produce on a large scale than antibodies. They can be synthesized (as opposed to antibodies, which must be expressed) and large amounts can be made using well-established technologies.

It has been shown that a range of specificities and affinities comparable to antibodies can be achieved using aptamers [54]. Aptamers have been demonstrated to be non-immunogenic [55,56]. They possess a high degree of solubility, being constructed from highly polar units. One approved aptamer therapy exists currently at the time of writing (Macugen® [Pfizer/OSI Eyetech], for macular degeneration) while a number of candidates are in clinical development (see Table 12.3).

TABLE 12.3 Aptamers in Various Stages of Development

Aptamer	Target	Clinical Phase	Developer
Pegaptanib (Macugen®)	VEGF/macular degeneration	Approved (2004)	Pfizer/OSI Eyetech
Edifoligide[a]	E2F/coronary/peripheral bypass surgery	Phase III (no improvement over placebo)	Anesiva
Avrina[a]	NF-kB/eczema	Phase III	Anesiva
AS1411	Nucleolin/oncology	Phase I/II	Antisoma
REG1	Factor IX/anticoagulant	Phase I (complete)	Regado Biosciences
ARC183	Thrombin/anticoagulant	Phase I (complete; on hold)	Archemix
NU172 (ARC2172)	Thrombin/anticoagulant	Preclinical	Nuvelo/Archemix

Source: Adapted from [80].

[a]Target mimetics.

One problem arising with aptamers is the duration of potency for the therapy. As aptamers are comprised of short oligonucleotide sequences, they often fall well within the size range of molecules efficiently sieved from the blood by the kidney and eliminated in the urine [57]. An additional problem when treating with aptamers is degradation by nucleases, which can result in clearance with a very rapid time scale [58]. These rapid clearances, when coupled with the need to administer aptamers by injection, may limit their therapeutic utility.

One strategy to improve the pharmacokinetics of aptamer therapies is the use of spiegelmers. An ordinary aptamer is constructed using D-oligonucleotides (with the chirality normally found in all living organisms). A spiegelmer (from the German *Spiegel*, or "mirror"), on the other hand, is an aptamer synthesized using L-nucleotides. The method for generating spiegelmers is as follows: First, the target epitope of interest is synthesized using L-amino acids, which effectively generates a mirror image of the native target peptide. Next an ordinary (D-) aptamer is identified with good binding properties for this mirror epitope. Finally, the identified aptamer sequence is synthesized using L-nucleotides, which should have good binding affinity for the native D-peptide. The extra step is needed because the polymerase enzymes used during aptamer panning, selection, and amplification can only operate on D-nucleotides. The final product has the significant advantage of not being recognized by native polynucleotide degradation enzymes, but carries the manufacturing liability inasmuch as it cannot be produced using normally arising enzymes. The in vitro stability of spiegelmers is in fact extraordinary; a 58-mer of D-RNA incubated in human serum displayed a half-life of less than 12 seconds, whereas an L-RNA spiegelmer with the same primary sequence showed no significant decay after 60 hours under the same conditions [58]. Finally, spiegelmers, similar to aptamers, have been shown to have low immunogenic risk [59].

Even if clearance by nuclease action can be neglected, an aptamer therapy may still be impractical from a dosing standpoint, as clearance by the kidneys still represents a significant hurdle to acceptable pharmacokinetics. Once again, PEGylation may represent a solution to preventing filtration by increasing molecular weight; one study [60] found that the terminal phase half life could be doubled or tripled with the addition of a 20 or 40kD PEG, respectively. This approach again comes with the warnings about reduction of potency by steric interference of the PEG and increased viscosity of the PEGylated therapeutic (see Section 12.4).

The dual approaches of PEGylation and the spiegelmer technique can be combined to generate novel therapeutics [61]. Pharmacokinetic modeling can give an estimate of the improvement in overall therapeutic half-life. In the extreme limiting case when both kidney filtration and nuclease degradation are completely abolished, the dominant route of clearance becomes fluid phase endocytosis, which gives the therapy an effective half-life of approximately one to three days. In one study [59] the pharmacological effects of a

PEGylated spiegelmer persisted for 48 hours, compared to 6 hours for a non-PEGylated but otherwise identical spiegelmer (at twice the dose). Potential concerns again arise with the buildup of therapeutic–ligand complexes. However, if these complexes have a low enough activity and the levels of the target and complex are small enough, this PEGylated spiegelmer strategy may be sufficient for weekly dosing, and represent a desirable modality for addressing certain conditions.

12.6 BIOMOLECULE-BASED THERAPIES

The next set of biotherapeutics to be considered includes "biomolecules," natural or slightly modified molecules such as hormones or signaling peptides that natively occur within the body. These molecules can be used therapeutically in a number of ways:

- Disease may occur when these molecules are not present at a sufficient level. For example, hypoinsulinemia is a characteristic of Type I diabetes, and stature deficiency is caused by lowered growth hormone levels. In these cases supplementing or replacing the natural production of the relevant biomolecules may provide a therapeutic gain.
- Superphysiological doses may confer a therapeutic benefit. A number of natural appetite-suppressing peptides are being investigated as treatments for obesity (see Table 12.4).

TABLE 12.4 Peptides under Investigation for Regulation of Appetite

Peptide	Effect on Food Intake
CCK	
Bombesin	
Gastrin-releasing peptide	
GIP	
Apolipoprotein A-IV	
GLP-1	Reduced
Amylin	intake
Exendin-4	
PYY_{3-36} (peripheral)	
Obestatin	
Enterostatin	
Oxyntomodulin	
Ghrelin	Increased
β-casomorphin	intake

Source: Adapted from [81].

- Acute administration may achieve a beneficial effect. For example, atrial natriuretic peptide (ANP) is utilized for increasing sodium excretion and decreasing blood pressure in hypertension or chronic heart failure [62].
- Treatment in combination with small molecules may result in synergistic benefits. Supplementing pioglitazone with glucagon-like peptide-1 (GLP-1) has been shown to increase glucose-lowering in diabetes [63].

Modification of these biomolecules may be performed to improve therapeutic response. For example, amide permethylation has been utilized to identify altered peptides with antimicrobial activity [64], and N-methylated derivatives of beta-amyloid fragments have been shown to be potentially useful as therapeutic agents to prevent amyloid formation in Alzheimer's disease [65]. These molecules may also come from nonhuman origin; exendin-4 (marketed synthetically as Byetta® [exenatide; Amylin Pharmaceuticals/Eli Lilly]), originally derived from Gila monster *Heloderma suspectum* venom, is a potent supplemental therapy for hyperglycemia in diabetic patients [66].

Biomolecules carry a low risk of toxicity or immunogenicity (at least at physiological levels) as these substances exist naturally within the human body. They possess a naturally arising specificity and affinity; their receptors have evolved specifically to recognize them. These molecules often have half-lives that are rather short but are appropriate when produced endogenously at suitable rates. For example, peptides involved in appetite regulation are often cleared in minutes [67,68], which is appropriate for managing a behavior that fluctuates on the order of hours (the postprandial production of a persistent anorectic agent could interfere with later feeding). One major difficulty with supplying these molecules exogenously is that these rapid clearances may necessitate frequent dosing to maintain the desired circulating levels. This requirement is made especially troublesome when injections are required for delivery of the therapeutic.

Often a major route for clearance of these biomolecules is proteolysis. If one particular protease is responsible for the bulk of the clearance, or if multiple proteases are involved but share a single recognition site on the molecule, altering the docking or cleavage site by mutation or chemical alteration may generate improved pharmacokinetics. Such altered molecules need to be tested to ensure that the functionality of the molecule is retained. One striking example of mutation to reduce clearance while maintaining potency is an altered form of human growth hormone (HGH) [69]. In this work, altering a single residue in HGH shifted the in vitro lifetime of the molecule in plasma from 20 minutes to 7 days, with a negligible shift in potency. In another example, oxyntomodulin, a peptide involved in regulating appetite, is normally cleared from human plasma (largely by DPP-4 protease activity) with a half-life of less than 12 minutes [67]. Mutants of oxyntomodulin, including some with substituted nonnatural amino acids have been identified, and they have significantly longer half-lives and retained bioactivity [70].

If no mutation strategy can be identified, or if the resulting increased lifetime is still not sufficient, alternate delivery strategies (other than injection) can be considered to make frequent dosing more acceptable. Testosterone can be delivered via subcutaneous implants (Organon Laboratories) that maintain appropriate circulating levels for four to five months, by transdermal patch (Andropatch®, GlaxoSmithKline) that is replaced daily or a gel applied to the skin (Testim® gel, Ipsen). Recently advances in formulation technologies have resulted in novel delivery mechanisms for previously injection-only therapies. For example, Exubera® (Pfizer/Nektar/Sanofi-Aventis) is a spray-dried fast-acting insulin formulation with a high glass transition temperature, yielding a powder with tight reproducible particle size and moisture content [71]. This powder is inhaled by the patient, reducing the need for injections of this biotherapeutic. Other formulations for insulin, including nasally delivered, have been tested in animals [72]. As technologies such as these continue to evolve, the attractiveness of biotherapies will continue to increase from both a pharmaceutical and patient standpoint.

12.7 ENGINEERED PROTEASE THERAPIES

A final biotherapeutics platform that is gaining in popularity is engineered proteases. Native proteases have evolved to effectively degrade their substrates. In a number of disease conditions where the causative agent has a reasonably nonpromiscuous protease, the natural enzyme (or one prepared recombinantly) may be useful as a therapeutic. Examples of natural proteases which are used therapeutically include Factor VIIa (NovoSeven®, Novo Nordisk) and Factor IX (BeneFIX®, Wyeth) for hemophilia, tissue-type plasminogen activator (Activase®, Genentech) for blood clots, activated protein C (Xigris®, Eli Lilly) for sepsis, and botulinum toxin type A (Botox®, Allergan) for cosmetics.

If no natural (known) protease exists for a given target, or if the native protease interacts with many targets (and therefore carries a significant risk of side effects when administered systematically), then mutation of native proteases may permit a therapeutic window. Strategies for altering natural proteases to achieve desired properties have been studied for some time. For example, the binding domain of trypsin has been altered to generate mutants with altered substrate specificity [73]. Mutants of activated protein C (a serine protease) have been generated that preserve the same substrate binding but have other altered properties that render them resistant to inactivation by protein C inhibitor and α1-antitrypsin [74]. Researchers have successfully altered the substrate specificity of a bacterial α-lytic serine protease (a protease-bearing homology to mammalian proteases) [75]. A general review of directed mutagenesis of enzymes in general (including proteases) with the goal of achieving "rational alteration of enzyme specificity and reactivity" is available [76].

An example of engineering of proteases to attack novel targets can be found in the approach of Catalyst Biosciences. This company is approaching the generation of engineered therapeutic proteases in a similar way to approaches used to identify antibodies or small-molecule therapies. The process begins with a library of natural proteases. A round of "rational mutagenesis" follows, along with combinatorial selection to build a greatly enhanced collection of proteases with a range of substrate binding properties and enzymatic activity. Once a target has been identified, the protease library is screened against the target to identify initial hits. These proteases then go through rounds of "evolution" in order to obtain the desired therapeutic properties [77].

The advantages of a protease-based therapy are numerous. The need for considering the buildup of target–therapeutic complexes is minimal, while the complex generated is designed to undergo proteolytic cleavage; therefore the target should retain no activity. The catalytic nature of proteases implies a need for lower (substoichiometric) doses. With a high-affinity, high-turnover protease a dose much lower than the target level may be sufficient to significantly lower the concentration of the target. Indeed this strategy may represent the only way to address problems with certain high-concentration targets.

A major concern with protease therapies is obtaining the (1) affinity, (2) specificity, and (3) catalytic activity needed to attack a particular target. A good affinity is needed in order to obtain a potent therapy. Specificity is absolutely critical to avoid destruction of nontarget proteins. The development of assays to determine any "off-target" proteolytic activity is required in order to validate the specificity of the protease; such assays present significant technical hurdles. A good catalytic activity is required to ensure that the target is in fact cleared; in the absence of any catalytic capacity, the protease is reduced to a simple binding factor for the target, build up target/therapeutic complex begins, and the dosing advantage gained by using a protease is lost.

One of the greatest challenges facing the development of protease therapies with these three properties is the avoidance of immunogenicity. As naturally occurring proteases are mutated repeatedly to get the required affinity, specificity, and catalytic activity for the new target of interest, the resulting protein begins to look less and less like the native (non-immunogenic) protein. The chance of generating an epitope that is capable of stimulating an immune response becomes more of a concern. Clearly, there is much opportunity and motivation for the development of techniques for obtaining the desired therapeutic properties while overcoming this hurdle.

12.8 CONCLUSION

The growing field of biologic therapeutics utilizes numerous strategies, including antibodies, aptamers, biomolecules, and engineered proteases. Each of these modalities has its own particular set of advantages and drawbacks that must be considered in the context of each particular target to select the best platform for the desired therapeutic goal. Mechanistic systems modeling of pharmacokinetics and pharmacodynamics can identify these concerns for general cases, provide estimates of the magnitude of the problem early in the discovery and development process for particular therapies, and suggest avenues for avoiding or mitigating them. A number of existing and novel discoveries are enabling the continual evolution of biologic therapeutics. As a final comment on the significant role that biotherapeutics will play in the future of the pharmaceutical industry, from 2007 to 2010 the forecast for biologic therapeutics is projected to grow by \$26 billion, representing 60% of revenue growth for the industry over that time period [78]. Modeling can make the process of generating these therapeutics more efficient, expedited, economical and can efficacious and can speed novel, quality, and safe therapies to the patients who need them.

REFERENCES

1. Aggarwal S. What's fueling the biotech engine? *Nat Biotechnol* 2007;25: 1097–104.
2. Filpula D. Antibody engineering and modification technologies. *Biomol Eng* 2007;24:201–15.
3. Cerchia L, De Franciscis V. Nucleic acid-based aptamers as promising therapeutics in neoplastic diseases. Meth *Mol Biol* 2007;361:187–200.
4. Almagro JC. Identification of differences in the specificity-determining residues of antibodies that recognize antigens of different size: implications for the rational design of antibody repertoires. *J Mol Recognit* 2004;17:132–43.
5. Koleba T, Ensom MH. Pharmacokinetics of intravenous immunoglobulin: a systematic review. *Pharmacotherapy* 2006;26:813–27.
6. Presta LG. Engineering of therapeutic antibodies to minimize immunogenicity and optimize function. *Adv Drug Deliv Rev* 2006;58:640–56.
7. Coffey GP, Fox JA, Pippig S, Palmieri S, Reitz B, Gonzales M, et al. Tissue distribution and receptor-mediated clearance of anti-CD11a antibody in mice. *Drug Metab Dispos* 2005;33:623–9.
8. Coffey GP, Stefanich E, Palmieri S, Eckert R, Padilla-Eagar J, Fielder PJ, et al. In vitro internalization, intracellular transport, and clearance of an anti-CD11a antibody (Raptiva) by human T-cells. *J Pharmacol Exp Ther* 2004;310:896–904.
9. McNulty R, Wang H, Mathias RT, Ortwerth BJ, Truscott RJ, Bassnett S. Regulation of tissue oxygen levels in the mammalian lens. *J Physiol* 2004;559:883–98.
10. Graff CP, Wittrup KD. Theoretical analysis of antibody targeting of tumor spheroids: importance of dosage for penetration, and affinity for retention. *Cancer Res* 2003;63:1288–96.
11. Del Giudice G, Pizza M, Rappuoli R. Mucosal delivery of vaccines. *Methods* 1999;19:148–55.

12. Garg S, Hoelscher M, Belser JA, Wang C, Jayashankar L, Guo Z, et al. Needle-free skin patch delivery of a vaccine for a potentially pandemic influenza virus provides protection against lethal challenge in mice. *Clin Vaccine Immunol* 2007;14:926–8.

13. Yang MX, Shenoy B, Disttler M, Patel R, McGrath M, Pechenov S, et al. Crystalline monoclonal antibodies for subcutaneous delivery. *Proc Natl Acad Sci USA* 2003;100:6934–9.

14. Wahl RL, Laino L, Fisher S, Schteingart M, Beierwaltes WH. Improved radio-immunolocalization of human tumor xenografts following subcutaneous delivery of monoclonal antibodies. *Eur J Nucl Med* 1988;13:530–6.

15. Chen D, Maa YF, Haynes JR. Needle-free epidermal powder immunization. *Exp Rev Vaccines* 2002;1:265–76.

16. Shah RB, Ahsan F, Khan MA. Oral delivery of proteins: progress and prognostication. *Crit Rev Ther Drug Carrier Syst* 2002;19:135–69.

17. Lund U, Rippe A, Venturoli D, Tenstad O, Grubb A, Rippe B. Glomerular filtration rate dependence of sieving of albumin and some neutral proteins in rat kidneys. *Am J Physiol Renal Physiol* 2003;284:F1226–34.

18. Maack T, Hyung Park C, Carmago MJF. Renal filtration, transport, and metabolism of proteins. In: Seldin DW, Giebisch G, eds. *The kidney: physiology and pathophysiology*. New York: Raven, 1992.

19. Lazzara MJ, Deen WM. Model of albumin reabsorption in the proximal tubule. *Am J Physiol Renal Physiol* 2007;292:F430–9.

20. Appelros S, Thim L, Borgstrom A. Activation peptide of carboxypeptidase B in serum and urine in acute pancreatitis. *Gut* 1998;42:97–102.

21. Sato K, Hirata Y, Imai T, Iwashina M, Marumo F. Characterization of immunoreactive adrenomedullin in human plasma and urine. *Life Sci* 1995;57:189–94.

22. Herington AC, Smith AI, Wallace C, Stevenson JL. Partial purification from human serum of a specific binding protein for human growth hormone. *Mol Cell Endocrinol* 1987;53:203–9.

23. John H, Hierer J, Haas O, Forssmann WG. Quantification of angiotensin-converting-enzyme-mediated degradation of human chemerin 145–154 in plasma by matrix-assisted laser desorption/ionization-time-of-flight mass spectrometry. *Anal Biochem* 2007;362:117–25.

24. Collett-Solberg PF, Nunn SE, Gibson TB, Cohen P. Identification of novel high molecular weight insulin-like growth factor-binding protein-3 association proteins in human serum. *J Clin Endocrinol Metab* 1998;83:2843–8.

25. Yamamura Y, Yamashiro K, Tsuruoka N, Nakazato H, Tsujimura A, Yamaguchi N. Molecular cloning of a novel brain-specific serine protease with a kringle-like structure and three scavenger receptor cysteine-rich motifs. *Biochem Biophys Res Commun* 1997;239:386–92.

26. Gurbaxani B. Mathematical modeling as accounting: predicting the fate of serum proteins and therapeutic monoclonal antibodies. *Clin Immunol* 2007;122:121–4.

27. Dautry-Varsat A. Receptor-mediated endocytosis: the intracellular journey of transferrin and its receptor. *Biochimie* 1986;68:375–81.

28. Dautry-Varsat A, Ciechanover A, Lodish HF. pH and the recycling of transferrin during receptor-mediated endocytosis. *Proc Natl Acad Sci USA* 1983;80:2258–62.

29. Bishop NE. Dynamics of endosomal sorting. *Int Rev Cytol* 2003;232:1–57.

30. Smith MW, Gumbleton M. Endocytosis at the blood–brain barrier: from basic understanding to drug delivery strategies. *J Drug Target* 2006;14:191–214.

31. Garg A, Balthasar JP. Physiologically-based pharmacokinetic (PBPK) model to predict IgG tissue kinetics in wild-type and FcRn-knockout mice. *J Pharmacokinet Pharmacodyn* 2007;34:687–709.

32. Rodewald R. pH-dependent binding of immunoglobulins to intestinal cells of the neonatal rat. *J Cell Biol* 1976;71:666–9.

33. Waldman TA, Strober W. Metabolism of immunoglobulins. *Prog Allergy* 1969;13: 1–110.

34. Maggon K. Monoclonal antibody "gold rush." *Curr Med Chem* 2007;14:1978–87.

35. Jain M, Kamal N, Batra SK. Engineering antibodies for clinical applications. *Trends Biotechnol* 2007;25:307–16.

36. Benhar I. Design of synthetic antibody libraries. *Expert Opin Biol Ther* 2007;7:763–79.

37. Ternant D, Paintaud G. Pharmacokinetics and concentration-effect relationships of therapeutic monoclonal antibodies and fusion proteins. *Expert Opin Biol Ther* 2005;5(suppl 1):S37–47.

38. Kuus-Reichel K, Grauer LS, Karavodin LM, Knott C, Krusemeier M, Kay NE. Will immunogenicity limit the use, efficacy, and future development of therapeutic monoclonal antibodies? *Clin Diagn Lab Immunol* 1994;1:365–72.

39. Hwang WY, Foote J. Immunogenicity of engineered antibodies. *Methods* 2005;36: 3–10.

40. Venturoli D, Rippe B. Ficoll and dextran vs. globular proteins as probes for testing glomerular permselectivity: effects of molecular size, shape, charge, and deformability. *Am J Physiol Renal Physiol* 2005;288:F605–13.

41. Haringman JJ, Gerlag DM, Smeets TJ, Baeten D, van den Bosch F, Bresnihan B, et al. A randomized controlled trial with an anti-CCL2 (anti-monocyte chemotactic protein 1) monoclonal antibody in patients with rheumatoid arthritis. *Arthritis Rheum* 2006;54:2387–92.

42. Ghetie V, Popov S, Borvak J, Radu C, Matesoi D, Medesan C, et al. Increasing the serum persistence of an IgG fragment by random mutagenesis. *Nat Biotechnol* 1997;15:637–40.

43. Raghavan M, Bjorkman PJ. Fc receptors and their interactions with immunoglobulins. *Ann Rev Cell Dev Biol* 1996;12:181–220.

44. Ward ES. Antibody engineering: the use of *Escherichia coli* as an expression host. *FASEB J* 1992;6:2422–7.

45. Kubetzko S, Balic E, Waibel R, Zangemeister-Wittke U, Pluckthun A. PEGylation and multimerization of the anti-p185HER-2 single chain Fv fragment 4D5: effects on tumor targeting. *J Biol Chem* 2006;281:35186–201.

46. Schwarz KB, Mohan P, Narkewicz MR, Molleston JP, Nash SR, Hu S, et al. Safety, efficacy and pharmacokinetics of peginterferon alpha2a (40kd) in children with chronic hepatitis C. *J Pediatr Gastroenterol Nutr* 2006;43:499–505.

47. Avramis VI, Sencer S, Periclou AP, Sather H, Bostrom BC, Cohen LJ, et al. A randomized comparison of native *Escherichia coli* asparaginase and polyethylene

glycol conjugated asparaginase for treatment of children with newly diagnosed standard-risk acute lymphoblastic leukemia: a Children's Cancer Group study. *Blood* 2002;99:1986–94.

48. Bailon P, Berthold W. Polyethylene glycol-conjugated pharmaceutical proteins. *Pharmaceut Sci Technol Today* 1998;1:352–6.

49. Bailon P, Palleroni A, Schaffer CA, Spence CL, Fung WJ, Porter JE, et al. Rational design of a potent, long-lasting form of interferon: a 40kDa branched polyethylene glycol-conjugated interferon alpha-2a for the treatment of hepatitis C. *Bioconjug Chem* 2001;12:195–202.

50. Pasut G, Veronese FM. PEGylation of proteins as tailored chemistry for optimized bioconjugates. *Adv Polym Sci* 2006;192:95–134.

51. Sadeghi H, Prior CP, Turner A. Modified transferrin-antibody fusion proteins. Needham, MA: BioRexis Pharmaceutical Corporation, 2003.

52. Nimjee SM, Rusconi CP, Sullenger BA. Aptamers: an emerging class of therapeutics. *Ann Rev Med* 2005;56:555–83.

53. Eulberg D, Jarosch F, Vonhoff S, Klussmann S. Spiegelmers for therapeutic applications—use of chiral principles in evolutionary selection techniques. In: Klussmann S, ed. *The aptamer handbook: functional oligonucleotides and their applications.* Hoboken, NJ: Wiley, 2006, p. 417–42.

54. Gebhardt K, Shokraei A, Babaie E, Lindqvist BH. RNA aptamers to S-adenosyl-homocysteine: kinetic properties, divalent cation dependency, and comparison with anti-S-adenosylhomocysteine antibody. *Biochemistry* 2000;39:7255–65.

55. Preclinical and phase 1A clinical evaluation of an anti-VEGF pegylated aptamer (EYE001) for the treatment of exudative age-related macular degeneration. *Retina* 2002;22:143–52.

56. Anti-vascular endothelial growth factor therapy for subfoveal choroidal neovascularization secondary to age-related macular degeneration: phase II study results. *Ophthalmology* 2003;110:979–86.

57. Borkowski S, Dinkelborg LM. Aptamers for in vivo imaging. In: Klussmann S, ed. *The aptamer handbook: functional oligonucleotides and their applications.* Hoboken, NJ: Wiley, 2006, p. 343–62.

58. Klussmann S, Nolte A, Bald R, Erdmann VA, Furste JP. Mirror-image RNA that binds D-adenosine. *Nat Biotechnol* 1996;14:1112–5.

59. Wlotzka B, Leva S, Eschgfaller B, Burmeister J, Kleinjung F, Kaduk C, et al. In vivo properties of an anti-GnRH Spiegelmer: an example of an oligonucleotide-based therapeutic substance class. *Proc Natl Acad Sci USA* 2002;99:8898–902.

60. Healy JM, Lewis SD, Kurz M, Boomer RM, Thompson KM, Wilson C, et al. Pharmacokinetics and biodistribution of novel aptamer compositions. *Pharm Res* 2004;21:2234–46.

61. Kobelt P, Helmling S, Stengel A, Wlotzka B, Andresen V, Klapp BF, et al. Anti-ghrelin Spiegelmer NOX-B11 inhibits neurostimulatory and orexigenic effects of peripheral ghrelin in rats. *Gut* 2006;55:788–92.

62. Cody RJ, Atlas SA, Laragh JH, Kubo SH, Covit AB, Ryman KS, et al. Atrial natriuretic factor in normal subjects and heart failure patients. Plasma levels and

renal, hormonal, and hemodynamic responses to peptide infusion. *J Clin Invest* 1986;78:1362–74.

63. Zander M, Christiansen A, Madsbad S, Holst JJ. Additive effects of glucagon-like peptide 1 and pioglitazone in patients with type 2 diabetes. *Diabetes Care* 2004;27:1910–4.

64. Ostresh JM, Husar GM, Blondelle SE, Dorner B, Weber PA, Houghten RA. "Libraries from libraries": chemical transformation of combinatorial libraries to extend the range and repertoire of chemical diversity. *Proc Natl Acad Sci USA* 1994;91:11138–42.

65. Hughes E, Burke RM, Doig AJ. Inhibition of toxicity in the beta-amyloid peptide fragment beta-(25–35) using *N*-methylated derivatives: a general strategy to prevent amyloid formation. *J Biol Chem* 2000;275:25109–15.

66. Mikhail N. Exenatide: a novel approach for treatment of type 2 diabetes. *South Med J* 2006;99:1271–9.

67. Schjoldager BT, Baldissera FG, Mortensen PE, Holst JJ, Christiansen J. Oxyntomodulin: a potential hormone from the distal gut. Pharmacokinetics and effects on gastric acid and insulin secretion in man. *Eur J Clin Invest* 1988;18: 499–503.

68. Drucker DJ. Biologic actions and therapeutic potential of the proglucagon-derived peptides. *Nat Clin Pract Endocrinol Metab* 2005;1:22–31.

69. Alam KS, Morimoto M, Yoshizato H, Fujikawa T, Furukawa K, Tanaka M, et al. Expression and purification of a mutant human growth hormone that is resistant to proteolytic cleavage by thrombin, plasmin and human plasma in vitro. *J Biotechnol* 1998;65:183–90.

70. Roy RS, Bianchi E, Pessi A, Ingallinella P, Marsh DJ, Eiermann G, et al. Oxyntomodulin derivatives. Merck and Co., Instituto di Richerche di Biologia Molecolare P. Angeletti S.P.A., 2007.

71. White S, Bennett DB, Cheu S, Conley PW, Guzek DB, Gray S, et al. Exubera: pharmaceutical development of a novel product for pulmonary delivery of insulin. *Diabetes Technol Ther* 2005;7:896–906.

72. Illum L, Farraj NF, Davis SS. Chitosan as a novel nasal delivery system for peptide drugs. *Pharm Res* 1994;11:1186–9.

73. Craik CS, Largman C, Fletcher T, Roczniak S, Barr PJ, Fletterick R, et al. Redesigning trypsin: alteration of substrate specificity. *Science* 1985;228:291–7.

74. Berg DT, Gerlitz B, Shang J, Smith T, Santa P, Richardson MA, et al. Engineering the proteolytic specificity of activated protein C improves its pharmacological properties. *Proc Natl Acad Sci USA* 2003;100:4423–8.

75. Bone R, Silen JL, Agard DA. Structural plasticity broadens the specificity of an engineered protease. *Nature* 1989;339:191–5.

76. Knowles JR. Tinkering with enzymes: what are we learning? *Science* 1987;236: 1252–8.

77. http://www.catalystbiosciences.com. 2007.

78. Datamonitor. http://www.datamonitor.com/~13a000cbe6344ecfa1934088bb6af6e9~ /industries/news/article/?pid=CA9BC1FB-BDDB-4DC8-BFEA-EEC628A73C2D &type=ExpertView. 22 Jun 2006.

79. Janeway CA, Travers P, Walport M, Capra JD. *Immunobiology: the immune system in health and disease*. New York: Garland, 1999.

80. Que-Gewirth NS, Sullenger BA. Gene therapy progress and prospects: RNA aptamers. *Gene Ther* 2007;14:283–91.

81. Nogueiras R, Caton SJ, Perez-Tilve D, Bidlingmaier M, Tschop MH. Gastrointestinal signalling peptides in obesity. *Drug Discov Today Dis Mech* 2006;3:463–70.

13

REGULATION OF GENE EXPRESSION BY SMALL, NON-CODING RNAs: PRACTICAL APPLICATIONS

ROMAN HERRERA AND ERIC TIEN

Contents

13.1 INTRODUCTION

Posttranscriptional regulation of gene expression is an important mechanism that is widely used to determine embryonic differentiation, development, and maturation. An ever-expanding and novel area of genetic control mediated

Drug Efficacy, Safety, and Biologics Discovery: Emerging Technologies and Tools,
Edited by Sean Ekins and Jinghai J. Xu
Copyright © 2009 by John Wiley & Sons, Inc.

by small RNAs offers practical applications that are adaptable as therapeutic modalities [1,2]. The world of RNA biology has expanded dramatically during the last decade. The identification of small non-coding RNA (18–28 nucleotides long) of diverse structure, function, and biogenesis in libraries made from *C. elegans*—small inhibitory RNA (siRNA), micro RNA (miRNA), tiny noncoding RNA (tnc-RNA), small modulatory double-stranded RNA (smRNA), repeat-associated small inhibitory RNA (rasiRNA), and PIWI associated small RNA (piRNA)—has prompted the search and characterization of similar structures in other organisms [3]. Important observations have already been made regarding the biological activities associated with two of the best characterized small RNAs: siRNA and miRNA [4,5].

miRNA are short single-stranded RNA nucleotides (19–25 nt long) encoded in independent transcriptional regions of the genome often from within introns. The maturation of the functional miRNA takes place both in the nucleus and in the cytosol. Thus, after they are transcribed as capped and polyadenylated molecules by RNA polymerase II, they adopt a structure that contains long hairpin loops. They are partially processed by an RNAase type III enzyme (named Drosha and its partner Pasha) to an intermediate hairpin structure (also know as stem loops precursors of 65 nucleotides or so in length) forming the pre-miRNA that has two nt 3′ overhanging ends. This molecule is transported to the cytosol (a process mediated by exportin 5/Ran-GTP) where it is processed by another type III nuclease (dicer) generating a 19 to 25 nt long double-stranded RNA molecule. The functional miRNA is contained within a protein complex known as RISC (composed of Dicer, tar-binding protein and argonaute-2 protein). The miRNA recognize complementary sequences in its target mRNA, and depending on whether it is a perfect or partial match, they regulate gene expression by preventing their translation or promoting their degradation [6] (Figure 13.1).

RNA interference (RNAi) is a method of posttranscriptional gene-silencing induced by double-stranded RNA (dsRNA) via a biologically well-conserved pathway that results in fragmentation of a specific target mRNA. RNAi was originally observed in plants where it appears to provide an inherent defense mechanism against viral pathogens. It was later demonstrated experimentally in *C. elegans*, and more recently has been performed in mammalian cells in culture as well in vivo in flies and in vertebrates.

The generation of siRNA follows a similar path to miRNAs. dsRNA (and double-stranded regions of short hairpin RNA; shRNA) are cleaved by Dicer to generate short dsRNA fragments 21 to 23 nucleotides in length with two base overhangs at each end. This siRNA is incorporated into the multisubunit RNA-induced silencing complex (RISC) where it is partially unwound, permitting base-specific hybridization with a complementary mRNA molecule. A RISC endonuclease subunit known as argonaute 2 (Ago2) then cleaves the target mRNA exactly 10 bases downstream of the 5′-terminus of the siRNA antisense strand. Since the siRNA antisense strand is not degraded in this step,

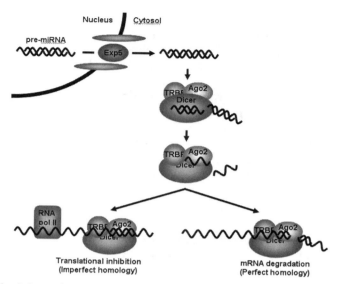

Figure 13.1 Schematic representation of the RNAi pathway. Exogenously administered siRNA or dsRNA produced by viral infection incorporate into the processing pathway at different steps to affect cellular signaling and gene expression. Ago2—argonaute 2; TRBP—tar-binding protein. (See color insert.)

the sequence-specific mRNA cleavage event is catalytic in the RISC/siRNA complex. Given the fact that siRNA can be obtained by direct supply of dsRNA to the RISC complex, it has become an important platform to develop tools and therapeutic strategies.

The advantages of RNAi over other existing technologies have led to its rapid acceptance as the method of choice for target validation and analysis of gene function [7,8]. Biotechnology companies have commercialized kits and reagents for preparing RNAi constructs and getting them into cells (Invitrogen Carlsbad, CA; Dharmacon, Boulder, CO; Qiagen, Valencia, CA). Synthetic siRNA as well as vector-based shRNA are used for screening thousands of potential drug targets in the human genome. The extension of RNAi to in vivo models also has proceeded rapidly. Compared to gene knockouts in mice that can take up to 9 months, target suppression using RNAi can produce answers in days or weeks; still target suppression is of a shorter duration and may be less than 100% (these properties actually may make RNAi a better model for small molecules than gene knockout mice).

While no therapeutic RNAi has yet reached the market, RNAi technologies have progressed rapidly and clinical trials are already underway [5]. The FDA approved an IND for Cand5 (Bevasirnamib, Acuity) in August 2004. Cand5 inhibits the production of VEGF and is intended for the treatment of age-related macular degeneration (AMD). It is currently undergoing phase II clinical evaluation for the treatment of wet AMD and diabetic macular edema. In September 2004 Sirna began clinical evaluation of Sirna-027, which targets VEGFR-1, also for treatment of AMD. Preclinical programs investigating RNAi are widespread across the biotech and large pharmaceutical companies encompassing antivirals (e.g., respiratory syncytial virus RSV, pandemic influenza, hepatitis C virus (HCV), human immunodeficiency virus (HIV), and severe acute respiratory symdrome (SARS)), neurological and genetic disorders (Huntington's disease, Parkinson's disease, amyotrophic lateral sclerosis (ALS), cystic fibrosis, and spinal cord injury), and cancer. Initial success is most likely to be associated with local, topical use of RNAi, similar to the experience with antisense.

13.2   POTENTIAL USE OF siRNA FOR THERAPEUTIC USE: CONSIDERATIONS

The largest obstacles to successful use of RNAi for pharmaceutical applications are generally considered to be:

- *Delivery.* The administration of RNAi in therapeutic quantities to patients represents a pharmaceutics challenge for several reasons. Native RNA is not a very stable molecule in vivo and is readily hydrolyzed by nucleases RNA is large and highly charged and therefore not orally bioavailable.
- *Pharmacokinetics.* Native siRNA is rapidly degraded in vivo (half-life, $t_{1/2}$, is on the order of minutes). Greater persistence is achievable through chemical modification of the siRNA itself and by formulation with a variety of vehicles. One or both of these approaches is likely to be required to achieve therapeutically useful exposures in vivo.
- *Safety and specificity.* In addition to general toxicity concerns, siRNA can trigger the innate immune system, producing what is referred to as a type-1 interferon response. In addition "off-target effects," namely hybridization to mRNAs that are not the intended targets, can occur. The potential for an imperfect match would induce the siRNA to behave like a miRNA.

13.2.1   Chemical Approaches to Improved RNAi

Native siRNA can be generated in vivo from shRNA that is transcribed from an engineered viral genome or a DNA plasmid. This approach to siRNA delivery builds on past experience in gene therapy. The main advantage of using biological vectors to deliver the siRNA is the potential for sustained production of the siRNA. This property is particularly attractive for the treatment of chronic diseases. Favored biological vectors include adenovirus-associated virus and lentivirus derived systems [9,10].

In contrast, synthetic siRNA exerts a relatively short duration effect in vivo, but it has the potential to be modified to address stability and pharmacokinetic weaknesses. In addition, targeting to specific tissues is possible in principle by conjugating the RNA to small molecules or macromolecules that bind to specific cell surface targets. The following sections will detail chemical modifications that been applied to improve the stability and duration of siRNA [11].

Modified Backbones   The most widely used modified oligonucleotides (ONs) are phosphorothioate oligonucleotides (PS) (Figure 13.2), in which one of the nonbridging oxygens of the phosphodiester is replaced by a sulfur atom [12]. PS oligonucleotides are readily prepared on laboratory scale by solid phase synthesis or by in vitro transcription. Their stability in serum is high versus unmodified siRNA (up to 72 h). Antisense PS oligodeoxynucleotides (PS ODNs) have been extensively studied. PS ODNs are more nuclease resistant than DNA ($t_{1/2}$ in human serum = 9–10 h vs. ~1 h for unmodified ODNs). They form regular Watson–Crick base pairs with RNA that can activate RNaseH. PS ODNs are the best-studied therapeutic ONs clinically. They display attractive pharmacokinetics, are well absorbed, and distribute broadly. The only

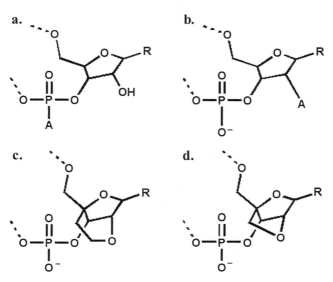

Figure 13.2   Potential chemical modifications to RNAi. A sample of chemical modifications to RNA molecules to increase stability/efficacy or avoid toxicity. (*a*) Phosphoro-substituted at position "A": Phosphothioate (S-), Boranophosphate (BH3-). (*b*) 2′ substitutions at position "A": F, *O*-methyl, methoxyethyl. (*c*) Ethylene bridged nucleic acid. (*d*) Locked nucleic acid. Position "R" represents base identity.

marketed antisense drug (Vitravene) is a PS ODN and several other PS ODNs are in advanced clinical studies. The disadvantages of PS ODNs are that they bind nonspecifically to certain proteins (e.g., heparin, which can cause toxicity), and they form less stable hybrids with RNA than does DNA (based on melting temperatures). PS siRNA is approximately half as effective as unmodified siRNA in inhibiting gene expression, with modifications in the antisense guide strand being more detrimental than modifications in the sense strand [13]. Similar to antisense, PS modifications do increase serum stability of siRNA.

A more recent innovation in the area of backbone modification is the introduction of boranophosphate siRNAs [14] (Figure 13.2). Boranophosphates also may be prepared by in vitro transcription albeit with lower yields than for phosphorothioates. Initial studies suggest that boranophosphates hybridize less tightly to RNA than does PS siRNA, but may possess greater stability toward nucleases than phosphorothioates and be more effective inducers of RNAi. A single group has demonstrated improved stability and cellular penetration with siRNA that was modified by partial alkylation of enzymatically prepared ON with 2,4-dinitrophenyl groups.

Modified Sugars   The 2′-OH of RNA is generally implicated in nuclease-mediated and hydrolytic cleavage through formation of a cyclic phosphate with expulsion of the 3′-nucleotide. Thus increased stability is conferred by deletion of the 2′-OH to produce DNA. However, replacing either the antisense strand or both strands of siRNA with deoxynucleotides completely abolishes RNAi activity. Abiotic modifications, such as introduction of 2′-deoxy-2′-fluoro ribose, and 2′-*O*-alkylation, also confer increased resistance to nucleases, as well as reduced toxicity and the formation of more stable double-strand hybrids. The most common *O*-alkyl modifications in antisense RNA are 2′-O-methyl and 2′-*O*-methoxymethyl (2′-*O*-acetoxyethyl orthoesters have also been investigated). Full *O*-alkyation leads to ONs that cannot induce RNaseH-mediate mRNA cleavage, thus these modifications are generally combined with ODN or PS modifications in a single strand (gapmers), with the *O*-alkyated nucleotides stabilizing the strand termini. The bulkiness of even a methyl group, however, appears to limit interactions between siRNA, target mRNAs and/or the RNAi machinery, when all nucleotides in either strand are 2-*O′*-alkylated. The decrease in potency is less pronounced with only partial methylation. In contrast, complete replacement of 2′-OHs with fluorines (in Cs and Us) and hydrogen (in As and Gs) is tolerated, and substitution of cytidine and uridine with 2′-F in the antisense strand alone provides modified siRNA with activity comparable to wild type. 2′-Fluorination stabilizes the C3′-*endo* conformation of the ribose ring, which is preferred for dsRNA. Moreover 2′-fluorination confers increased serum stability, especially when it is performed on both RNA strands. Interestingly, substantially *enhanced* activity (>500-fold) has been reported for siRNA with all 2′-OH groups alternately replaced with fluoro- or *O*-methyl [15].

13.2.2   Delivery of siRNA; In vitro and In vivo Approaches

Liposomes   The development of "lipoplex" methodologies has yielded formulations to achieve enhanced cellular uptake of RNA [8,16]). In general, these formulations are composed of a cationic lipid and sometimes a helper lipid. The cationic lipid usually is either N-(1-(2, 3-dioleoyloxy)propyl)-N,N,N-trimethylammonium chloride (DOTAP), 3β[N-(N,N'-dimethylaminoethane) carbamoyl]-cholesterol (DC-CHOL), or ceramide carbomoyl spermine (CCS). Each lipid combination is capable of existing in two forms—either large unilamellar vesicles (~100 nm LUV) or unsized heterolamellar vesicles (UHV). Comparative in vitro studies using anti-sense oligonucleotides have shown that CCS lipoplexes (UHV-derived) produced a maximal 50-fold improvement in antisense efficacy compared to treatment with free oligonucleotide.

An increase in the efficiency and reduction in toxicity of liposome-siRNA complexes has been achieved by generation of cationic liposomes derived from cardiolipin analogues. This observation suggests that careful design of naturally occurring lipid analogues may provide an advantage for systemic delivery of siRNA. An example of this approach is the use of a 1, 2-dioleoyl-sn-glycero-3-phosphatidylcholine liposome to explore the synergistic effects of siRNA and chemotherapy for the treatment of cancer in animal models. A choline-derived liposome was shown to be 10-fold more efficient than a liposome made of DOTAP [17].

Additional variation to the liposome approach involves the combination of cationic, neutral, and fusogenic lipids that serve to encapsulate the nucleic acid, forming stable nucleic acid lipid particles (SNALPs). Thus *APOB*-specific siRNAs encapsulated in SNALPs and administered by intravenous injection to cynomolgus monkeys at doses of 1 or 2.5 mg kg^{-1} resulted in dose-dependent silencing of *APOB* messenger RNA expression in the liver 48 hours after administration, with maximal silencing of >90% [18]. Significant reductions in ApoB protein, serum cholesterol, and low-density lipoprotein levels were observed as early as 24 hours after treatment and lasted for 11 days at the highest siRNA dose.

A frequently cited example of reduced plasma clearance of a modified siRNA involves the conjugation of siRNA to cholesterol [11,19]. The conjugation of cholesterol to the 3′ end of the sense strand of a siRNA molecule by means of a pyrrolidine linker did not result in a significant loss of gene-silencing activity in cell culture and enhanced siRNA binding to albumin. Following i.v. injection, this conjugate improved in vivo pharmacokinetic properties as compared to unconjugated siRNAs. After i.v. injection in rats at 50 mg kg^{-1}, radioactively labeled chol-siRNAs had an elimination half-life ($t_{1/2}$) of 95 minutes and a corresponding plasma clearance (C_L) of 0.5 ml min^{-1}, whereas unconjugated siRNAs had a $t_{1/2}$ of 6 minutes and C_L of 17.6 ml min^{-1}. Treatment of mice with this chol-siRNA resulted in a 25% reduction in HDL particle concentration. Furthermore treatment of mice with chol-apoB-1 siRNA resulted in an almost 50% reduction of chylomicron levels and an approximately 40% reduction in LDL levels, whereas VLDL levels were not altered. These findings are comparable to the changes observed in KO mice and validate the principle. A limitation of this approach could be in the doses required to achieve activity. When the same gene was targeted using liposome-mediated delivery, the dose required to achieve similar efficacy was reduced 10-fold.

Antibody and Peptide-Mediated Targeting   Increased selectivity in the delivery of siRNA can be accomplished by conjugation to antibodies. Examples have been described in animal studies. In one study, a tumor expressing the gp160 of HIV envelope protein was targeted by conjugating an anti–gp120 Fab fragment protamine and mixing this conjugate with several siRNA directed against endogenous genes expressed in the tumor. The delivery was either i.v. or via direct injection into the tumor and surrounding tissues. Intratumoral injection of siRNA was slightly more efficient than i.v. delivery [20].

An example of peptide-mediated delivery of siRNA is the use of siRNA/atelocollagen complexes. To test whether atelocollagen-mediated siRNA delivery accomplished gene silencing in vivo, animal experiments were performed on mice bearing a luciferase-producing melanoma [21]. Mice administered with a luciferase-siRNA/atelocollagen complex showed relatively strong and sustained inhibition of luciferase expression. In contrast, liposome-mediated delivery was effective for only up to 3 days postinjection. Inhibition of tumor growth by a siRNA/atelocollagen complex also was inhibited by treatment with human HST-1/FGF-4 -siRNA complexed with atelocollagen. At 21 days following treatment, the tumor volume in mice treated with siRNA complexed with atelocollagen was smaller than in the control mice treated with atelocollagen alone. Atelocollagen may offer additional advantages for siRNA delivery: the complex of siRNA/atelocollagen becomes solid when transplanted and remains solid for a defined period in vivo. In addition an atelocollagen complex can be delivered as microparticles for intravenous injection.

Nanotechnology: Nanoparticles and Nanotubes   The delivery of siRNA can be greatly enhanced by the use of nanotechnology. A few representative examples will be described. In one study the polysaccharide chitosan was used to create nanoparticles containing siRNA. Formation of chitosan/siRNA nanoparticles was accomplished by mixing chitosan (114 kDa) and siRNA at low (250 μg/ml) and high (1 mg/ml) concentrations of chitosan. Pulmonary RNA interference was demonstrated using daily nasal administration in a mouse transgenic model. Mice dosed with nanoparticles containing siRNA showed reduced numbers of epithelial cells expressing the GFP transgene (43% compared to untreated control mice) in the bronchioles [22].

Another approach involves making stable aqueous suspensions of short single-walled carbon nanotubes (SWNTs) by noncovalent adsorption of phospholipid molecules with poly(ethylene glycol) (PL-PEG, MW of PEG = 2000) chains and terminal amine or maleimide groups (PL-PEG-NH$_2$ or PL-PEG-maleimide). The amine or maleimide terminal on the PL-PEG immobilized on SWNT can then be conjugated with a wide range of biological molecules. In one, SWNTs were used to deliver siRNA into antigen presenting dendritic cells (DCs) in vivo. The positively charged SWNTs could absorb siRNA to form SWNT/siRNA complexes. These SWNT/siRNA complexes were preferentially taken up by splenic CD11c+ DCs, CD11b+ cells and also Gr-1+CD11b+ cells comprising DCs, macrophages and other myeloid cells to silence the targeting gene. In addition the system demonstrated, via repression of suppressor of cytokine signaling 1 (*SOCS1*), that it was possible to delay the growth of established B16 tumor in mice, indicating the potential for in vivo immunotherapeutics using a SWNT-based siRNA transfer system. Carbon nanotubes therefore represent novel molecular transporters that are promising for various applications including gene and protein therapy [23].

Ligand-Mediated Targeting   The basic principle of ligand-mediated targeting is to link siRNA to a small molecule that confers higher cellular or tissue uptake, as well as possibly reduced renal clearance. The design of nanoparticles (NPs) that are specifically taken up by the targeted cells represents a significant challenge. Nanoparticles containing specific ligands have been described. For example, a combination of cationic RNA-binding polymer (PEI), a neutral "coating molecule" (e.g., PEG) and a ligand (e.g., transferrin or an RDG peptide) constitute the basic system. This concept is illustrated by TargeTran, the carrier system in the ICS-283 siRNA delivery technology [24]. In the prototype, 25 kDa branched-PEI, 3.5 kDa bifunctional PEG bearing an *N*-hydroxysuccinimide ester for coupling the targeting peptide and a vinylsulfone group for coupling to the PEI, and RGD-2C were combined in a molar ratio of 1:40:40. The cationic charges of the polyamine interact electrostatically with the negative charges of the nucleic acids, leading to complex formation. The charge ratio determines the particle characteristics, such as surface charge and size. Nanoplexes are prepared by mixing equal volumes of aqueous solutions of cationic polymer and nucleic acid to give a net molar excess of ionizable nitrogen (polymer) to phosphate (nucleic acid) over the range of 2 to 6 with average particle size distribution of about 100 nm.

In the TargeTran system, 3.4-kD PEG chains are conjugated to the PEI to reduce opsonization in vivo. The steric stabilization capacity of PEG is governed by two main factors: molecular weight and density. To induce uptake by target cells, targeting ligands are coupled to the PEG terminal ends. In TargeTran the RGD sequence is used to mediate interaction with the integrin cell adhesion proteins. A good target tissue is the surface of activated endothelial cells during angiogenesis. An added level of specificity and differential affinity is achieved by cyclization of the peptide, thus modulating the specific interaction of the particles with the particular subset of integrin receptors expressed on the target tissue/cell. In summary, the RGD-PEG-PEI structure accomplishes the following:

- PEI—complexation for siRNA binding, nuclease protection, reduction of renal excretion, and promoting endosomal escape.
- PEG—promoting colloidal stability, reduction of surface charge, and reduction of nonspecific cell uptake.
- RGD—targeting activated endothelial cells during angiogenesis.

The potential for modifications to this basic strategy could, in principle, allow the production of an array of similar nanoparticles that, depending on the selection of the ligand, would provide a variety of cell type specificities.

Aptamer-Mediated Targeting   The first example of delivery vehicle using RNA aptamers for targeting comprised two components: a biodegradable and biocompatible polymer suitable for clinical use (poly(D,L-lactic-*co*-glycolic acid) (PLGA), and a surface functionalized with nucleic acid moieties for targeted delivery. The chosen cargo was a chemotherapeutic agent currently in clinical use for the management of prostate cancer, Docetaxel. Using nuclease-stabilized A10 2′-fluoropyrimidine RNA aptamers that recognize the extracellular domain of the prostate-specific membrane antigen (PSMA) it was shown that NP-Apt conjugates were differentially bound and taken up by LNCaP prostate epithelial cells that express the PSMA protein efficiently and with high specificity. In contrast, there was no uptake in PC3 prostate epithelial cells, which do not express the PSMA protein. The concept of using aptamers as targeting motifs has now been extended to siRNA [25]. A chimeric RNA was prepared comprising the targeting domain (aptamer) and the silencing domain (siRNA), which gets released by enzymatic processing via Dicer. As above, the aptamer was targeted to the prostate specific antigen PSMA. The interfering RNA was designed to target survival genes such as BCL2. The in vivo experiment used mice bearing tumors of LNCaP or PC-3 cells (cells that do not express the antigen). Intratumoral injections of the chimeric RNA resulted in inhibition of tumor growth and tumor regression in a xenograft model [26].

Novel and improved systemic delivery options will be required to increase the commercial and therapeutic appeal of siRNA. The combination of chemical modifications of the RNA and its incorporation into carriers (liposomes, nanoparticles, hybrid derivatives using ligand-specific targeting, etc.) is fertile ground for technical development.

13.3   SAFETY OF OLIGONUCLEOTIDE-BASED THERAPEUTICS

Small molecule based therapeutics have been a staple of pharmaceutical development. The difficulty in identifying good targets and developing compounds with useful therapeutic indexes has lead to exploratory work in the potential of oligonucleotide-based therapeutic strategies. The functionality of

RNAi and similar technologies such as antisense oligonucleotides and aptamer RNA offers up a wide array of potential therapeutic uses. However, safety is a critical component for assessing the therapeutic index of a treatment strategy, and RNAi presents its own challenges in this regard. There are three major safety issues concerning the use of RNAi: stimulation of severe immune response in the form of interferon and cytokine production, repression and inhibition of unintended target RNA sequences, and induction of necrosis and apoptosis of cells in the liver. These potential toxicities represent significant hurdles in the safety as well as effectiveness of RNAi as a viable human therapeutic. The exact mechanisms behind each of these toxicities are at varying stages of discovery and remain extremely active areas of research.

13.3.1 Antisense versus RNAi

While antisense oligonucleotides have not become a mainstay of biotherapeutics and pharmaceutical development, a great deal of the information learned from the difficulties with antisense, have been found to be applicable to RNAi technology as well. This therefore provides an excellent starting point for tackling inherent safety issues surrounding RNAi. Many of the chemical modifications that have been effective in circumventing immunostimulation of RNAi were originally discovered in relation to antisense oligonucleotide safety. Thus the potential safety of current RNAi technology has advanced at a tremendous pace given the favorable starting position for the field.

Like RNAi, antisense involves the targeting of specific RNA sequences for degradation to affect protein function. While excellent in principle, antisense oligonucleotides present their own safety challenges. A primary toxicity issue with antisense is the activation of the complement and coagulation cascades (reviewed in [27]). There are several non–sequence-related issues as well. Antisense molecules are immunostimulatory, can regulate undesired RNA molecules through sequence complementarity, and even interact with cellular proteins through so-called aptamer effects leading to altered protein function ([28]; reviewed in [29]). These issues aside, antisense therapeutics have been targeted for treatment of viral infections such as HIV/AIDS and related conditions.

As summarized in Table 13.1, antisense oligonucleotides and RNAi present many similar technical and safety issues, and as noted earlier, many of these problems may have similar potential solutions. While antisense and RNAi share some similarities, it is worth noting that RNA aptamer technology is predicated upon a different mechanistic approach, and therefore they do not share some of the same safety concerns.

13.3.2 Immunostimulation

Similar to antisense technology, the introduction of foreign RNA molecules into the cell has the potential to stimulate mechanisms for sensing viral and/or

TABLE 13.1   Brief Comparison of Current Oligonucleotide-based Therapeutic Strategies

Technology	Antisense	RNA Aptamer	RNAi
Advantages	Easily synthesized	Easily synthesized Easily modified Low immunostimulation	Easily synthesized Low amount for effect
Disadvantages	Short half-life Very difficult delivery High amount for effect	Rapid clearance Nuclease sensitivity Fewer targets	Very short half-life Difficult delivery
Toxicity	Immunostimulation Off-target effects Activation of complement	Low to none	Immunostimulation Off-target effects Liver toxicity
Site of effect	Nucleus	Target dependent	Cytosol
Current therapeutic targets	Oncogenes Viruses	Viruses Coagulation eye	Eye lung

bacterial genomes as evidenced by the activation of cytokine (interleukins, IL; tumor necrosis factor, TNF) and interferon (IFN) production by transcription factors such as nuclear factor kappa B (NFκB) seen in whole animals and human cells (both cell lines and primary cells). A major player in cellular detection of these stimuli is the toll-like receptor (TLR) family of receptors. Three members of this family, TLR3, TLR7, and TLR8 function as RNA sensing receptors (reviewed in [30]). TLR3, however, does not recognize single-stranded RNA (ssRNA), leading to the suggestion that TLR3 may not have a significant role in immune response to siRNA [31]. Conversely, TLR7 can bind ssRNA, so it has become a main focus of RNAi immunostimulatory research [32]. Binding of RNA to TLR7 is sequence dependent. High U/G content can promote a higher binding level and increase immune stimulation, thus making sequence composition an important factor in receptor recognition [33]. The retinoic acid inducible gene 1 (RIG-1) is an anti-viral and double-stranded RNA (dsRNA) sensor that is also capable of inducing immune response after exposure to RNA molecules ([34], reviewed in [35]). Activation of immune response by RIG-I is higher for blunt-ended dsRNA molecules, suggesting that dsRNAs with overhanging ends may be able to dampen or even circumvent this signaling pathway [36]. The dsRNA-dependent protein kinase (PKR) also senses foreign RNA [37]. Activation of PKR leads to phosphorylation of the translation initiation factor EIF2α and general cellular suppression of protein synthesis that can result in cellular apoptosis [38,39].

As evidenced by the work done with TLR7, imunostimulation can also be caused by RNAi sequence. As demonstrated by Judge et al., inclusion of a

5′-UGUGU-3′ sequence will elicit immunostimulation [40], while Hornung et al. also implicated 5′-GUCCUUCAA-3′ [41] as immunostimulatory. Thus avoidance of these motifs adds another significant consideration during RNAi sequence selection. Table 13.2 offers an abbreviated summary of published RNAi sequences and their concomitant immunostimulatory effects. It is clear that not all RNAi sequences are created equal, and it is of particular importance to note that two sequences designed for different regions of the same gene (TLR9) have diametrically opposite immunostimulatory effects, strongly hinting that sequence selection must be done with great care and that all sequences must be thoroughly evaluated. In addition the fact that one gene can contain a sequence that is immunostimulatory and one that is not immunostimulatory would also suggest that, delivery difficulties aside, virtually all genes may contain viable target sequences.

While immunostimulation is a major issue with RNAi-based therapies, many strategies have emerged to dampen or completely avoid this problem. Many of the chemical modifications identified, as discussed at length elsewhere in this chapter, that are effective for antisense technology have also proved to be beneficial for RNAi molecules.

13.3.3 Off-target Effects of RNAi

Antisense oligonucleotide and RNAi-based therapies have similar problems concerning off-target effects. Off-target effects can be classified into two major categories: binding to nontarget sequences and effects not related to the sequence of the oligonucleotides. There are an enormous multitude of suggestions for design and sequence selection for RNAi molecules, though no unifying set of rules currently exists. The length of the target sequence selected becomes an issue with concern to RNAi because sequences over 21 nucleotides in length can stimulate the aforementioned immune response. Conversely, being limited to shorter sequence length means greater difficulty in choosing truly selective target sequences. RNAi-based silencing follows the same general processing as endogenous microRNA (miRNA) for silencing of genes, and it yields clues for effective sequence selection. It has been estimated that every miRNA molecule can recognize as many as 200 distinct target genes [42]. With such promiscuity it makes sense that multiple miRNAs can work together to target an RNA molecule for degradation [43]. Thus, utilizing multiple, short RNAi molecules to target a particular RNA for degradation may be a possible avenue for greater sequence specificity and target selectivity.

RNAi sequences can be partitioned into three simple categories. Canonical sequences that exhibit excellent complementarity along the length of the sequence, "seed" sequences with excellent 5′ matching but poorer 3′ matching, and compensatory sequences that have excellent 3′ matching and poorer 5′ matching (reviewed in [44]). Clearly, canonical sequences would be ideal but in the cell comprise a small portion of known miRNAs [45]. Conversely, 5′ complementarity in the "seed" region has been shown to be truly critical for

TABLE 13.2 Immunostimulatory Effects of Varied RNAi Sequences

Gene	Sequence	Immunostimulation	Reference
TLR9	5′-AGCUUAACCUGUCCUUCAAdTdT-3′	Increase IFNα	[41]
HIV U5	5′-GCCCGUCUGUUGUGUGACUC-3′	Stimulate TNFα, IL12, IL6 and IFNα	[32]
MMP9	5′-CCAACUAUGACCAGGAUAA-3′	Stimulate TNFα and IL6	[58]
Luciferase	5′-GAAACGAUAUGGGCUGAAUAC-3′	Increase IFNα and IFNβ	[59]
COX-2	5′-AACTGCTCAACACCGGAAT-3′	Increase STAT1 phosphorylation	[36]
TLR9	5′-UGGACGGCAACUGUUAUUAdTdT-3′	No stimulation of IFNα	[41]
Nonsense	5′-GAACUGAUGACAGGGAGGC-3′	No stimulation TNFα or IL6	[58]
HIV U6	5′-GGGTGCGAGAGCGTCAAUAUUA-3′	No stimulation of IFNβ or target genes	[60]
MARV-NP	5′-CAGUUCUCGAGUUCAUCUUdTdT-3′	No stimulation of OAS or PKR	[39]
PTENb	5′-CCAGUCAGAGGGCGCUAUGUdTdT-3′	Low stimulation of IFN regulated genes	[61]

proper target recognition, even if 3′ complementarity is less than ideal [46]. Thus 5′ complementarity would likely be the best starting point for selecting effective and specific RNAi target sequences.

Careful sequence selection, however, has proved to be insufficient to prevent off-target degradation of mRNA in every case. Multiple examples exist of low complementarity, resulting in the degradation of non–target mRNA sequences [47–49]. It has been shown; however, that modification of the second base in the siRNA sequence with a 2′ or 5′-O-methylation can help to significantly reduce these off-target effects [50,51]. It should be noted, however, that off-target effects were not completely eliminated with these base modifications. Thus the target selection process will likely need to be a combination of sequence analysis for seed region complementarity and base modification followed by careful titration of the RNAi molecule to ensure the lowest level of off-target effects possible. Table 13.3 summarizes known RNA sequences and their off-target effects. It is notable that highly modified RNA molecules are able to minimize off-target effects.

The potential exists also for off-target RNAi toxicity, which is unrelated to the RNA molecule itself, in particular with regard to delivery agents and delivery mechanisms for RNAi molecules. There are a wide range of different options available for targeted and systemic delivery of RNAi from liposome coating to nanoparticles to polymer conjugates. All these delivery systems must be considered when evaluating the potential toxicity of RNAi, even though these toxicities may have no relation to the RNA molecules. In cell-based cytotoxicity assays, both lipid and nanoparticle based delivery methods exhibited varying levels of toxicity as evidenced by cell death [52]. While the mechanisms for these toxic effects are unclear at the moment, delivery method toxicity remains of concern when developing therapeutically useful RNAi technology.

TABLE 13.3 Target Sequences and Their "Off-target" Effects

Target	Sequence	Off-Target	Reference
MAPK14	5′-CCUACAGAGAACUGCGGUU-3′	KPNB3 RPA2	[48]
ICAM-1	3′-CACCGGAAGUCGUCCUCGA-5′	TNFR1	[47]
PIK3CB	3′-GAGGAUUAUACUUAGGATA-5′	YY1	[51]
GRK4	5′-GACGUCUCUUAGGCAGUU-3′	HIF1-α	[49]
Luc19	5′-TCCCGCTGAATTGGAATCC-3′	miR-122	[54]
CCR5	5′-AACGCTTCTGCAAATGCTGTTCTATTT-3′	miR-30A	[55]
FVII	5′-GGA**UCAUCUC**AAG**UCUUA**CTT-3′	None	[40]
Luc	5′-cuuAcGcuG**AG**uAcuucGAT*T-3′	None	
scap	5′-Gcuu**A**AuGGuucccuuGAuT*T-3′	None	
ApoB-2	5′-GG**AA**UCuuAuAuuuG**A**UCcA*A-3′	None	

Note: 2′O-Methyl modified nucleotides are in lower case, 2′-F modified nucleotides are in bold, and phosphorothioate linkages are denoted by asterisks.

13.3.4 RNAi-Induced Liver Toxicity

A large portion of RNAi introduced into the body accumulates in the liver [53]. Thus possible liver toxicity is a major concern with regard to RNAi safety. Overt liver toxicity and necrosis after viral vector based delivery of RNAi in mice has been observed [54]. These mice developed dose-dependent liver toxicity which ultimately leads to a high rate of mortality. The cause of this effect was determined to be an oversaturation of endogenous miRNA processing pathways. Endogenous miRNA processing requires export of the molecule from the nucleus by the protein exportin 5. RNAi that has been delivered through the use of viral vectors must also be processed and exported from the nucleus by exportin 5. However, viral expression results in such a high level of exogenous siRNA expression that this export pathway becomes overwhelmed and export of endogenous miRNAs is drastically reduced. Thus the authors observed a significant decrease in endogenous miRNA expression. The decrease in miRNA in the liver concomitantly affects the functionality of the miRNA pathways and the misregulation of a wide range of genes. This conclusion is supported by another study showing that overexpression of exportin 5 enhances RNAi effectiveness [55]. In addition it has been shown that using a very strong viral promoter (U6) to drive siRNA production in the cell can induce cytotoxicity whereas using a relatively weaker (H1) promoter will not further support the concept of overwhelming endogenous processing pathways [26]. Thus maintaining a proper, controlled expression of exogenous siRNA in the cell may be critical to avoidance of liver toxicity. Interestingly, other studies have been published that show no liver toxicity after long-term viral delivery of RNAi [32] possibly though lower expression of virally introduced siRNA. Regardless, it is not clear at this point whether liver toxicity and mortality due to viral delivery of RNAi and oversaturation of miRNA trafficking is a global issue for this method of RNAi delivery, and much more work is needed to determine why some virus constructs will elicit this problem if one wishes to use viral technology as a primary delivery mechanism.

Given the severity of the effect seen in the previous report [54], if overt liver toxicity in mice due to RNAi administration is due to oversaturation of exportin 5 dependent nuclear export, it stands to reason that preprocessed RNAi molecules such as siRNA will not have the same effect. To date no liver toxicity has been reported in other studies utilizing liposome based or naked RNA delivery methods, suggesting that viral vectors, while efficacious, may not be safe enough for human-based therapies. One can imagine a multitude of possible solutions to this problem such as coupling the RNAi to an RNA aptamer targeted for a different nuclear export pathway to circumvent exportin 5 and avoid blocking normal miRNA processing. Liver toxicity in mice, however, also begs the question of whether rodent-based models will be effective for predicting human toxicity concerning RNAi therapies. There are instances where overt toxicity or carcinogenicity in rodents does not appear to accurately model toxicity for humans [56,57]. With this in mind, caution must be taken when evaluating the potential hepatic toxicity of RNAi in humans.

13.4 SUMMARY

RNA interference offers numerous possibilities as a new class of therapeutic drugs. The challenges to implementing this technology are significant as evidenced by the surrounding issues concerning stability, delivery, efficacy, and safety of these molecules. Chemical modifications to the base pair constituents of the RNA molecules can potentially alleviate many of the problems surrounding stability while careful target sequence selection and evaluation can help provide maximal efficacy. A wide range of options to deliver RNAi to target tissues, including ligand-mediated delivery, liposomal coating, and nanoparticle conjugation are being studied and tested as possible solutions to this issue. Last, much of the work developed with regard to antisense toxicity has provided a solid base to begin assessing and circumventing the toxicity concerns of oligonucleotide-based therapeutics like RNAi.

The potential to theoretically affect any gene in the genome with a RNA molecule provides encouragement that formerly unreachable targets can now be beneficially modulated. Overall, the use of RNAi technology as a novel therapeutic agent has progressed at a very rapid rate. There are already examples of successful implementation of RNAi in whole animals that serve as an encouraging sign that this technology will be widely used for the development of therapeutics in the future.

REFERENCES

1. Costa FF. Non-coding RNAs, epigenetics and complexity. *Gene* 2008;410:9–17.

2. Filipowicz W, Bhattacharyya SN, Sonenberg N. Mechanisms of post-transcriptional regulation by microRNAs: are the answers in sight? *Nat Rev Genet* 2008; 9:102–14.

3. Kato M, Slack FJ. MicroRNAs: small molecules with big roles—*C. elegans* to human cancer. *Biol Cell* 2008;100:71–81.

4. Chapman EJ, Carrington JC. Specialization and evolution of endogenous small RNA pathways. *Nat Rev Genet* 2007;8:884–96.

5. Novobrantseva TI, Akinc A, Borodovsky A, de Fougerolles A. Delivering silence: advancements in developing siRNA therapeutics. *Curr Opin Drug Discov Devel* 2008;11:217–24.

6. Shyu AB, Wilkinson MF, van Hoof A. Messenger RNA regulation: to translate or to degrade. *EMBO J* 2008;27:471–81.

7. Behlke MA. Progress towards in vivo use of siRNAs. *Mol Ther* 2006;13:644–70.

8. de Fougerolles AR. Delivery vehicles for small interfering RNA in vivo. *Hum Gene Ther* 2008;19:125–32.

9. Fewell GD, Schmitt K. Vector-based RNAi approaches for stable, inducible and genome-wide screens. *Drug Discov Today* 2006;11:975–82.

10. Grimm D, Kay MA. Therapeutic short hairpin RNA expression in the liver: viral targets and vectors. *Gene Ther* 2006;13:563–75.

11. Nawrot B, Sipa K. Chemical and structural diversity of siRNA molecules. *Curr Top Med Chem* 2006;6:913–25.

12. Chen X, Dudgeon N, Shen L, Wang JH. Chemical modification of gene silencing oligonucleotides for drug discovery and development. *Drug Discov Today* 2005; 10:587–93.

13. Chiu YL, Rana TM. siRNA function in RNAi: a chemical modification analysis. *RNA* 2003;9:1034–48.

14. Hall AH, Wan J, Shaughnessy EE, Ramsay Shaw B, Alexander KA. RNA interference using boranophosphate siRNAs: structure-activity relationships. *Nucleic Acids Res* 2004;32:5991–6000.

15. Zhang HY, Du Q, Wahlestedt C, Liang Z. RNA Interference with chemically modified siRNA. *Curr Top Med Chem* 2006;6:893–900.

16. Aigner A. Nonviral in vivo delivery of therapeutic small interfering RNAs. *Curr Opin Mol Ther* 2007;9:345–52.

17. Landen CN, Jr, Chavez-Reyes A, Bucana C, Schmandt R, Deavers MT, Lopez-Berestein G, et al. Therapeutic EphA2 gene targeting in vivo using neutral liposomal small interfering RNA delivery. *Cancer Res* 2005;65:6910–8.

18. Zimmermann TS, Lee AC, Akinc A, Bramlage B, Bumcrot D, Fedoruk MN, et al. RNAi-mediated gene silencing in non-human primates. *Nature* 2006;441: 111–4.

19. Wolfrum C, Shi S, Jayaprakash KN, Jayaraman M, Wang G, Pandey RK, et al. Mechanisms and optimization of in vivo delivery of lipophilic siRNAs. *Nat Biotechnol* 2007;25:1149–57.

20. Song E, Zhu P, Lee SK, Chowdhury D, Kussman S, Dykxhoorn DM, et al. Antibody mediated in vivo delivery of small interfering RNAs via cell-surface receptors. *Nat Biotechnol* 2005;23:709–17.

21. Minakuchi Y, Takeshita F, Kosaka N, Sasaki H, Yamamoto Y, Kouno M, et al. Atelocollagen-mediated synthetic small interfering RNA delivery for effective gene silencing in vitro and in vivo. *Nucleic Acids Res* 2004;32:e109.

22. Howard KA, Rahbek UL, Liu X, Damgaard CK, Glud SZ, Andersen MO, et al. RNA interference in vitro and in vivo using a novel chitosan/siRNA nanoparticle system. *Mol Ther* 2006;14:476–84.

23. Yang X, Zhang Z, Zhang Y, Wang S, Cai Z, Yang R, et al. Single-walled carbon nanotubes-mediated in vivo and in vitro delivery of siRNA into antigen-presenting cells. *Gene Ther* 2006;13:1714–23.

24. Schiffelers RM, Storm G. ICS-283: a system for targeted intravenous delivery of siRNA. *Exp Opin Drug Deliv* 2006;3:445–54.

25. Cheng J, Teply BA, Sherifi I, Sung J, Luther G, Gu FX, et al. Formulation of functionalized PLGA-PEG nanoparticles for in vivo targeted drug delivery. *Biomaterials* 2007;28:869–76.

26. McNamara JO, 2nd, Andrechek ER, Wang Y, Viles KD, Rempel RE, Gilboa E, et al. Cell type-specific delivery of siRNAs with aptamer-siRNA chimeras. *Nat Biotechnol* 2006;24:1005–15.

27. Levin AA. A review of the issues in the pharmacokinetics and toxicology of phosphorothioate antisense oligonucleotides. *Biochim Biophys Acta* 1999;1489:69–84.

28. Villa AE, Guzman LA, Poptic EJ, Labhasetwar V, D'Souza S, Farrell CL, et al. Effects of antisense c-myb oligonucleotides on vascular smooth muscle cell proliferation and response to vessel wall injury. *Circ Res* 1995;76:505–13.

29. Jason TL, Koropatnick J, Berg RW. Toxicology of antisense therapeutics. *Toxicol Appl Pharmacol* 2004;201:66–83.

30. Sioud M. Innate sensing of self and non-self RNAs by Toll-like receptors. *Trends Mol Med* 2006;12:167–76.

31. Alexopoulou L, Holt AC, Medzhitov R, Flavell RA. Recognition of double-stranded RNA and activation of NF-kappaB by Toll-like receptor 3. *Nature* 2001;413:732–8.

32. Heil F, Hemmi H, Hochrein H, Ampenberger F, Kirschning C, Akira S, et al. Species-specific recognition of single-stranded RNA via Toll-like receptor 7 and 8. *Science* 2004;303:1526–9.

33. Heil F, Ahmad-Nejad P, Hemmi H, Hochrein H, Ampenberger F, Gellert T, et al. The Toll-like receptor 7 (TLR7)-specific stimulus loxoribine uncovers a strong relationship within the TLR7, 8 and 9 subfamily. *Eur J Immunol* 2003;33: 2987–97.

34. Yoneyama M, Kikuchi M, Natsukawa T, Shinobu N, Imaizumi T, Miyagishi M, et al. The RNA helicase RIG-I has an essential function in double-stranded RNA-induced innate antiviral responses. *Nat Immunol* 2004;5:730–7.

35. Bowie AG, Fitzgerald KA. RIG-I: tri-ing to discriminate between self and non-self RNA. *Trends Immunol* 2007;28:147–50.

36. Marques JT, Devosse T, Wang D, Zamanian-Daryoush M, Serbinowski P, Hartmann R, et al. A structural basis for discriminating between self and nonself double-stranded RNAs in mammalian cells. *Nat Biotechnol* 2006;24:559–65.

37. Clarke PA, Mathews MB. Interactions between the double-stranded RNA binding motif and RNA: definition of the binding site for the interferon-induced protein kinase DAI (PKR) on adenovirus VA RNA. *RNA* 1995;1:7–20.

38. Scheuner D, Patel R, Wang F, Lee K, Kumar K, Wu J, et al. Double-stranded RNA-dependent protein kinase phosphorylation of the alpha-subunit of eukaryotic translation initiation factor 2 mediates apoptosis. *J Biol Chem* 2006;281: 21458–68.

39. Sledz CA, Holko M, de Veer MJ, Silverman RH, Williams BR. Activation of the interferon system by short-interfering RNAs. *Nat Cell Biol* 2003;5:834–9.

40. Judge AD, Sood V, Shaw JR, Fang D, McClintock K, MacLachlan I. Sequence-dependent stimulation of the mammalian innate immune response by synthetic siRNA. *Nat Biotechnol* 2005;23:457–62.

41. Hornung V, Guenthner-Biller M, Bourquin C, Ablasser A, Schlee M, Uematsu S, et al. Sequence-specific potent induction of IFN-alpha by short interfering RNA in plasmacytoid dendritic cells through TLR7. *Nat Med* 2005;11:263–70.

42. Krek A, Grun D, Poy MN, Wolf R, Rosenberg L, Epstein EJ, et al. Combinatorial microRNA target predictions. *Nat Genet* 2005;37:495–500.

43. Doench JG, Sharp PA. Specificity of microRNA target selection in translational repression. *Genes Dev* 2004;18:504–11.

44. Ghosh Z, Chakrabarti J, Mallick B. miRNomics-The bioinformatics of microRNA genes. *Biochem Biophys Res Commun* 2007;363:6–11.

45. Nielsen CB, Shomron N, Sandberg R, Hornstein E, Kitzman J, Burge CB. Determinants of targeting by endogenous and exogenous microRNAs and siRNAs. *RNA* 2007;13:1894–910.

46. Lai EC. Micro RNAs are complementary to 3′ UTR sequence motifs that mediate negative post-transcriptional regulation. *Nat Genet* 2002;30:363–4.

47. Clark PR, Pober JS, Kluger MS. Knockdown of TNFR1 by the sense strand of an ICAM-1 siRNA: dissection of an off-target effect. *Nucleic Acids Res* 2008;36(4):1081–97.

48. Jackson AL, Bartz SR, Schelter J, Kobayashi SV, Burchard J, Mao M, et al. Expression profiling reveals off-target gene regulation by RNAi. *Nat Biotechnol* 2003;21:635–7.

49. Lin X, Ruan X, Anderson MG, McDowell JA, Kroeger PE, Fesik SW, et al. siRNA-mediated off-target gene silencing triggered by a 7 nt complementation. *Nucleic Acids Res* 2005;33:4527–35.

50. Chen PY, Weinmann L, Gaidatzis D, Pei Y, Zavolan M, Tuschl T, et al. Strand-specific 5′-O-methylation of siRNA duplexes controls guide strand selection and targeting specificity. *RNA* 2008;14:263–74.

51. Jackson AL, Burchard J, Leake D, Reynolds A, Schelter J, Guo J, et al. Position-specific chemical modification of siRNAs reduces "off-target" transcript silencing. *RNA* 2006;12:1197–205.

52. Weyermann J, Lochmann D, Zimmer A. Comparison of antisense oligonucleotide drug delivery systems. *J Control Release* 2004;100:411–23.

53. Braasch DA, Paroo Z, Constantinescu A, Ren G, Oz OK, Mason RP, et al. Bio-distribution of phosphodiester and phosphorothioate siRNA. *Bioorg Med Chem Lett* 2004;14:1139–43.

54. Grimm D, Streetz KL, Jopling CL, Storm TA, Pandey K, Davis CR, et al. Fatality in mice due to oversaturation of cellular microRNA/short hairpin RNA pathways. *Nature* 2006;441:537–41.

55. Yi R, Doehle BP, Qin Y, Macara IG, Cullen BR. Overexpression of exportin 5 enhances RNA interference mediated by short hairpin RNAs and microRNAs. *RNA* 2005;11:220–6.

56. Olson H, Betton G, Robinson D, Thomas K, Monro A, Kolaja G, et al. Concordance of the toxicity of pharmaceuticals in humans and in animals. *Regul Toxicol Pharmacol* 2000;32:56–67.

57. Yang Q, Nagano T, Shah Y, Cheung C, Ito S, Gonzalez FJ. The PPAR{alpha}–humanized mouse: a model to investigate species differences in liver toxicity mediated by PPAR{alpha}. *Toxicol Sci* 2008;101:132–9.

58. Sioud M. Induction of inflammatory cytokines and interferon responses by double-stranded and single-stranded siRNAs is sequence-dependent and requires endosomal localization. *J Mol Biol* 2005;348:1079–90.

59. Kariko K, Bhuyan P, Capodici J, Weissman D. Small interfering RNAs mediate sequence-independent gene suppression and induce immune activation by signaling through toll-like receptor 3. *J Immunol* 2004;172:6545–9.

60. Cave E, Weinberg MS, Cilliers T, Carmona S, Morris L, Arbuthnot P. Silencing of HIV-1 subtype C primary isolates by expressed small hairpin RNAs targeted to gag. *AIDS Res Hum Retroviruses* 2006;22:401–10.

61. Mise-Omata S, Obata Y, Iwase S, Mise N, Doi TS. Transient strong reduction of PTEN expression by specific RNAi induces loss of adhesion of the cells. *Biochem Biophys Res Commun* 2005;328:1034–42.

PART III

FUTURE PERSPECTIVE

14

FUTURE PERSPECTIVES OF BIOLOGICAL ENGINEERING IN PHARMACEUTICAL RESEARCH: THE PARADIGM OF MODELING, MINING, MANIPULATION, AND MEASUREMENTS

JINGHAI J. XU, SEAN EKINS, MICHAEL MCGLASHEN, AND DOUGLAS LAUFFENBURGER

Contents

Drug discovery and development needs to be more like engineering.
—Janet Woodcock, FDA, PharmaDiscovery Conference, May 10, 2006

14.1 INTRODUCTION

The success of pharmaceutical discovery to a great extent hinges on providing satisfying answers to two fundamental questions:

1. What is the key biological target(s) that will change the disease outcome?
2. How much of the biological target(s) can my drug afford to perturb without causing intolerable harm to the patient population being treated?

The first question relates to the selection of drug targets that can be validated as impacting the disease and in turn to translate into a clinical disease-modifying outcome. The second question relates to the selection of drug molecules and their dosage such that it has a sufficient therapeutic index. Providing satisfying predictions to both of these fundamental questions prior to costly and time-consuming large-scale human clinical trials is a critical mission of modern pharmaceutical research.

The answers to the first question depend on a deep understanding of disease mechanisms and pathways from a clinical perspective. What lie beneath a common disease phenotype can be sub-types of diseases, each with distinct upstream pathway defects but overlapping downstream pathway defects. Careful selection and prioritization of targets critical to the clinical disease outcome requires a new breed of translational researcher with both bench biology and clinical backgrounds.

The answers to the second question depend on a deep understanding of toxicology and mechanisms and pathways of drug-induced toxicity. The human body, the major recipient of modern pharmaceuticals, has in many cases adapted to distribute, respond to, metabolize, and excrete drugs and xenobiotics. Selecting a potential drug with a sufficient therapeutic index involves seeking a fine balance between robust drug efficacy and manageable drug risk, both of which require a fundamental appreciation of the complexity of the human body acquired through the millennia of evolution.

The human body is also a highly integrated system or complex network. Even after the completion of the human genome, the functional interrogations of the various functions of each of the gene products, namely proteins, are far from complete. In fact investigation of how the various proteins and protein pathways interact to produce what we call "physiological homeostasis" have merely started in the postgenomic era. Since the knowledge gathering for major pathways important in human diseases is expected to accelerate in the coming decade, it is only fitting to contemplate in this chapter what paradigm(s) we will use to interrogate this vast body of emerging knowledge in the years ahead.

14.2 BIOLOGICAL ENGINEERING: A QUANTITATIVE APPROACH TO COMPLEX BIOLOGICAL SYSTEMS

The ancient Chinese viewed the human body as several interrelated *Qi*'s (also known as *Chi* or *Ki*). This philosophy guided them well in generations of practice in Chinese medicine, mostly through trial and error. Our postgenomic view of the human body is a series of increasingly large biological pathways, from single cells to multiple cell–cell interactions to tissues, organs, and ultimately the whole body. This system is dynamic, integrated, and subject to feedback and feedforward controls. In view of such a dauntingly complex system, how can we quantitatively predict the therapeutic index of new drug therapy a priori?

Biological engineering, applies *engineering* principles to biological systems for the purpose of understanding living systems and to bring solutions to various problems associated with these systems. It exploits new developments in molecular biology, biochemistry, microbiology, cell metabolism, systems biology, and engineering principles and applies them to answer specific biological questions that have not been resolved before. So what are some of the key engineering principles? *Modularity* is probably the most fundamental principle of good engineering design. A large system can be analyzed by looking at increasingly smaller (though no less important) *subsystems* (i.e., body, organ, tissue, cell, nucleus, DNA). All subsystems should have well-defined, robust state transition rules. The *interfaces* between these subsystems should be clearly specified (feedback, feedforward, etc.). All interfaces are *quantifiable* and *simulatable* by mathematics. Therefore all engineering *predictions* (quantity changes or state transitions) are verifiable by well-designed experimental testing.

Biological engineering utilizes quantitative mathematical representations of a system's state and flux in the form of ordinary differential equations (ODEs), partial differential equations (PDEs), reaction kinetics, and mass action balances. In cases where biological parameters are not readily available, it applies computational approaches to "scan" through all of the biologically possible parameter values to provide estimates in terms of experimentally measurable outcomes. In cases where biological noise is known to exist (e.g., with a large patient population), the effects can also be modeled by standard mathematical approaches such as Monte Carlo simulation [1,2]. Hence biological engineering can provide a quantitative perspective to understanding complex biological systems. Its relevance to the two fundamental questions of pharmaceutical discovery described above is obvious. If all the key knowledge about a human disease can be represented mathematically, predictions about the clinically relevant outcome upon perturbation of a particular target or

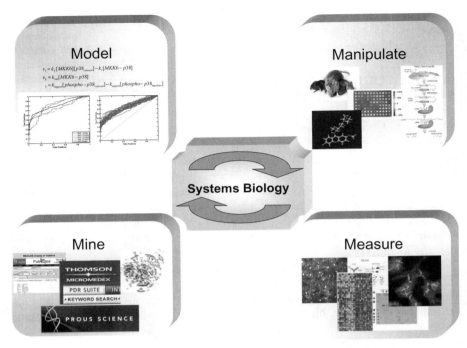

Figure 14.1 Schematic of the model, mine, measure, and manipulate (4M) paradigm. (See color insert.)

pathway can be made quantitatively, and then ultimately verified experimentally. If all of the key data about a drug's effects in human cells and tissues can be captured in a human physiology-based algorithm, the drug's therapeutic index can also be simulated and predicted (i.e., a bottom-up approach).

We therefore can perhaps reasonably view biological engineering as the cornerstone of the modern pharmaceutical research endeavor. Any successful pharmaceutical research program should find ways of integrating biological engineering principals into its drug research and development program. In the remainder of this chapter we will elaborate on the four practical pillars of biological engineering, namely modeling, mining, manipulation, and measurements (4M, Figure 14.1). We will describe both how each of these is being applied to pharmaceutical research currently and how emerging technologies in each of these four areas are and will continue transforming pharmaceutical research into the future.

14.3 MODELING

Modeling in the context of biological engineering is defined as using mathematical principals and concepts to represent, simulate, and predict the behaviors of a complex system. These can involve the level of the molecule, protein, pathways, cell, cell–cell, organ, and/or the complete organism (Figure 14.2). Besides the pharmaceutical industry, many other industrial fields such as the chemical engineering, aerospace, and defense industries have all routinely and successfully adopted and applied mathematical modeling [3] and

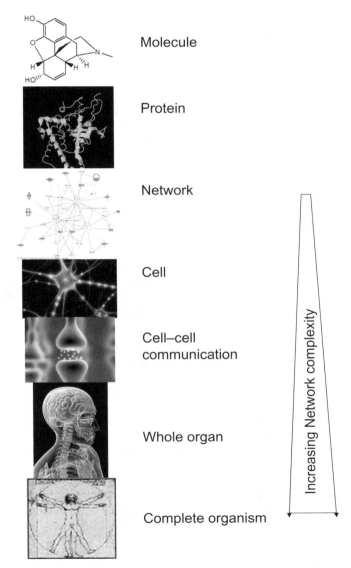

Figure 14.2 Schematic of the different levels at which models can be generated and the influence of networks. (See color insert.)

computer-aided design (CAD). For example, before the construction of large-scale chemical plants, chemical engineers utilize both mathematical modeling and experimentation in small-scale models to optimize the design of the final chemical production process. Before the launch of any new NASA spacecraft, teams of NASA scientists simulate and predict the likely behaviors of such spacecraft under a variety of atmospheric conditions to identify the most suitable engineering direction; similar steps are taken with airplanes, missiles, and automobiles. Even consumer products feel the trickle-down effects of CAD both in terms of design and usability testing.

In the life sciences in general, and pharmaceutical research in particular, mathematical modeling can help scientists select targets, identify leads, select dose, and simulate clinical trials and beyond [3]. Modeling should become indispensable at all stages of drug discovery and development from the idea stage to lead to identification, optimization, and clinical trial success [4].

The idea stage is when both the target or pathway to modulate or perturb the outcome of a disease and the amount of modulation needed to impose on that target are characterized. Of course, a target (or targets) almost always interacts with others in the form of pathways in a biological system, so modeling provides a comprehensive and quantitative analysis of targets (or pathways). It is also important to remember that target selection is not just disease driven but dependent on cost of goods, prior publications, novelty, number, and size of clinical trials required [3]. In the future, modeling should provide both novel target identification and quantitative predictions of how much affinity one should design into a drug molecule in order to afford sufficient efficacy. It should be noted that computational approaches could also be used for selecting molecules for use with combination devices to ensure they have desirable physicochemical properties before in vivo testing [5].

14.3.1 Modeling Approaches in Lead Identification

Currently computational modeling is an integral part of drug design and lead identification. Two recent reviews [6,7] have briefly described the history of in silico pharmacology that encompasses computational lead identification and lead optimization. This includes the use of quantitative structure–activity relationships, similarity searching, pharmacophores, homology models and other molecular modeling, structure-based design, machine learning, data mining, network analysis, and data analysis tools that all use a computer interface. Several other reviews of success stories in computer-aided design [8–11] have been published and describe in detail these technologies and specific applications to targets such as enzymes, receptors, ion channels, and transporters.

There has been relatively less modeling of protein–protein interactions, which are key components of cellular signaling cascades. The potential for blocking protein–protein interactions represents a sought after approach to treat various diseases [12]. These represent difficult targets for in silico methods to suggest small molecules due to the shallowness of their binding sites. For example, the G-protein $G\beta\gamma$ complex can regulate a number of signaling proteins via protein–protein interactions. Using FlexX docking and consensus scoring, nine compounds were identified with IC_{50} values from 100 nM to 60 μM as inhibitors of the $G\beta_1\gamma_2$-SIRK peptide to be used for further substructure searching [13]. Application of virtual screening to finding inhibitors of the HIV-1Nef–SH3Hck protein–protein interaction started with the NCI diversity set of 1990 molecules and after drug-like filtering and docking with FlexX/GF score, resulted in 10 hits [14]. Only one molecule of those tested was active. For comparison, high-throughput screening of the same library of molecules resulted in seven actives, and the best ($K_d = 1.8$ μM) was identical to that found by computational methods. Similarity searching with this hit in a database of over 400,000 molecules resulted in discovery of a slightly more potent molecule ($K_d = 0.98$ μM) [14]. Novel fragment compounds against the phosphotyrosine pocket of v-Src SH2 domain were described in one study using FlexX docking of a filtered library of roughly 13,000 available molecules, followed by NMR screening and thermodynamic evaluation ($K_d \sim 100$ μM) [15]. A virtual screen of over 17,700 compounds with FLO_QXP docking resulted in 22 molecules, of which 3 were confirmed binders to disrupt the β-catenin and Tcf/LEF interaction and one by $K_d = 450$ nM [16]. These represent some of the recently published examples of using docking and other methods to derive active molecules for protein–protein interactions.

In the future, computational modeling is likely to be more widely used to identify novel modes of interaction with drug targets such as allosteric inhibitors. For example, a ligand-based pharmacophore has been generated for the allosteric antagonists of the GPCR metabotropic glutamate receptor 5 (mGluR5) [17]. An alignment of 7 molecules was used to search 20,000 drug like molecules from the Asinex library by CATS3D similarity searching. Nine out of 27 molecules had activities under 100 μM [17]. The same group has used six mGluR1 allosteric antagonists as search queries for the Asinex Gold library of over 200,000 molecules, whereby 23 molecules were tested and 7 molecules with IC_{50} values less than 15 μM were retrieved [18]. A coumarine derivative with $IC_{50} = 0.36$ μM was used as a lead for further optimization and ultimately resulted in one with $IC_{50} = 60$ nM. These molecules were also docked in a homology model of mGluR1 [18]. A search for allosteric inhibitors of the SARS virus has used flexible docking and 2D similarity searching of over one million molecules to suggest potential inhibitors for testing [19]. A combination of docking with MOE-Dock and a genetic algorithm was used to optimize peptide design and search for noncompetitive inhibitors of the enzyme quinoprotein glucose dehydrogenase in order to validate an in silico approach [20]. It is likely that these successes will encourage others to use computational modeling to derive leads for difficult targets.

14.3.2   Modeling Approaches in Lead Optimization

In lead optimization some of the most difficult issues are about surmounting cardiac or hepatic toxicity. Two separate proteins, namely the human ether-a-go-go-related gene (hERG) potassium channel and the receptor 5-HT$_{2B}$, have raised particular concern because of their association with potassium channel blockade or cardiac valve disease, respectively. Unintended activity at either of these two proteins independently by several drugs has prompted their sudden withdrawal from the market. Early identification and elimination of molecules that pose toxicity risks can save time, money, and lives. One way to do this is by computational modeling of toxicity-related proteins [21].

Many classes of drugs have been shown to prolong the QT interval, a slowing of repolarization of the ventricular myocardium [22,23] by which excessive prolongation can lead to the potentially life-threatening ventricular tachyarrhythmia, *torsade de pointes*. Inhibition of the potassium channels in cardiac tissue is associated with QT interval prolongation [24,25]. The most common potassium channel linked to drug-induced QT interval prolongation is also responsible for the rapid component of the delayed rectifier potassium current (I_{Kr}). The focus of considerable research is hERG, which is believed to encode the protein that underlies the delayed rectifier potassium current I_{Kr} [26,27]. Many drugs associated with QT interval prolongation have been found to block hERG [28–30], and several drugs in the last decade have been withdrawn from the market in part due to cardiovascular toxicity associated with undesirable blockade of this channel (e.g., cisapride, terfenadine, astemizole, sertindole, and grepafloxacin). Since 2002 there have been many studies that have described individual quantitative structure activity relationship (QSAR) models, statistical models, or pharmacophores for hERG [31–44]. These different studies have encompassed a wide range of data generation and modeling techniques as well as an array of molecules for model building and testing [39]. There are some gross similarities in the suggested requirements for hERG inhibitors, such as the requirement for hydrophobic features surrounding a positive ionizable/basic nitrogen feature. The focus to date has been primarily on "global" models consisting of structurally diverse molecules across therapeutic targets (antipsychotics, antihistamines, antibiotics, etc.) although "local" models have also been generated around narrow structural series [34]. These ligand-based computational models, along with a growing number of homology models [45,46], have provided insights that complement experimental studies such as site-directed mutagenesis [47,48]. One such study compared multiple modeling approaches, including Kohonen map, Sammon map, and recursive partitioning, with the same training set to assess whether a single approach or a combination of approaches is preferable [48]. The descriptors selected for the qualitative mapping methods showed how the structural features of hERG inhibitors compared with those generated by other available methods, suggesting that molecular shape or topological characteristics are also important for hERG inhibitors. A more recent study used an additional series of shape-based descriptors to confirm the importance of molecular shape for interactions with hERG [49].

Serotonin is found in many physiological systems from the CNS to the intestinal wall and, in concert with its many receptors, has a major regulatory function in cardiovascular morphogenesis. The $5\text{-}HT_2$ receptor, family of G-protein coupled receptors, including $5\text{-}HT_{2B}$, is expressed in cardiovascular, gut, and brain tissues as well as in human carcinoid tumors [50]. In recent years this receptor has been implicated in valvular heart disease defects (VHD) caused by the now withdrawn "fen-phen" and pergolide [51–54]. The primary fenfluramine metabolite, norfenfluramine, potently stimulates $5\text{-}HT_{2B}$ [55,56]. Computational modeling of this receptor has been very limited to date but is urgently needed to identify drugs that may bind this receptor. Computational modeling of $5\text{-}HT_{2B}$ has encompassed a traditional QSAR study used a small number of tetrahydro-β-carboline derivatives as antagonists with the rat $5\text{-}HT_{2B}$ contractile receptor in the rat stomach fundus [57]. A 3D-QSAR with GRID-GOLPE using 38 (aminoalkyl)benzo and heterocycloalkanones as antagonists of the human receptor resulted in very poor model statistics, possibly due to the limited range of activity measured and the complexity of the functional response [58]. Homology models based on the bacteriorhodopsin as well as rhodopsin X-ray structures have been used for the mouse and human $5\text{-}HT_{2B}$ receptor and combined with site-directed mutagenesis. The models based on bacteriorhodopsin proved more reliable and confirmed an aromatic box hypothesis for ligand interaction along transmembrane domains 3, 6, 7 with serotonin [59]. A more recent $5\text{-}HT_{2B}$ homology model with the rhodopsin-based model of the rat $5\text{-}HT_{2A}$, together with molecular dynamics simulations, was used to determine the sites of interaction for norfenfluramine. Site-directed mutagenesis showed that Val 2.53 was implicated in high-affinity binding through van der Waals interactions and the ligand methyl groups [60].

Recently machine learning methods were used to generate classification models with shape-based descriptors for this receptor, and the results were generally better than for classification models of hERG data [49]. Also, in using a pharmacophore alignment of pergolide and norfenfluramine, it is possible to overlay the shape of the active ligand pergolide (Figure 14.3) and then use this for rapid searching of 3D databases of molecules likely to interact with $5\text{-}HT_{2B}$. For example, a set of 182 $5\text{-}HT_{2B}$ binders and nonbinders was used to validate this simple model. Of the 22 molecules that were mapped, 12 were known to have activities up to the tens of nM for this receptor. A similar search of a database of FDA-approved drugs retrieved 43 molecules (including pergolide and two known low μM molecules); the remainder were selected for future testing.

Although there have been many attempts at addressing cardiotoxicity by way of computational approaches, there have been far fewer efforts to predict hepatotoxicity [61,62] (see Chapter 6 by Ekins and Scheiber in this book). A recent study used 33 molecules associated with idiosyncratic hepatoxicity and

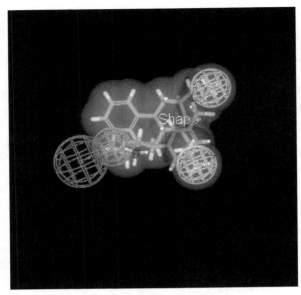

Figure 14.3 A shape feature HIPHOP pharmacophore model (Discovery Studio 2.0 Catalyst, Accelrys, San Diego, CA) of pergolide and norfenfluramine. Purple sphere = hydrogen bond donor, blue spheres = hydrophobic features, gray shape = van der Waals surface around pergolide. (See color insert.)

a similar number with no associated toxicities to generate classification models, namely in the form of linear discriminant analysis, artificial neural networks, and a decision tree [63]. One of the difficulties with this small training set is that our knowledge of molecules that involved in idiosyncratic hepatotoxicity is severely limited and our predictions for most molecules will generally be well outside of the range of the training set (see below). In this published study 11 molecules were used in a test set and 9 predictions were acceptable for those within the range of the training set [63]. This model represents a useful starting point for further expansion perhaps using some of the other approaches outlined earlier (Chapter 6).

One of the disadvantageous of using a computational models such as a QSAR is that predictions may be performed for molecules that are structurally more diverse than those in the training set of a narrow homologous series of molecules (local model) or a more structurally diverse range of molecules (global model). Poor predictions may result without a sense of how close the molecule is to the training set of the model in question. Several groups have started to address the applicability domain of models and develop methods to address this issue [64,65]. One approach has been to use molecular similarity to training set compounds as a reliable measure for prediction quality for a test molecule [66]. In an earlier study with hERG data [67], the similarity of the molecules in the test set to those in the recursive partitioning model were assessed using the Accord software molecule descriptors and the Tanimoto similarity coefficient [68]. In this case a value of one indicated the molecule was identical to one in the training set. As this value decreased, the less similar was the test molecule to molecules in the training set. Analysis of a 35 molecule test set using quantitative predictions derived from the recursive partitioning model resulted in a low though statistically significant correlation ($r^2 = 0.33$, Spearman $\rho = 0.55$, $p = 0.0006$). Next from a Tanimoto similarity analysis of the test set molecules, it was found that the log difference between the observed and predicted Log10 IC_{50} increased as the Tanimoto similarity declined. Therefore a Tanimoto similarity index under 0.77 was found to contain molecules with Log10 IC_{50} that were over 1 log unit different from the observed data. Compared with the whole test set, these 18 remaining molecules alone produced dramatically improved test set correlation statistics ($r^2 = 0.83$, Spearman $\rho = 0.75$, $p = 0.0003$).

In a recent study with Biopharmaceutics Drug Disposition Classification System data [69], we ascertained the distribution of training and test molecules in molecular descriptor space using a principal component analysis (PCA). The first three principal components of the training and test set explained 69.3% and 69.8% of the variance, respectively. Some test set molecules were well outside the descriptor space of the training set molecules. Consequently PCA analysis provided a convenient method for identifying outliers or molecules that are far removed from the training set descriptor field, and provided lower confidence in their predictions. We tried the same approach with data for the blood–brain barrier [70]. We followed with a study using similarity measures in the form of Euclidean distances, between pairs of molecules, that suggested significant structural differences between the training set and a test set for the 5-HT_{2B} receptor [49].

We also estimated the confidence in predictions for various ADME/Tox models derived with K-PLS algorithms using approaches called novelty detection and margin detection, which are two complementary methods [71]. Reliable confidence estimates enable uncertain predictions to be screened out so that only the high-confidence predictions remain. The goal of novelty detection is to identify compounds that are significantly different from those seen previously in the training set. Novelty detection can be implemented by any algorithm that can learn the distribution of the training set—a compound is considered novel if it falls outside of that distribution. Our implementation used the One-Class Support Vector Machine (SVM) algorithm [72,73] to learn a boundary around the training set distribution. In contrast, margin detection does not require the assumption that predictions on novel compounds be less reliable but instead uses the margin to directly measure the confidence of a prediction. In a classification task the margin is the distance of the prediction from the decision boundary—a larger margin implies higher confidence. These approaches were used with CYP3A4 and CYP2D6 inhibitor, blood–brain barrier permeation, and human fraction absorbed datasets. A clear improvement could be made in the classifications with the K-PLS models [71]. The applicability domain of other types of computational models (e.g., for target proteins) has not been addressed to any great extent to date. Applicability domain methods might eventually become commonly used alongside in silico lead optimization models in a seamlessly automated manner.

14.3.3 Modeling Approaches in Clinical Trial Design

The cost of bringing a molecule through drug discovery and development is undoubtedly high in the clinical trials. Therefore, if we could accurately model how a molecule is going to behave in vivo, we could ensure that only the molecules with a high probability of success would proceed through human dosing. While there have been some attempts at modeling human pharmacokinetic data [74–76], these datasets are generally small. The simulation of populations of patients with a disease and their controls [77–79] offers another way to crash-test the molecule or hypotheses before significant financial investment. Different types of computational models are widely used in postmarketing clinical trials that look at safety, cost effectiveness, and efficacy issues and lead to improved labeling or indications [80].

Currently clinical dose selection is based largely on allometry scaling and experimental verification by trial and error. PBPK modeling [81–83] (See Chapter 7 by Zhang, Tan, Bhattacharya, and Andersen in this book) will soon become the norm as it is being used increasingly for risk assessment [84]. Real-time clinical trial adjustment or adaptive research will likely also become a standard method, along with clinical trial modeling and simulation integrated in personalized medicine.

The development of computational models and informatics tools will likely mimic the supply chains in other industries in which parts are provided just in time (JIT), as needed, with computational models serving as a part of drug discovery or development. For example, if a model is needed for a project in early discovery, it could be created JIT from in-house data, literature data, or collaborator data when required. As a project progresses, the required models will become more specific and develop in parallel with experimental data generation (e.g., in understanding the pathways inhibited by a molecule and the effects on disease), progressing through multiple automated iterative loops of building and testing. The process of drug discovery and development could be treated as a computational model that can be tweaked and adjusted from idea to clinic and beyond.

14.4 KNOWLEDGE MINING AND REPRESENTATION (KMR)

The development of systems biology models in the pharmaceutical industry relies on knowledge of drug targets in their biological context that has been codified and assembled from prior research studies reported in the literature.

The exponential growth of heterogeneous, globally distributed biological data and information sources, combined with short timelines for pharmaceutical research and development projects, makes a manual approach to assembling this knowledge impractical, if not impossible. Alternatively, the costs of missing critical information or recreating key experimental data in the laboratory can be expensive. Deriving biological meaning and insight further requires tools to visualize and analyze the assembled knowledge, detect aberrant patterns, and infer causal relationships.

Emerging knowledge mining and representation (KMR) capabilities are already proving their potential in the practice of systems biology. Knowledge mining comprises extraction of essential facts (e.g., concentrations, kinetics, stoichiometries) and relationships (e.g., protein A, phosphorylates, protein B) from databases, journals, patents, secondary literature, "pathway" resources, or published models. Knowledge mining employs natural language processing, rich thesauri of biological and chemical terminology, and algorithms for recognizing and disambiguating biological and chemical entities and relationships. Applications of systems biology have recently been reviewed [85,86] as in silico technologies for drug target identification and validation.

Knowledge representation (KR) methods are used to transform the extracted facts and relationships into a logical representation that accelerates human- or machine-based reasoning, and the generation of testable hypotheses. Additionally KR plays a pivotal role in systems biology by providing a framework to identify, merge, and manage data, information, and knowledge. Taken together, KMR provides an ability to "identify and connect the dots," paving the way for the rapid assembly of systems biology models, and the discovery of new knowledge. Below, we describe KMR trends, and outline a vision for how advances in KMR concepts and applications will enable fundamental breakthroughs in systems biology.

14.4.1 KMR Trends

Scientific Communication   The Internet and associated technologies continue to dramatically reshape scientific communication, and biomedical research. Some of the biggest changes involve the format of published literature, including the growing trend toward the publication of data, models, and multimedia in conjunction with traditional journal articles, rich bidirectional linking between journals and associated data, and increasingly interactive figures and applications. In parallel, sophisticated search, navigation, and mining techniques are rapidly evolving to exploit these new media formats, and they will have a profound impact on our abilities to extract biological knowledge from published literature or their components (e.g., from the results section of a document, or from figures [87], tables [88–90], or multimedia).

Another important trend is the rapidly increasing availability of machine-level access to biomedical literature, including the growing movement toward "open access" publishing and the development of application programming interfaces (APIs) in the commercial publishing industry [91]. While the vast majority of high-impact scientific journal titles are still provided by commercial publishers, recent legislation regarding open access to NIH-funded research [92,93] will likely accelerate the open access trend. The traditionally conservative scholarly publishing industry is also developing APIs that enable direct machine-to-machine querying, parsing, and mining of its subscription content. The digitization of library collections of secondary literature [94] and the electronic publication of manuscripts, models, and associated media are already creating unprecedented opportunities to mine the higher order collective knowledge of the biomedical research community.

Another parallel development is the increasing access to biological knowledge that has been effectively "locked away" inside corporate firewalls. The integration of knowledge mining tools with enterprise search technologies is enabling pharmaceutical workers to fully exploit the rich legacy of proprietary research that, to date, has been dispersed in myriad reports and in various tightly secured repositories [95,96]. These mining methods are critical for pharmaceutical companies who must preserve document-level security while harvesting the knowledge that is generated in their own laboratories and that is often impossible to find in the public domain. Public calls for earlier access to clinical trial results [94] are expected to yield further opportunities to exploit KMR in the service of translational medicine.

Knowledge Representation   Encoding scientific knowledge empowers scientists by allowing them to search, share, compare, analyze, correct, and connect scientific knowledge via a wide variety of computational techniques, and it is changing the practice of systems biology. Codification and classification of biological knowledge has a long history [97], but its most recent, striking example is the Human Genome Project. Codification of nucleic acid protein sequences and chemical structures is now relatively standardized, and many bioinformatics tools are available to leverage these powerful resources.

In contrast, current methods to develop standardized representations of more complex forms of biological and medical knowledge remain relatively immature. For example, molecular biologists have painstakingly assembled hundreds of pathways that are, by now, well established (p53, NF-kB, B-catenin signaling networks, transcriptional regulatory networks, and many known metabolic routes), and a wide variety of commercial and open-access "pathway" resources are now available (Ingenuity, Ariadne, BioBase, GeneGo, KEGG, HPRD, etc.). Some of the challenges associated with using these resources arise from the fact that they are typically derived from manual curation of the literature for the purpose of answering frequently asked questions. This poses two problems: First, manual curation does not scale well, so the knowledge contained in any given resource is incomplete. Second, the knowledge contained in these resources is static, and may not be captured and organized at the level of granularity required to answer specific systems biology questions (e.g., "How does this pathway vary by cell type?", or "how does phosphorylation of amino acid X of domain Y affect its biological activity relative to phosphorylation at other sites?"). For biological molecules, context is embedded in a host of specific details, including oligonucleotide or protein sequence, primary–secondary–tertiary–or quaternary structure, posttranslational modifications, or the formation of multimeric complexes. A relevant context may further include knowledge about a given molecule's local interactions or participation in cellular processes, such as compartmentalization; developmental or cell cycle stage, or differentiation state; signaling among cells, tissues, or organs; and the health of the organism under study. Accordingly flexible KMR tools are needed to allow researchers to interrogate and assemble pertinent knowledge on the fly, while preserving the detailed biological context that is relevant for systems biology and pharmaceutical decision-making.

Another critical need is a high-throughput method to validate molecular pathways against the collective scientific knowledgebase, including experimental data. High-throughput biological profiling is changing the landscape of pharmaceutical research. Its ability to measure molecular activities at the cellular level and in genome-wide fashion is opening the door to the exploration of fundamental questions about physiological and pathological cellular processes. This flood of new data has pointed to the need for developing knowledge representation methods to map specific molecular interactions to our existing knowledgebase of cell structure and behavior, physiology, and disease. In principle, it is possible to "reverse engineer" a biological network by processing high-throughput data, using a complex set of computational algorithms to infer gene–gene, gene–protein, or protein–protein interactions; however, it is challenging to compare such networks against canonical pathways with the currently available resources.

Emerging knowledge mining and representation methods can provide a systematic, unbiased "shortcut" to this task. By marrying high-throughput biological data to KMR tools, researchers are systematically developing and exploiting large-scale networks of interactions among cellular entities more than one interaction at a time. The inferred networks of molecular interactions can produce a more holistic view of the fragmented knowledge than can a random list of genomic, proteomic, or metabonomic pieces. KMR researchers have made enormous progress in extracting and disambiguating biological entities, and their complex interrelationships in order to construct detailed networks, and pathways [98,99]. An even bigger challenge is mapping molecular-level knowledge to larger more complicated processes, such as cell division, intercellular communication, and disease phenotypes. KMR methods have been used identify key genes involved in hepatocellular carcinoma (HCC), and work has begun toward reverse-engineering key signaling pathways and assessing their impact on HCC-related phenotypes [91].

14.4.2　Future KMR Capabilities

Current KMR methods are challenging for most bench scientists to use. Increasing human–computer interaction will result in greater tool interoperability and tighter integration with normal workflows of systems biologists. Future KMR practices will allow incorporate novel data models, architectures, and sophisticated version control to support workflows that are integrated into the very fabric of the systems biology process. We outline some key aspects of future KMR tools and practices below.

Intelligent Knowledge Mining　Knowledge mining capabilities will be highly distributed, and we see richer ways of interacting with a federated network of data and knowledge that is unbound by the traditional document model. New kinds of scholarly publications will combine the strengths of traditional journals with the analytical capabilities of databases, the interactivity of blogs and wiki's, and other emerging capabilities offered by the Semantic Web. Future knowledge mining tools will identify relevant information sources, extract essential facts, and assemble models semiautomatically, making well-reasoned, transparent decisions about the accuracy and validity of the information contained therein. Biologists won't have to be trained as computer scientists to ask complex, important questions. For example, a discovery scientist will be able to pose questions like the following to the network: Find all human disease-relevant proteins where:

1. there is no known precedent (small-molecule, peptides, or antibodies with activity against this target have not advanced past phase II clinical trials);
2. germline mutations of the target caused primary human disease phenotypes;
3. selective reference compounds, reagents, and assays for executing a research project are readily available;
4. The target is expressed in therapeutically-accessible tissues;
5. Where there are known clinical biomarkers;
6. Clinical trials are expected to last less than 6 months;
7. Relevant patient populations are easy to recruit;
8. The resulting product is likely to be a first in class therapy in the marketplace.

Accelerating Systems Biology: From Knowledge to Models　Systems biology models both consume knowledge, in the form of the context or parameters with which they are supplied, and yield knowledge, in the form of the interpretations or hypotheses as a product of their execution. Models incorporate assumptions about real-world phenomena that are the subject of experimentation. Experimental data, in turn, are often inaccurate or noisy. Given the assumptions and simplifications entailed in model building, and noisy and inaccurate data, it is rare that the initial model behaves precisely as the real-world system does. For example, the model behavior may correspond to the experimental domain, but only over a limited set of inputs, or perhaps as a result of a different mechanism, or it may be an imprecise implementation of the theory it is intended to represent.

Humans will always be needed for analysis and tuning of systems biology models, and tighter integration of experimentation and modeling methods will drive the need for a fluid knowledge representation that can be utilized by both human and computational resources. For routine troubleshooting, KMR methods will increasingly be used to determine the correspondence between model output and experimental domain behavior. Encoded scientific knowledge will be increasingly analyzed computationally, before any experimentation or modeling. Users will be able to easily visualize, evaluate, and test interacting networks, automatically identify logic conflicts between coded representations, accumulated data, and the KMR system's suggestions to arrive at a resolution, or conduct further experimental work to resolve such conflicts.

KMR will also play an essential role in helping scientists map new knowledge to existing models and in developing new models from existing knowledge. Future KR methods can be expected to accommodate multiple levels of biological abstraction, from cellular pathways to higher level disease processes, to allow scientists from different fields to understand and learn from each other's solutions, and ultimately acquire a set of widely applicable complex problem solving capabilities, based on the use of a generic modeling approach, in much the same way that they now use generic tools and algorithms in chemistry and mathematics.

Accelerating Systems Biology: From Models to Hypotheses Future KMR methods can be expected to incorporate semantic Web capabilities that will integrate theoretical, computational, and experimental knowledge with the capabilities to probe leverage points in key pathways that are associated with disease. Knowledge-based systems (KBSs) [100], originally developed in the artificial intelligence community, will increasingly be used to interpret experimental results, and to semi-automatically generate new research hypotheses. KBSs are comprised of a reasoning engine or problem-solving process coupled with a domain-specific knowledge base (a way to store and manipulate the physical symbols that represent entities in a domain of interest; e.g., the targets, metabolites, and other elements in a pharmaceutically relevant pathway or network). KBSs can analyze chains of causal reasoning to generate, and evaluate hypotheses regarding possible causes of experimental observations e.g., using semantic reasoners: FaCT++, Pellet, Jena, etc.). Components of a KBS include:

1. a knowledge mining system (generally with human review and validation);
2. a knowledge representation scheme that codifies observations about a given domain;
3. algorithms and tools for manipulating, searching and visualizing graphs; and
4. an expert system for reasoning over the knowledge base,

The W3C have developed specific recommendations and a suite of tools and standards is evolving rapidly, (OWL-DL, RDF [triples], SPARQL, etc.); however, literature reports of systems biology applications are still fairly limited. We think that this field will accelerate rapidly and bring a powerful, simple, computationally efficient, and effective means for hypothesis generation into the mainstream of pharmaceutical research and development. Hypotheses generated using KBSs will likely be used to suggest experimental and modeling studies that inform target and modality choice, identify target/mechanism and efficacy biomarkers, and segment human populations and thus enable safe and efficient clinical trials.

14.5   MANIPULATION

Advances in modern medicine are heavily dependent on evidence from experimental approaches, and pharmaceutical research in the new millennium is no exception. What is new is the realization that any experimental system is at best an approximation of the ultimate goal of medicine: treating a diverse group of patients suffering from a devastating disease in the real-world setting. For example, in a recent article [100] it was suggested "what is efficacious in randomized clinical trials is not always effective in real-world day-to-day practice." This is due to the combination of several factors: (1) some of the strict and rigid inclusion and exclusion criteria used in randomized clinical trials are not realistic in the real-world setting; (2) the controlled experimental conditions typical of today's randomized clinical trials are not necessarily good models of the wide variability in patient types and severity, the complex dynamic and interactive nature of treatments, and increasingly popularity of polypharmacy used in the real world; and (3) patient compliance issues in the real world. This is not to say that randomized evidence-based medicine is not needed in establishing the *potential* of efficacy of an experimental medicine. One should indeed remember the inherent limitations of any experimental system even in human controlled clinical trials, as any experimental system is subject to one form of manipulation or another, often by experimental design and by necessity.

Of course, any experimental system is by design, a manipulation (or many manipulations) to answer a specific scientific question. Scientific rigor and human insights are needed to step from one manipulated system to another, to inch closer to the goal of providing both efficacious and safe medications to benefit humankind as bespeaks the arduous journey of today's pharmaceutical discovery. The scientist cannot afford to be a blind optimist proceeding without close scrutinization with the types of manipulations and detailed experimental protocols used to discover drugs. Nowadays, the types of manipulations in the life sciences span from the idea stage, to lead identification, to lead optimization, and to clinical trial success; In the future, the types of manipulations used (and the measurements performed) in each of these stages will be much more sophisticated and representative of the complexities in the real-world disease setting.

The most common approach to system manipulation is genetic, using DNA- or RNA-based knockout or knockdown of gene products in animals or cells derived to probe the effects of altered molecular pathways. Conditional knockouts are generally required for exploration of pathophysiology and prospective therapeutics in mature tissues, and tissue-specific regulation of the genetic effect is often employed toward narrowing the scope of the study. RNAi libraries are already available on a genome-wide basis for many organisms, enabling high-throughput screening of drug effects over a full scope of gene product knockdowns.

However, influence of the genetic manipulation typically propagates broadly beyond the pathway of concern, since the necessarily long time period required for the gene or message reduction to transpire following activation of the knockout or knockdown technology permits up-regulation and down-regulation of various mechanisms in consequence—whether compensatory for (often inappropriately termed "redundancy") or exacerbating of the initial manipulation. Thus it must be appreciated that a substantial portion of the observed changes of the manipulated biological system in response to prospective therapeutics is more an epi-phenomenon that is only indirectly related to the genetic alteration.

An alternative approach, certainly complementary rather than competitive, is to pursue manipulation as driving the responses of the biological system across a broad landscape of contexts, for example, as diverse combinations of medium and substrate components. Take the study of embryonic stem cell differentiation across a landscape of 16 contexts comprising various combinations of extracellular matrix factors and growth factors. Such study enabled discernment of the particular conditions under which a protein kinase inhibitor gives a significant affect compared to other conditions under which it did not [101]. This result has been buttressed by other similar studies [102–104]. The important implication is that screening the effects of any drug candidate on the background of any genetic manipulation(s), no matter how specific, may be of limited value if undertaken in only one or a small number of contexts.

This alternative view of biological system manipulation opens an avenue of hope toward relating in vitro studies to in vivo studies, at least within a comparable animal species. Any particular in vitro setting is unlikely to resemble in vivo physiology, although new tissue-engineered ex vivo constructs are making significant progress in this direction [105]. If the in vitro assay is undertaken across a broad landscape of contexts, there is a strong possibility that the state of intracellular molecular network activity under a representative in vivo circumstance will be interpolatively comprehended within the range of cell network states generated over the context landscape. Thus there can be envisioned a networkwide measurement capability developed for mRNA, protein, and phosphorylated protein levels for in vivo tissue as well as for the same compendium of molecular activities across a broad landscape of in vitro assay contexts, and then to employ computational modeling methods to relate the network state to phenotypic behavior in both the in vivo setting and the in vitro landscape. A very substantive hypothesis can then be tested, whether the network state to phenotypic behavior relationship that is predictive of drug effects across the in vitro landscape can then similarly predict the drug effects in an interpolated in vivo situation. As noted above, genetic knockout and knockdown technologies can be used in complementary fashion to extend the scope of conditions for which network states and consequent phenotypic responses are measured.

14.6   MEASUREMENT

Even though mining and modeling can provide in silico predictions of drug effects, the efficacy and safety of any medicine need to be established experimentally, with increasingly complex and realistic experimental systems. "Measurement" is defined as quantitative determinations of a panel of parameters from a complex system. These parameters span the amount, rate of change, frequency, and localization of molecules. They include chemicals and biologics, gene sequences and copy numbers (genetics), gene transcripts (genomics), proteins (proteomics), metabolites (metabonomics), kinase activities (kinomics), lipid biochemistries (lipidomics), phenotypic responses, imaging data (e.g., cytomics and noninvasive in vivo imaging modalities), besides glycomics (see Chapter 11 by Sasisekharan and Viswanathan in this book). The various high-throughput methodologies, when applied to measurements, enable a vast number of biological parameters to be measured in a highly parallel fashion at an unprecedented speed, as highlighted in the various chapters of this book.

Other advances in measurement technology will likely come from various engineering fields such as nanotechnology (see Chapter 10 by Bhavsar, Jain, and Amiji this book), material sciences, and sensitive detection technologies. Emerging technologies in these fields will push the boundary of the traditionally more conservative field of clinical measurements, and make high content clinical measurements more real-time, noninvasive, and accessible to the masses (i.e., ordinary people). Imagine a picture in which an ordinary person can sit at their dinner table and put their finger in a small electronic device. The device sends a micro-scale laser to puncture the skin of the finger and retrieves a few microliters of blood. Then the device will measure a panel of clinically important parameters including blood sugars, insulin, major electrolytes, inflammatory markers, and other diagnostic markers from major organs such as liver, kidney, and heart. If certain combinations of biomarkers are in the abnormal range for a predefined period of time, the device will automatically send a warning signal to the person's primary care physician. The availability of such theoretical home electronic devices will provide a new standard of care to patients and a whole new meaning to the field of preventative medicine.

In addition to providing a real-time warning, the availability of such early noninvasive biomarker measurements will provide a plethora of data for both statistical modeling (i.e., what combinations of biomarkers are predictive of a later disease outcome), disease pathway mining (i.e., better understanding of the early pathogenesis of a human disease before it becomes an emergency), and drug therapy monitoring (e.g., does the drug cause intended therapeutic effects without causing undue toxicities in the liver, heart, or kidney?). Drug therapy monitoring could bring evidence-based medicine to a whole new level. Coupled with individual genome sequencing, it could provide for on-time delivery of personalized medicines and other therapeutic options.

In the realm of preclinical and in vitro measurements, emerging fields such as nanotechnology and tissue engineering promise to provide in vitro human cells and tissues with differentiated functions that more closely mimic the in vivo situation. In particular, stem cell technology promises to deliver reliable sources of mammalian cells of any tissue and organ (also see Chapter 8 by Davila, Stedman, Engle, Pryor, and Vacanti in this book). Tissue engineering applies engineering approaches to tissue culture and co-culture techniques with the promise to deliver well-controlled three-dimensional culture apparatus to maintain the normal tissue function and tissue–tissue interactions for a sustained period of time, making in vitro measurements more relevant to the in vivo situation.

The "human body on a chip" for drug testing is currently a goal that encapsulates permeability (e.g., Caco-2 cell line), metabolic stability (e.g., hepatocytes), efficacy (e.g., drug target cell types), and key toxicity organs (e.g., heart, kidney, liver), all to be cultured in defined compartments on a silicon chip sized device with defined flow in and out of each compartment (mimicking "blood flow" in and out of each of these organs). Access ports into this in vitro system can be engineered in between each of these compartments. To date, there have been some positive movements in this direction [106–109]. A myriad of drug response data can be retrieved from this system, by making both real-time (longitudinal) and final (end-stage) measurements. Such a device will provide a new "one-stop shopping" approach for drug screening toward any particular therapeutic target, with the only changing module being the target cell compartment (for different disease end points and therefore requiring different disease target cell types and their flow characteristics in vivo). More important, this or similar chip devices will aim to provide both in vivo relevant potency data and therapeutic index data all in one go.

In essence, the future of measurements will likely be captured by one central theme: increased application of multifactorial measurements to capture a more complete picture of the underlying biology. On the one hand, ever more sophisticated cell culture models will become a reality as stem cell and tissue-engineering technology matures and delivers. Meanwhile an increasing number of biomedical laboratories will be equipped with knowledge and expertise to measure functional readouts from genomics, proteomics, kinomics (or phosphoproteomics), metabonomics, lipidomics, glycomics, phenotypic responses, and morphometric multiparametric imaging data. These data will in turn be presented in a dynamic pathway view of the changing biology, with the cause and effect relationship more clearly identified than before.

14.7 CONCLUSION

In the future the diagnosis, treatment, response, and prognosis of human diseases will be optimized at the individual level with the help of technological advances described in this book. The research-based pharmaceutical industry will continue to be at the forefront, turning promising laboratory research into clinical reality in terms of more efficacious and safe medicines to extend human lifespan and enhance the quality of life. However, the desire for more efficient technologies and processes indicates a need for more iterative use of the 4M paradigm (Figure 14.1).

The development of computational tools that can bridge the gap between the expert and nonexpert modeler, providing some confidence in the predictions while facilitating an improvement in hypothesis generation and testing, will continue to form the pillars of modeling and mining. The tasks of integrating modeling, mining, manipulation, and measurement falls to a new breed of systems biologists (Figure 14.1). These scientists will be trained in an interdisciplinary manner and have a fundamental understanding of engineering principles and at least one field of biology (pharmacology, toxicology, etc.).

All the endeavors described in this chapter are aimed at providing a better answer to the fundamental question of any drug therapy: Does there exist a sufficient therapeutic window?

REFERENCES

1. Bertoldo A, Sparacino G, Cobelli C. "Population" approach improves parameter estimation of kinetic models from dynamic PET data. *IEEE Trans Med Imag* 2004;23:297–306.

2. Jayawardhana B, Kell DB, Rattray M. Bayesian inference of the sites of perturbations in metabolic pathways via Markov chain Monte Carlo. *Bioinformatics* 2008;24:1191–7.

3. Swaan PW, Ekins S. Reengineering the pharmaceutical industry by crash-testing molecules. *Drug Discov Today* 2005;10:1191–200.

4. Ekins S. *Computer applications in pharmaceutical research and development.* Hoboken, NJ: Wiley, 2006.

5. Hupcey MAZ, Ekins S. Improving the drug selection and development process for combination devices. *Drug Discov Today* 2007;12:844–52.

6. Ekins S, Mestres J, Testa B. In silico pharmacology for drug discovery: applications to targets and beyond. *Br J Pharmacol* 2007;152:21–37.

7. Ekins S, Mestres J, Testa B. In silico pharmacology for drug discovery: methods for virtual ligand screening and profiling. *Br J Pharmacol* 2007;152:9–20.

8. Kubinyi H. Success stories of computer-aided design. In: Ekins S, ed. *Computer applications in pharmaceutical research and development.* Hoboken, NJ: Wiley, 2006. p. 377–424.

9. Kurogi Y, Guner OF. Pharmacophore modeling and three-dimensional database searching for drug design using catalyst. *Curr Med Chem* 2001;8:1035–55.

10. Guner O, Clement O, Kurogi Y. Pharmacophore modeling and three dimensional database searching for drug design using catalyst: recent advances. *Curr Med Chem* 2004;11:2991–3005.

11. Fujita T. Recent success stories leading to commercializable bioactive compounds with the aid of traditional QSAR procedures. *Quant Struct Act Relat* 1997;16: 107–12.

12. Tesmer JJG. Hitting the hot spots of cell signaling cascades. *Science* 2006;312: 377–8.

13. Bonacci TM, Mathews JL, Yuan C, Lehmann DM, Malik S, Wu D, et al. Differential targeting of Gbetagamma-subunit signaling with small molecules. *Science* 2006;312:443–6.

14. Betzi S, Restouin A, Opi S, Arold ST, Parrot I, Guerlesquin F, et al. Protein protein interaction inhibition (2P2I) combining high throughput and virtual screening: Application to the HIV-1 Nef protein. *Proc Natal Acad Sci USA* 2007;104:19256–61.

15. Taylor JD, Gilbert PJ, Williams MA, Pitt WR, Ladbury JE. Identification of novel fragment compounds targeted against the pY pocket of v-Src SH2 by computational and NMR screening and thermodynamic evaluation. *Proteins* 2007;67: 981–90.

16. Trosset JY, Dalvit C, Knapp S, Fasolini M, Veronesi M, Mantegani S, et al. Inhibition of protein-protein interactions: the discovery of druglike beta-catenin inhibitors by combining virtual and biophysical screening. *Proteins* 2006;64: 60–7.

17. Renner S, Noeske T, Parsons CG, Schneider P, Weil T, Schneider G. New allosteric modulators of metabotropic glutamate receptor 5 (mGluR5) found by ligand-based virtual screening. *ChemBioChem* 2005;6:620–5.

18. Noeske T, Jirgensons A, Starchenkovs I, Renner S, Jaunzeme I, Trifanova D, et al. Virtual screening for selective allosteric mGluR1 antagonists and

structure-activity relationship investigations for coumarine derivatives. *ChemMed-Chem* 2007;2:1763–73.

19. Plewczynski D, Hoffmann M, von Grotthuss M, Ginalski K, Rychewski L. In silico prediction of SARS protease inhibitors by virtual high throughput screening. *Chem Biol Drug Des* 2007;69:269–79.

20. Yagi Y, Terada K, Noma T, Ikebukuro K, Sode K. In silico panning for a non-competitive peptide inhibitor. *BMC Bioinform* 2007;8:11.

21. Ekins S, Swaan PW. Computational models for enzymes, transporters, channels and receptors relevant to ADME/TOX. *Rev Comp Chem* 2004;20:333–415.

22. Tan HL, Hou CJ, Lauer MR, Sung RJ. Electrophysiologic mechanisms of the long QT interval syndromes and torsade de pointes. *Ann Intern Med* 1995;122:701–14.

23. Thomas SH. Drugs, QT interval abnormalities and ventricular arrhythmias. *Adv Drug React Toxicol Rev* 1994;13:77–102.

24. Barry DM, Xu H, Schuessler RB, Nerbonne JM. Functional knockout of the transient outward current, long-QT syndrome, and cardiac remodeling in mice expressing a dominant-negative Kv4 alpha subunit. *Circ Res* 1998;83:560–7.

25. Jeron A, Mitchell GF, Zhou J, Murata M, London B, Buckett P, et al. Inducible polymorphic ventricular tachyarrhythmias in a transgenic mouse model with a long Q-T phenotype. *Am J Physiol Heart Circ Physiol* 2000;278:H1891–8.

26. Trudeau MC, Warmke JW, Ganetzky B, Robertson GA. HERG, a human inward rectifier in the voltage-gated potassium channel family. *Science* 1995;269:92–5.

27. Warmke JW, Ganetzky B. A family of potassium channel genes related to eag in Drosophila and mammals. *Proc Natl Acad Sci USA* 1994;91:3438–42.

28. Curran ME, Splawski I, Timothy KW, Vincent GM, Green ED, Keating MT. A molecular basis for the cardiac arrhythmia: HERG mutations cause long QT syndrome. *Cell* 1995;80:795–803.

29. Rampe D, Murawsky MK, Grau J, Lewis EW. The antipsychotic agent sertindole is a high affinity antagonist of the human cardiac potassium channel HERG. *J Pharmacol Exp Ther* 1998;286:788–93.

30. Suessbrich H, Schonherr R, Heinemann SH, Attali B, Lang F, Busch AE. The inhibitory effect of the antipsychotic drug haloperidol on HERG potassium channels expressed in *Xenopus* oocytes. *Br J Pharmacol* 1997;120:968–74.

31. Tobita M, Nishikawa T, Nagashima R. A discriminant model constructed by the support vector machine method for HERG potassium channel inhibitors. *Bioorg Med Chem Lett* 2005;15:2886–90.

32. Roche O, Trube G, Zuegge J, Pflimlin P, Alanine A, Schneider G. A virtual screening method for the prediction of the hERG potassium channel liability of compound libraries. *ChemBioChem* 2002;3:455–9.

33. Pearlstein RA, Vaz RJ, Rampe D. Understanding the structure-activity relationship of the human ether-a-go-go-related gene cardiac K+ channel. A model for bad behavior. *J Med Chem* 2003;46:2017–22.

34. Pearlstein RA, Vaz RJ, Kang J, Chen X-L, Preobrazhenskaya M, Shchekotikhin AE, et al. Characterization of HERG Potassium channel inhibition using CoMSiA 3D QSAR and homology modeling approaches. *Bioorg Med Chem* 2003;13:1829–35.

35. O'Brien SE, de Groot MJ. Greater than the sum of its parts: combining models for useful ADMET prediction. *J Med Chem* 2005;48:1287–91.

36. Kesuru GM. Prediction of hERG potassium channel affinity by traditional and hologram QSAR methods. *Bioorg Med Chem Lett* 2003;13:2773–5.

37. Ekins S, Crumb WJ, Sarazan RD, Wikel JH, Wrighton SA. Three dimensional quantitative structure activity relationship for the inhibition of the hERG (human ether-a-gogo related gene) potassium channel. *J Pharmacol Exp Thera* 2002;301: 427–34.

38. Ekins S. Predicting undesirable drug interactions with promiscuous proteins in silico. *Drug Discov Today* 2004;9:276–85.

39. Ekins S. In silico approaches to predicting metabolism, toxicology and beyond. *Biochem Soc Trans* 2003;31:611–4.

40. Cianchetta G, Li Y, Kang J, Rampe D, Fravolini A, Cruciani G, et al. Predictive models for hERG potassium channel blockers. *Bioorg Med Chem Lett* 2005;15: 3637–42.

41. Cavalli A, Poluzzi E, De Ponti F, Recanatini M. Toward a pharmacophore for drugs inducing the long QT syndrome: insights from a CoMFA study of HERG K+ channel blockers. *J Med Chem* 2002;45:3844–53.

42. Bains W, Basman A, White C. HERG binding specificity and binding site structure: evidence from a fragment-based evolutionary computing SAR study. *Prog Biophys Mol Biol* 2004;86:205–33.

43. Aronov AM, Goldman BB. A model for identifying HERG K+ channel blockers. *Bioorg Med Chem* 2004;12:2307–15.

44. Aptula AO, Cronin MT. Prediction of hERG K+ blocking potency: application of structural knowledge. *SAR QSAR Environ Res* 2004;15:399–411.

45. Osterberg F, Aqvist J. Exploring blocker binding to a homology model of the open hERG K+ channel using docking and molecular dynamics methods. *FEBS Lett* 2005;579:2939–44.

46. Rajamani R, Tounge BA, Li J, Reynolds CH. A two-state homology model of the hERG K+ channel: application to ligand binding. *Bioorg Med Chem Lett* 2005;15:1737–41.

47. Fernandez D, Ghanta A, Kauffman GW, Sanguinetti MC. Physicochemical features of the HERG channel drug binding site. *J Biol Chem* 2004;279:10120–7.

48. Sanguinetti MC, Mitcheson JS. Predicting drug-hERG channel interactions that cause acquired long QT syndrome. *Trends Pharmacol Sci* 2005;26:119–24.

49. Chekmarev DS, Kholodovych V, Balakin KV, Ivanenkov Y, Ekins S, Welsh WJ. Shape signatures: new descriptors for predicting cardiotoxicity in silico. *Chem Res Toxicol* 2008;21:1304–14.

50. Nebigil CG, Choi DS, Dierich A, Hickel P, Le Meur M, Messaddeq N, et al. Serotonin 2B receptor is required for heart development. *Proc Natal Acad Sci USA* 2000;97:9508–13.

51. Roth BL. Drugs and valvular heart disease. *N Engl J Med* 2007;356:6–9.

52. Schade R, Andersohn F, Suissa S, Haverkamp W, Garbe E. Dopamine agonists and the risk of cardiac-valve regurgitation. *N Engl J Med* 2007;356:29–38.

53. Zanettini R, Antonini A, Gatto G, Gentile R, Tesei S, Pezzoli G. Valvular heart disease and the use of dopamine agonists for Parkinson's disease. *N Eng J Med* 2007;356:39–46.

54. Jahnichen S, Horowski R, Pertz HH. Agonism at 5-HT2B receptors is not a class effect of the ergolines. *Eur J Pharmacol* 2005;513:225–8.

55. Fitzgerald LW, Burn TC, Brown BS, Patterson JP, Corjay MH, Valentine PA, et al. Possible role of valvular serotonin 5-HT(2B) receptors in the cardiopathy associated with fenfluramine. *Mol Pharmacol* 2000;57:75–81.

56. Rothman RB, Baumann MH, Savage JE, Rauser L, McBride A, Hufeisen SJ, et al. Evidence for possible involvement of 5-HT(2B) receptors in the cardiac valvulopathy associated with fenfluramine and other serotonergic medications. *Circulation* 2000;102:2836–41.

57. Singh P, Kumar R. Quantitative structure-activity relationship study on tetrahydro-beta-carboline antagonists of the serotonin 2B (5HT2B) contractile receptor in the rat stomach fundus. *J Enzyme Inhib* 2001;16:491–7.

58. Brea J, Rodrigo J, Carrieri A, Sanz F, Cadavid MI, Enguix MJ, et al. New serotonin 5-HT(2A), 5-HT(2B), and 5-HT(2C) receptor antagonists: synthesis, pharmacology, 3D-QSAR, and molecular modeling of (aminoalkyl)benzo and heterocycloalkanones. *J Med Chem* 2002;45:54–71.

59. Manivet P, Schneider B, Smith JC, Choi DS, Maroteaux L, Kellermann O, et al. The serotonin binding site of human and murine 5-HT2B receptors: molecular modeling and site-directed mutagenesis. *J Biol Chem* 2002;277:17170–8.

60. Setola V, Dukat M, Glennon RA, Roth BL. Molecular determinants for the interaction of the valvulopathic anorexigen norfenfluramine with the 5-HT2B receptor. *Mol Pharmacol* 2005;68:20–33.

61. Cheng A, Dixon SL. In silico models for the prediction of dose-dependent human hepatotoxicity. *J Comput Aided Mol Des* 2003;17:811–23.

62. Clark RD, Wolohan PR, Hodgkin EE, Kelly JH, Sussman NL. Modelling in vitro hepatotoxicity using molecular interaction fields and SIMCA. *J Mol Graph Model* 2004;22:487–97.

63. Cruz-Monteagudo M, Cordeiro MN, Borges F. Computational chemistry approach for the early detection of drug-induced idiosyncratic liver toxicity. *J Comput Chem* 2007.

64. Tetko IV, Bruneau P, Mewes HW, Rohrer DC, Poda GI. Can we estimate the accuracy of ADME-Tox predictions? *Drug Discov Today* 2006;11:700–7.

65. Dimitrov S, Dimitrova G, Pavlov T, Dimitrova N, Patlewicz G, Niemela J, et al. A stepwise approach for defining the applicability domain of SAR and QSAR models. *J Chem Infor Model* 2005;45:839–49.

66. Sheridan RP, Feuston BP, Maiorov VN, Kearsley SK. Similarity to molecules in the training set is a good discriminator for prediction accuracy in QSAR. *J Chem Info Comput Sci* 2004;44:1912–28.

67. Ekins S, Balakin KV, Savchuk N, Ivanenkov Y. Insights for human ether-a-go-go-related gene potassium channel inhibition using recursive partitioning, Kohonen and Sammon mapping techniques. *J Med Chem* 2006;49:5059–71.

68. Willett P. Similarity-based approaches to virtual screening. *Biochem Soc Trans* 2003;31:603–6.

69. Khandelwal A, Bahadduri P, Chang C, Polli JE, Swaan P, Ekins S. Computational models to assign biopharmaceutics drug disposition classification from molecular structure. *Pharm Res* 2007;24:2249–62.

70. Kortagere S, Chekmarev DS, Ekins S, Welsh WJ. A novel generalized predictive blood brain barrier model using molecular and shape based descriptors. *Pharm Res* 2008;25:1836–45.

71. Ekins S, Embrechts MJ, Breneman CM, Jim K, Wery J-P. Novel applications of Kernel-partial least squares to modeling a comprehensive array of properties for drug discovery. In: Ekins S, ed. *Computational toxicology: risk assessment for pharmaceutical and environmental chemicals.* Hoboken, NJ: Wiley-Interscience, 2007. p. 403–32.

72. Scholkopf B, Platt JC, Shawe-Taylor J, Smola AJ, Williamson RC. *Estimating the support of a high-dimensional distribution.* Cambridge, MA: Microsoft Research, 1999.

73. Chang CC, Lin CJ. *LIBSVM: A library for support vector machines.* 2001. http://www.csie.ntu.edu.tw/~cjlin/libsvm

74. Hirono S, Nakagome I, Hirano H, Matsushita Y, Yoshi F, Moriguchi I. Non-congeneric structure-pharmacokinetic property correlation studies using fuzzy adaptive least-squares: oral bioavailability. *Biol Pharm Bull* 1994;17:306–9.

75. Hirono S, Nakagome I, Hirano H, Yoshi F, Moriguchi I. Non-congeneric structure-pharmacokinetic property correlation studies using fuzzy adaptive least squares: volume of distribution. *Biol Pharm Bull* 1994;17:686–90.

76. Gobburu JVS, Shelver WH. Quantitative structure-pharmacokinetic relationships (QSPR) of beta blockers derived using neural networks. *J Pharm Sci* 1995;84:862–5.

77. Michelson S. Assessing the impact of predictive biosimulation on drug discovery and development. *J Bioinform Comput Biol* 2003;1:169–77.

78. Kansal AR. Modeling approaches to type 2 diabetes. *Diabetes Technol Ther* 2004;6:39–47.

79. Musante CJ, Lewis AK, Hall K. Small- and large-scale biosimulation applied to drug discovery and development. *Drug Discov Today* 2002;7:S192–6.

80. Arnold RJ. Cost-effectiveness analysis: should it be required for drug registration and beyond? *Drug Discov Today* 2007;12:960–5.

81. Charnick SB, Kawai R, Nedelman JR, Lemaire M, Niederberger W, Sato H. Perspectives in pharmacokinetics: physiologically based pharmacokinetic modeling as a tool for drug development. *J Pharmacokinet Biopharm* 1995;23:217–29.

82. Gerlowski LE, Jain RK. Physiologically based pharmacokinetic modeling: principles and applications. *J Pharm Sci* 1983;72:1103–27.

83. Blesch KS, Gieschke R, Tsukamoto Y, Reigner BG, Burger HU, Steimer JL. Clinical pharmacokinetic/pharmacodynamic and physiologically based pharmacokinetic modeling in new drug development: the capecitabine experience. *Invest New Drugs* 2003;21:195–223.

84. Knaak JB, Dary CC, Power F, Thompson CB, Blancato JN. Physicochemical and biological data for the development of predictive organophosphorus pesticide QSARs and PBPK/PD models for human risk assessment. *Crit Rev Toxicol* 2004;34:143–207.

85. Ananiadou S, Kell DB, Tsujii J. Text mining and its potential applications in systems biology. *Trends Biotechnol* 2006;24:571–9.

86. Jensen LJ, Saric J, Bork P. Literature mining for the biologist: from information retrieval to biological discovery. *Nat Rev Genet* 2006;7:119–29.

87. Hearst MA, Divoli A, Guturu H, Ksikes A, Nakov P, Wooldridge MA, et al. BioText search engine: beyond abstract search. *Bioinformatics* 2007;23:2196–7.

88. Rodriguez-Esteban R, Iossifov I, Rzhetsky A. Imitating manual curation of text-mined facts in biomedicine. *PLoS Comput Biol* 2006;2:e118.

89. Rodriguez-Esteban R, Rzhetsky A. Six senses in the literature. The bleak sensory landscape of biomedical texts. *EMBO Rep* 2008;9:212–5.

90. Rodriguez-Esteban R, McGlashen M. Personal communication.

91. McGlashen M. *Personal communication*.

92. H.R. 2764: http://thomas.loc.gov/cgi-bin/bdquery/z?d110:h.r.02764:

93. Division G, Title II, Section 218 of PL 110-161 (Consolidated Appropriations Act, 2008).

94. http://books.google.com/

95. McGlashen M. Knowledge management for science and technology R&D. Infonortics Search Engine Conference, 2003.

96. McGlashen M. Knowledge mining and representation in systems biology. Linguamatics Users Conference. Boston, 2007.

97. Linnaeus C. *Systema naturae*. Nieuwkoop, Netherlands: De Graaf, 1735.

98. Santos C, Eggle D, States DJ. Wnt pathway curation using automated natural language processing: combining statistical methods with partial and full parse for knowledge extraction. *Bioinformatics* 2005;21:1653–8.

99. Oda K, Kim JD, Ohta T, Okanohara D, Matsuzaki T, Tateisi Y, et al. New challenges for text mining: mapping between text and manually curated pathways. *BMC Bioinform* 2008;9(Suppl3):S5.

100. Westfall JM, Mold J, Fagnan L. Practice-based research—"Blue Highways" on the NIH roadmap. *JAMA* 2007;297:403–6.

101. Prudhomme W, Daley GQ, Zandstra P, Lauffenburger DA. Multivariate proteomic analysis of murine embryonic stem cell self-renewal versus differentiation signaling. *Proc Nat Acad Sci USA* 2004;101:2900–5.

102. Janes KA, Albeck JG, Gaudet S, Sorger PK, Lauffenburger DA, Yaffe MB. A systems model of signaling identifies a molecular basis set for cytokine-induced apoptosis. *Science* 2005;310:1646–53.

103. Miller-Jensen K, Janes KA, Brugge JS, Lauffenburger DA. Common effector processing mediates cell-specific responses to stimuli. *Nature* 2007;448:604–8.

104. Kumar N, Afeyan R, Kim HD, Lauffenburger DA. Multipathway model enables prediction of kinase inhibitor cross-talk effects on migration of Her2-overexpressing mammary epithelial cells. *Mol Pharmacol* 2008;73:1668–78.

105. Sivaraman A, Leach JK, Townsend S, Iida T, Hogan BJ, Stolz DB, et al. A microscale in vitro physiological model of the liver: predictive screens for drug metabolism and enzyme induction. *Cur Drug Metab* 2005;6:569–91.

106. Lee MY, Park CB, Dordick JS, Clark DS. Metabolizing enzyme toxicology assay chip (MetaChip) for high-throughput microscale toxicity analyses. *Proc Nat Acad Sci USA* 2005;102:983–7.

107. Sin A, Chin KC, Jamil MF, Kostov Y, Rao G, Shuler ML. The design and fabrication of three-chamber microscale cell culture analog devices with integrated dissolved oxygen sensors. *Biotechnol Prog* 2004;20:338–45.

108. Fang Y, Offenhaeusser A. ADMET biosensors: up-to-date issues and strategies. *Med Sci Monit* 2004;10:MT127–32.

109. Zieziulewicz TJ, Unfricht DW, Hadjout N, Lynes MA, Lawrence DA. Shrinking the biologic world—nanobiotechnologies for toxicology. *Toxicol Sci* 2003;74:235–44.

INDEX

RETURN TO: CHEMISTRY LIBRARY

100 Hildebrand Hall · 510-642-3753

LOAN PERIOD 1	2 *1 Month* 3	
4	5	6

ALL BOOKS MAY BE RECALLED AFTER 7 DAYS.

Renewals may be requested by phone ~~or, using GLADIS, type~~ **inv**
~~followed by your patron ID number.~~

DUE AS STAMPED BELOW.

~~FEB 14~~		

FORM NO. DD 10
3M 7-08

UNIVERSITY OF CALIFORNIA, BERKELEY
Berkeley, California 94720–6000